This exciting ethnographic account of the measles epidemic in Pakistan focuses on the ultimate causes of vaccination resistance. While biomedical and global public health officials point to "backward" cultural beliefs and behaviors and the irrational embrace of conspiracy theories (e.g., vaccination is a plot to achieve Muslim sterilization), Inayat Ali reveals the fundamental role of socioeconomic inequality, locally, nationally, and globally, in fueling the measles epidemic in his country. Moreover, Ali mobilizes the social insights of Foucault on the social distribution of power, and the ideas of various medical anthropologists, to affirm measles vaccination avoidance in Pakistan as an expression of resistance.

—Merrill Singer, *University of Connecticut, USA*

A credible research resource, addressing a public health issue through an anthropological lens, for public health professionals, practitioners, and policy makers particularly relevant to Pakistan in the Covid-19 pandemic-affected health care systems and vaccination programs. Inayat Ali has examined the issues surrounding measles in the larger context of the fragile health system and inequitable social structures of Pakistan. He illustrates that the disease outbreaks are indeed the outcome of competing narratives, inequalities, and social conflicts. This dimension is largely missing in the public health professionals' dialogues. His work is guided by theoretical and methodological frameworks that have relevance to other public health problems. The author argues the need for a comprehensive effective governance approach to deal with the global Covid-19 pandemic as well as draw upon a deep understanding of vaccine hesitancy to improve the vaccination programs. A must read for public health professionals.

—Saima Hamid, *Fatima Jinnah Women University, Pakistan*

Contesting Measles and Vaccination in Pakistan

This book explores issues surrounding measles and vaccination in Pakistan. Drawing on long-term ethnographic research, it focuses on two major outbreaks in Sindh province and on Pakistan's vaccination campaigns. The chapters examine the responses to outbreaks and vaccination from various stakeholders including local people, the Pakistani Government, and the WHO. Inayat Ali reflects on the competing agendas, differing conceptualizations of measles and vaccination, and the factors that lie behind these contestations. Situating outbreaks within the institutionalized form of disparities, he analyzes the rituals used to deal with measles and local resistance to vaccines in Pakistan. The distinct imaginaries and practices related to measles and vaccination are considered in both national and global contexts, and the book makes a valuable contribution to the development of an anthropology of vaccination and medical anthropology of Pakistan.

Inayat Ali is in charge of the Department of Public Health and Allied Sciences and Assistant Professor in the Department of Anthropology at Fatima Jinnah Women University, Rawalpindi, Pakistan. He is also Research Fellow in the Department of Social and Cultural Anthropology at the University of Vienna, Austria.

Routledge Studies in Health and Medical Anthropology

https://www.routledge.com/Routledge-Studies-in-Health-and-Medical-Anthropology/book-series/RSHMA

Contesting Measles and Vaccination in Pakistan

Cultural Beliefs, Structured Vulnerabilities, Mistrust, and Geo-Politics

Inayat Ali

Routledge
Taylor & Francis Group

LONDON AND NEW YORK

First published 2025
by Routledge
4 Park Square, Milton Park, Abingdon, Oxon OX14 4RN

and by Routledge
605 Third Avenue, New York, NY 10158

Routledge is an imprint of the Taylor & Francis Group, an informa business

© 2025 Inayat Ali

The right of Inayat Ali to be identified as author of this work has been asserted in accordance with sections 77 and 78 of the Copyright, Designs and Patents Act 1988.

British Library Cataloguing-in-Publication Data
A catalogue record for this book is available from the British Library

ISBN: 9781032151939 (hbk)
ISBN: 9781032182711 (pbk)
ISBN: 9781003253716 (ebk)

DOI: 10.4324/9781003253716

Typeset in Sabon
by codeMantra

I dedicate this book to my loving family!

Contents

Preface

Merrill Singer

In May 2022, UNICEF released a disconcerting announcement: during the first two months of the year, the number of reported measles cases worldwide increased by 79% compared to the same time the previous year. This jump in measles is seen by UNICEF and other public health institutions as a very worrying sign of a more general global increase in risk from the spread of several highly contagious viruses and other vaccine-preventable diseases. The cause of this brewing crisis has been described as a perfect storm that involves the intersection of Covid-related disruptions, increasing inequalities in access to vaccines, and the diversion of resources from routine immunization. In 2020, 23 million children missed out on all basic childhood vaccines. This is the highest number of missed vaccines since 2009 and 3.7 million more than in 2019. But the picture is more complex still. Looking through an on-the-ground ethnographic lens at two towns in Sindh province in Pakistan with high rates of measles but no biomedical facilities, in combination with multi-sited research at various levels in the local, national, and global public health domain, Inayat Ali reveals the key social forces driving the spread of measles.

Ali, a rising star in medical anthropology, is Assistant Professor in the Department of Anthropology of Fatima Jinnah Women University in Rawalpindi, Pakistan. Additionally, he is Research Fellow in the Department of Social & Cultural Anthropology at the University of Vienna, and Academic/Associate Editor for *PLOS Global Public Health*. To his study of measles, he brings a background in the study of Covid vaccination, vaccination resistance, vaccination preparedness, vaccination conspiracy theories, and Covid syndemics, all based on research in Pakistan.

As Ali makes clear, epidemics are biosocial events that produce and reflect both biological and social urgencies. While governments at all levels as well as public health institutions—especially once vaccines are available—tend to treat infectious diseases as primarily biological conditions, a long history of anthropological, sociological, and other social science research challenges this assumption. Ali's account makes a significant contribution to our comprehension of the social structures, relationships, and motivations that put many Pakistani children at risk for measles.

To achieve his illuminating insights on the measles epidemic, Ali makes good use of several concepts and perspectives in the arsenal of medical anthropology and beyond, including structural violence, social suffering, social drama, critical events, global assemblages, and meaning-centered and critical medical anthropology. In his holistic analysis, he views measles in Pakistan in the context of measles globally, reviews the history of medical anthropology in Pakistan, details the help-seeking behaviors of rural Pakistanis, explores medical pluralism in the country and the respective beliefs about disease etiology and related therapeutic practices of existing healing modalities, examines the history of vaccination in Pakistan within the context of trust and distrust, and analyzes the global anti-vaxx movement. This broad approach enables Ali to view measles simultaneously as a disease in need of addressing and a clarifying window on the fault lines of Pakistani society and the place of his country in the world political economy.

To further his contrast of the perspectives and actions of various stakeholders, Ali introduces the concepts of "local and global [disease] containment" and analyzes the efforts of actors at various levels from the public health sector to denigrate local customs and beliefs as primitive. Local Muslim actors, in turn, who view measles as a sacred disease of childhood and resort to local—often Hindu—healers, see anti-Muslim conspiracies in global containment campaigns like vaccination. This conception and the clash/negotiations among multiple competing narratives were reinforced by the "fake" vaccination campaign launched by the CIA in its hunt for Osama bin Laden. As part of his critical analysis, Ali identifies local opposition to measles vaccination as a form of resistance to subordination by external forces from the West. In this, he affirms Foucault's analysis of the complex distribution of power in society as an unequal but not a wholly top-down affair. This discussion opens wide a window on the ways social and economic inequality—rather than local cultural practice, including vaccination resistance—are the most responsible drivers of the spread of measles in Pakistan. This discussion leads Ali, a vaccination supporter, to call for the creation of an "anthropology of vaccination" that draws on anthropology's strengths in the effort to construct effective and socially acceptable vaccination approaches.

Overall, this book embodies an insightful and distinctly medical anthropology approach to the crises of infectious disease in a world of inequality and injustice and makes a major contribution to understanding health as an undeniably biosocial phenomenon.

Prologue

"You could have died"—An Autoethnographic Account of Measles as a Sacred Illness and Systemic Disparities

Measles has been reported to infect humans from as early as the sixth century BCE (Düx et al. 2020) and continues to challenge the world, including Pakistan, where two consecutive measles outbreaks occurred in 2012 and 2013, mainly in its Sindh province. These two outbreaks are the focus of this book, *Constructing and Negotiating Measles: Cultural Beliefs, Structured Vulnerabilities, Mistrust, and Geo-Politics in Pakistan.* I was intrigued by the question of why measles still causes outbreaks, in which thousands of children, especially those who belong to low-income families, contract the virus and suffer accordingly. Herein I ask, what are those factors that impede the progress of Pakistan's Expanded Programme on Immunization (EPI), which was started as early as 1978? How do different stakeholders conceptualize and deal with measles?

I began my quest for answers by accumulating secondary data through different media sources and from information shared by my family, friends, and acquaintances. This preliminary information pointed to competing interpretations of issues surrounding measles and vaccination programs in the country. These competing narratives highlight social conflict, as measles and vaccination are perceived differently by diverse stakeholders. Many in Sindh province see measles as a necessary sacred illness, while others consider it to be a harmful infectious disease that should be avoided via vaccination. Likewise, the meaning of vaccination varies as well: some perceive it as a lifesaving endeavor while others interpret it as a "Western plot."

At the outset of this project, the phenomena of measles as a necessary sacred illness, in which the Hindu goddess *Mātā* manifests, and of vaccination as a "Western plot" to sterilize women in order to control the Muslim population, were already familiar to me due to my upbringing in the country. I have experienced both phenomena: measles afflicted me when I was an infant, and (by my choice) I received the hepatitis vaccine during my teenage years.

According to my mother, not only I but also my siblings contracted measles. She told me:

[In *Serāikī*] *Hik Ddīhan, Māī Meharbān Waddā Bār Rakhyā Taiddy Mathun*. One day, the kind goddesses showed high intensity over you.[1] Your eyes stuck in one place. You were fainting. This state made us highly worried. I was crying. Then our grandmother chanted *Lolī* [lullaby, which is a Hindu religious song called *Bhajjan*]. She already performed *Katchā Chandā* [in which a local woman—a healer—chants specific verses and pours drops of milk on the face of a child who has contracted measles; further details are provided in Chapter 3]. Not only you had measles, but in our extended family there were a few more children; thus, she could not perform the *Pakā Chandā* as it is performed once *Māī Meharbān* (kind goddess) cools down every contract child and returns. We played *Bhajjan* on the stereo that your *Nānā* (my mother's father) brought from a Hindu family. Our grandmother, my mother, your father's mother, and I were continually sitting beside you to look after you. My parents, your father's parents, and your father were coming repeatedly to check your state. It was very critical. We thought you would not survive. Despite chanting *Lolī*, you could not sleep the entire night, but in the early morning, finally, when you woke up, *Māī Meharbān* (kind goddess) decreased the intensity, as she showed her kindness.

However, after your recovery, the situation of your cousin, Rameez (a pseudonym), deteriorated. He was a few weeks younger than you, and the elder son of your *Māmā* [a term used for "mother's brother" in the *Serāikī, Sindhī, Punjābī* and Urdu languages]. Although he also had measles, he was all right. Each family member was worried about you. Suddenly, his health became critical, as it is always the case—whenever the kind goddess shows benevolence to one, she manifests intensity on another. Thus, after showing kindness over you, *Māī Meharbān* increased the intensity of pain on Rameez.

Your *Māmā* (the father of Rameez) was in *Karāchī* to do a governmental job. Rameez's situation continually deteriorated; hence, we had no choice but to bring him to a Hindu *Hakīm*. There was a famous *Hakīm*, called *Nāru*, whose clinic was at a distance of 8–10 kilometers. We already consulted him for you and Rameez. To bring Rameez there, your *Nānā* (my mother's father) made the oxcart ready, as we had no other transport. Your *Nānā* and *Nānī*, your *Māmī* [*Māmā*'s wife], I, you (to seek some treatment for you, too) and Rameez got on the oxcart to reach the *Hakīm*. There was no paved road available. Hence, your *Nānā* took the bank of the canal. Without caring about the heat of the day and dust of the bank, we continued our journey.

Unfortunately, Rameez's health was not improving. We were singing *Lolī* in the cart, and putting a piece of cloth wet with goat milk over his forehead. Instead of improving, his situation continually became more critical. We were almost halfway through our journey; his eyes stopped blinking. Your *Nānā* started beating the oxen to run and reach quickly.

Despite every effort, we were perhaps still 4–5 kilometers short. We were helpless and could not save Rameez, as he took his last breath in the lap of your *Māmī*. His sudden death broke us. We started crying and returned the oxcart home. Nobody anticipated that Rameez would die: everyone thought that Inayat Ali would not survive. After his death, your *Māmī* was not in her senses, as Rameez was her first child and then a son. We managed to deliver this tragic news to your *Māmā*, which broke him entirely. He could not see Rameez for the last time, as Karachi was quite far away. We had already buried Rameez when your *Māmā* arrived. The death of Rameez shook every family member because he was charming. Thereafter, your *Māmā* cried too much and resigned from his government job. Rameez's pain exerted a profound effect on his mind. Despite our constant push to continue the job, he did not listen to anyone. Instead of resuming his government job in Karachi, he preferred to work as daily wage labor. This is because he wished to stay close to his family.

This anecdote illustrates not merely my painful and firsthand relationship with measles but also reveals my firsthand experiences of structured disparities. I was fortunate enough to survive, but not everyone survives, as in the case of Rameez. However, when I applied for a PhD scholarship and reached Vienna to pursue this degree, this was not the topic on my mind. I had another proposal concerning exploring how people of the Thar Desert of Sindh deal with health and illness, as basic needs, such as food and clean water, are scarce and necessary facilities such as schools and biomedical hospitals are scant there. I wanted to explore verbal healing and herbal medicine.

Nonetheless, just as I was planning to reach Vienna at the end of 2012, measles caused an outbreak in Pakistan. Yet another consecutive outbreak occurred in 2013. Both outbreaks affected thousands of children countrywide, of which a few hundred died.

At that time, I was already at the Department of Social and Cultural Anthropology, University of Vienna, and attending a colloquium on "Rethinking Ethnography," offered by Ayse Caglar, for which every participant had to present their project. After attending a few presentations, I became interested in working on measles. To develop the project, I further accumulated information from various sources, including the media, academic literature, family members, friends, and acquaintances. These preliminary data, including my autoethnographic account, highlighted the magnitude and diversity of the matter and that a dispute among perceptions and measures regarding measles and vaccination is underway between positions that frame measles as a necessary and inevitable sacred illness or as an infectious disease, and vaccination as a "Western plot" or as necessary to eliminate infectious diseases.

These diverse perspectives may all be viewed as valid within their sociocultural contexts. Therefore, it was indispensable to situate these views within a historical background of the critical sociocultural, economic, and (geo)political events that have shaped these views and their contexts, which I have done in this book.

During further seminar discussions, Ayse suggested that working on the "making of vaccination" in Pakistan could be a promising "entry point" to understand these events. Her suggestion nurtured my idea to work further on infectious diseases. My concept matured during repeated meetings with my PhD supervisor, Bernhard Hadolt. At that time, I preferred not to directly study vaccination due to the ongoing (geo-)politics (see Chapters 10 and 11) revolving around vaccination in Pakistan. For example, in 2012, a "fake" vaccination program was used by the American CIA to find Osama bin Laden. As a result, many vaccination teams faced assaults, and multiple vaccinators were killed. The critical state of this lifesaving endeavor frightened me, and this anxiety has remained with me. I thought that it would be too risky to conduct research on vaccination in Pakistan. My anxiety had much to do with the Pakistani Government since, in Pakistan, many critical thinkers and protestors who try to "speak truth to power," have gone "missing"—abducted and killed. Thus, researching the political "hot potato" topic of vaccination in Pakistan carries significant risks for the researcher and has strong roots in contemporary and past critical events.

To comprehend this interplay, in this book I employ a few critical anthropological concepts, such as "structural violence" (Farmer 1996), "social suffering" (Kleinman, Das, and Lock 1997), and "critical events" (Das 1996). With these concepts, I index all those factors and events that have played pivotal roles in shaping and configuring the particular sociocultural, political, and economic structures in Pakistan today, while including a wide range of stakeholders at local, national, and global levels. Particularly dwelling on the concept of "critical events," as Das has used it to trace the state of present-day India as the result of an interplay of several historical factors, mainly colonization, I discuss several economic and geopolitical critical events (such as the invasion by the Union of Soviet Socialist Republics [USSR] of Afghanistan and the production of the *Tālibān* in Pakistan to fight in Afghanistan in the 1980s), which have significantly shaped the present situation of Pakistan.

Given the risky nature of researching Pakistan's vaccination program, to ward off risks to myself yet still to contribute to Pakistani society, I chose to work on measles from two perspectives: (1) measles as a disease; and (2) measles as an analytical entry point to study the role of those critical events and structures that have had significant impacts on current Pakistan, including on its EPI to control and eliminate infectious diseases from the country.

The abovementioned theoretical concepts also beg a brief note. Not only with measles and vaccination, I also have direct experience that enables me to understand and operationalize these theoretical concepts. I have experienced how structured types of inequalities affect an individuals life (Ali, n.d.). Although my autoethnographic account of measles above vividly demonstrates the implications of these institutionalized forms of disparities, I briefly elaborate on these effects while providing another personal experience:

My younger sister Reema—a more brilliant student than all of us—prematurely died when she was about to enter her teenage years due to an improper diagnosis of chronic liver disease. For many years, we, especially I, brought her to different doctors—from local towns to the federal hospital—but no doctor could diagnose her disease. At the final stages of her disease, she became unconscious and my family—as I was in Islamabad for my Master's degree—brought her to a district-level hospital. My parents were profoundly worried about the money to pay the hospital bills. Yet with economic support from relatives and friends, they decided to visit a private hospital where a famous specialist doctor was practicing. This doctor used to practice at several places across the province. We had consulted him previously a few times, when Reema was physically okay. However, this doctor could not diagnose the disease earlier; he only finally diagnosed it when my sister was already unconscious. I reached this hospital the very next day after travelling for around 18 hours by bus, as I could not afford air travel. She never regained consciousness and passed away after two nights at the hospital; we certainly never anticipated that Reema would leave us so early.

This vignette reveals various levels of chronic disparities and their serious effects: (a) the lack of proper and affordable healthcare services and a dearth of qualified doctors; (b) the unavailability of economic resources to afford effective treatment and travel; and (c) the social stigma that disclosing critical symptoms may generate a bad social image about the family, and especially about Reema, who might have faced severe consequences had she lived, via the social stigma that she would have suffered.

This book has distinct contours. It is related to me, and is not limited to the present, as it has strong roots in history, current affairs, and (geo-)politics. I did not limit my orientation only to anthropology but also read non-anthropological literature. This interdisciplinary orientation was necessary in order to have a thorough lens through which to view my project, as health has profoundly been shaped by historical experiences, events, and structures that are interrelated with economic regimes, political affairs, technological advancements, and travel of the microorganisms that cause outbreaks.

Considering that there is always room for improvement, I end this prologue by noting that research can be a never-ending process, and there comes a time where the researcher is compelled by several factors, especially time and resource constraints, to stop and write up the results of his/her work, even if that is only a momentary endpoint.

Note

1 All translations are mine unless otherwise indicated.

Introduction

This book primarily addresses measles and vaccination programs in Sindh province, Pakistan. Almost seven years before the Covid-19 pandemic, measles caused outbreaks revealing what Victor Turner (1974, 37) called "social drama" in the country as multiple stakeholders started negotiating it. In 2012 and 2013, two measles outbreaks occurred in Pakistan, in which over 25,000 children contracted the virus, and around 500 died (World Health Organization 2013a). These overwhelming outbreaks significantly affected Sindh province, which reported around 300–400 deaths (M.H. Khan 2014), thereby receiving the attention of multiple local and global stakeholders to search for its explanation. This complex array of stakeholders, which included local people, Hindu *Hakīm* (Hindu herbalists who mostly follow *Ayurvedā*), vaccinators, government officials, politicians, and global stakeholders such as the World Health Organization (WHO), conceptualized measles differently, enacted their authority in various ways, and displayed their interwoven yet competing agendas around it.

Local people in Sindh, including local Hindu *Hakīm*, believe that measles is a necessary and inescapable sacred illness in which *Mātā*, a Hindu goddess, manifests herself. Hence, they deal with it by performing various rituals, and consider that contracting measles is a natural means of immunization. Along with ritualistic treatments at home, they may also take their ill child to a local healer. Their conceptions and practices draw on culturally specific beliefs about measles' origins and etiology, risk perception, and attitudes toward those infected, which are passed down through families and acquired through enculturation. I call such dealings "local rituals of containment" (Ali 2021). A growing number of local people are suspicious of vaccination and mistrust vaccinators and those who give/donate vaccines.

In contrast, a biomedical doctor or a WHO official interprets measles as a potentially deadly infectious disease that puts patients and other unimmunized persons (nationally or internationally) at risk. Unlike the local people of Sindh and other rural provinces, such officials, along with biomedical doctors, consider eradicating measles to be a necessity.

In contrast, there is an emphasis on the biological and physical aspects of a disease by various other stakeholders who practice the "universal" biomedical model of disease causation and cure. They rely on science and logical

DOI: 10.4324/9781003253716-1

positivism while considering an individual as a biological organism that contains various parts, and sees illness as a result of malfunctioning in one or more of these parts. For example, the doctors, public media, government officials, and representatives of the WHO consider measles as a potentially lethal disease that needs to be controlled and eliminated through vaccination. Thus, they tend to blame local people for adhering to "rural customs" and "classical taboos" from the "Stone Age," insisting that these cultural practices significantly hinder the elimination of the virus. The WHO also tends to blame the Pakistani Government for lack of "political will" to properly implement what I call *global rituals of containment*, that is, vaccination programs. Meanwhile, local people have their own socioculturally and politically based reasons for not vaccinating their children.

Measles still prevails in Pakistan, the most recent infections occurred in 2022. Governments and global stakeholders are extremely concerned about vaccine preventable diseases (VPDs), including measles, as the coronavirus pandemic has overstretched health services and disrupted routine vaccination drives (I. Ali 2020c).

Negotiations and contestations around measles and vaccination can occur at a microlevel, for example, between/among a local person and a vaccinator, and at a macro-level, for example, between the government and global stakeholders. In this way, measles involves domestic and international politics that occur via bargaining (indirectly) between a layperson and a WHO official, or among diverse stakeholders situated in distinct locations simultaneously. A parent's refusal of vaccination entails negotiations with the vaccinator, the government, and global stakeholders. For instance, for vaccinating her children, an economically poor woman, *Nazul,* negotiates with the vaccinator to receive proper attention and medicine at a hospital, and she negotiates with the government to receive a card from the Benazīr Income Support Program (BISP) (see Chapter 11). For another example, a parent can refuse vaccination, and that refusal, combined with many others, may force government officials to reformulate vaccination programs. In this way and others, seemingly powerless individuals can turn vaccination into a politically charged issue.

Thus, measles and vaccination in Pakistan are encompassed by multiple competing narratives that are constructed, negotiated, and interact to justify interventions and responses to them. Arguing that these phenomena reveal ongoing social conflicts and tensions, which further reveal institutionalized forms of sociocultural, economic, and political inequalities that are appropriated at the local, national, and global levels, this book is based on a long-term ethnographic project that focused on the complex issues surrounding measles and vaccination programs in Pakistan, primarily in its rural Sindh province. This book extensively explores and elaborates on the multiple imaginaries, beliefs, and practices of multiple stakeholders, from the local to the global.

Herein, I elucidate those competing narratives, inequalities, and social conflicts that have created a conducive environment for infectious diseases, including measles, to cause outbreaks. Thus, this book provides in-depth analyses of the present inequalities and the historical contexts (especially the pre- and post-*Tālibān* events) of the country that have played a significant role in shaping people's current views concerning measles and vaccination. I show how parents express the impacts of structured inequalities that are a result of the government's policies and disparities, which themselves are a product of global geopolitical and economic regimes. I aim to elucidate the impacts of global-level inequalities as they multiply national-level disparities and ultimately inflict suffering on local people in several forms, including outbreaks of infectious diseases, such as measles.

The project's locale is multi-sited, ranging from two villages in Sindh to the WHO headquarters in Geneva. Yet my fieldwork has mainly focused on two villages, *Rahīmpur* and *Rāmpur*, in the *Sakhar* and *Tharpārkar* districts of Sindh province, respectively.[1] I view measles from two perspectives: as a disease and as an analytical window on the world of relationships where inequalities are produced, exercised, and experienced. Measles is the micro-story that illuminates the macro interplay between historical (geo)politics and economic regimes, especially the USSR invasion of Afghanistan in the 1980s; the Pakistan–US relations that produced the *Tālibān*; and in the more recent past, the CIA's "fake" 2011 vaccination campaign designed to ferret out Osama bin Laden (see Chapters 10 and 11).

Some of the central questions addressed in this book include: why does measles still prevail in the country, mainly in Sindh province? How and why do different stakeholders situated in diverse locations deal with measles differently? Why is measles as a single phenomenon attributed different meanings by different stakeholders? How do they deal with it? How can measles serve as a window on a world in which disparities are generated and appropriated, and how can measles help us to understand these institutionalized forms of vulnerabilities? Why are some populations seemingly more vulnerable to contracting measles than others? And, what can anthropology teach us about the occurrences of measles and the failures of vaccination programs through its unique perspectives?

Measles Outbreaks and Structural Inequalities

As the coronavirus pandemic has made eminently clear, microorganisms have long held a distinct place in the human imagination, beliefs, and practices, as they consistently and significantly challenge us. Microorganisms have regularly been shaping our sociocultural, politico-economic, and biological history. They repeatedly cause outbreaks, epidemics, and pandemics, and challenge not solely our physical bodies, but also social, political, and economic bodies. They shape cultural beliefs and myths, and affect our economic and political structures. Prior to the invention of the microscope, humans were suspicious about the existence of microorganisms. Some scientists suspected their existence, ultimately confirmed by microscopic investigation, which initiated exploration of the relationships among micro- and macro-species, most notably humans, especially when the former were finally recognized to cause large-scale morbidities and mortalities in the latter.

Measles is one among them. The present measles outbreak has multiple historical precedents. As is currently understood, the measles virus began infecting humans in large numbers around the sixth century BCE as part of the process of early urbanization (Düx et al. 2020). Since then, measles has spurred discussions and debates on its primary causes in the past (Morley 1969; Furuse, Suzuki, and Oshitani 2010; Rāzī 1848; Koplik 1962) when, along with smallpox and other infectious diseases, measles ravaged populations (Cunha 2004). Nowadays, measles has re-emerged as a subject of debate and contestation in public discourse. This is because, despite enormous global efforts such as the Measles and Rubella Initiative (M&RI), the virus still prevails in various regions, including Pakistan, and still causes outbreaks worldwide. For instance, in 2017, measles caused around 90,000 deaths globally (WHO 2017), and in 2018, measles-related deaths increased to 110,000 (Lindmeier 2018). One year later, the *Agence France-Presse* (AFP) (2018) reported a 30% rise in measles infections across the globe. During 2019, the media also informed us about several measles epidemics. To name but a few: during February of 2019, a measles outbreak occurred in the Philippines and killed around 30 people; in April, measles broke out in New York City, where the mayor declared an emergency; and in May, two children died in Switzerland due to measles (Hein 2019). In 2018, the newspaper *Dawn* (2018)—Pakistan's renowned English daily[2]—reported a measles outbreak in several districts of Sindh province, mainly in the *Thattā* and *Sijāwal* districts, in which some children died. In 2019, Pakistan reported that around 2,000 people had contracted measles (WHO 2019d) while by June 2020, around 2,000 Pakistanis had contracted the virus, and other suspected cases totaled approximately 3,000 (WHO 2020a). Standing among the top five countries with a considerable number of children who did not receive a measles vaccine in 2021 (Rana et al. 2021), Pakistan reported the second highest toll of measles cases—3,780—along with Nigeria, which reported 5,380 cases (CDC 2021).

For many decades, national and global stakeholders have been constantly engaged in order to eradicate measles from the country. As a United Nations (UN) signatory, Pakistan began to implement the WHO's Expanded Programme on Immunization (EPI) as early as 1978 to eliminate several infectious diseases, including measles. Despite that program, the WHO's (2019c, 2019e) data from 1981 to 2019 show two major infectious diseases—pertussis and measles—as still highly problematic in Pakistan. Over this period, both diseases infected around 400,000 and 280,000 people, respectively (ibid.). In an accumulative figure of all infections caused by communicable diseases, which is approximately 841,400, those two diseases account for around 80% (ibid.).

Historically, the most severe outbreak of measles in Pakistan occurred in 1988, infecting around 55,550 people (ibid.). Yet despite the vaccination program that resulted, more current data from 2010 onward demonstrate an increase in measles, which has infected around 30,000 people, and a decrease in pertussis, which only infected 575 people in Pakistan. As previously noted, in 2012 and 2013, there were two consecutive measles outbreaks (this book's primary subject of study) that significantly challenged Pakistan: over 25,000 children were infected (WHO 2013a), and around 500 died (Azeem 2013). These outbreaks significantly affected Sindh province, which, again, reported around 300–400 of those 500 deaths (M.H. Khan 2014).

Consequently, measles remained a prominent topic of debate, especially in the Pakistani media. As noted above, these outbreaks gathered huge attention from diverse stakeholders, ranging from local to global, who dealt with them distinctively. This complex array of stakeholders enacted their authority and wove different competing agendas around measles—the manifestation of the goddess *Mātā* that needs reverent attention, or a potentially lethal disease that requires aggressive measures—to justify interventions and responses in a complex process of negotiation and contestation that revealed several institutionalized forms of sociocultural, economic, and political inequalities.

Those stakeholders (e.g., government officials and representatives of INGOs) who consider measles as a potentially lethal disease, instead of talking about the crucial economic and political factors that underlie measles outbreaks yet are easily obscured, blame local people for their "rural customs," "classical Stone Age taboos," and their refusals and resentments of vaccination, which adversely affect the elimination of the virus.

For instance, the newspaper *Dawn* (2014) reported that when measles occurs in a child in rural areas, the family members follow "superstitions" to deal with the condition because they consider it a "Hindu" disease, and believe that only a Hindu faith healer knows the proper way to handle it. Similarly, the *Express Tribune* (2012)—another English daily of Pakistan—published an interview with Sindh's Provincial Health Secretary, who criticized local people because most parents are still reluctant to allow doctors to check their ailing children, as they fear the wrath of Hindu goddess *Mātā Rani* [Queen Goddess; in Hinduism, she is believed to be one Goddess—*Mātā* or *Devī*, *Durga*, called *"Māhādevī"* (Great Goddess)—who manifests in different forms (Dowson 2000, 90–1)]. Even Muslim families interpret measles in terms of Hindu mythology and believe that fever and red spots are signs of this goddess, who has possessed the children.

In this book, I argue that it is easy to "blame" measles outbreaks on "the locals" and their "primitive" beliefs. It is harder, yet essential, to contextualize measles outbreaks within historical, socio-structural, economic, and political factors and their resulting inequities and inequalities. This fault-finding has roots in colonization and in a common perception among biomedical practitioners, especially in "developed" nations and for agents of "development," that low-income countries are vulnerable to measles epidemics due to several interrelated factors. For instance, David Morley (1969)—who was a British pediatrician and started early trials of measles vaccines—in his articles, "Severe Measles in the Tropics. I & II," claimed that in several "developing" countries, those who lack economic resources and live in villages deliberately delay recognizing measles due to their strong beliefs. He tried to blame the beliefs that people hold about measles but left the economic and political reasons unattended, though these factors considerably contribute to the specific views being held and to the spread of measles.

The new economic and political regimes, I argue, have also purposefully overemphasized the sociocultural factors. This overemphasis is a deliberate effort of specific countries to coin the concept of "development" to divide the world into "developed" and "underdeveloped." According to this categorization, those who cling to sociocultural norms and values are "backward." Thus, they urgently need external intervention from countries in the "developed" category to change their "backwardness" via education and modernization.

I extend my argument that sociocultural reasons are neither the main nor the sole factors behind measles outbreaks to note that these outbreaks stem more from various gross economic and political inequalities that occur at global, national, and local levels. Outbreaks can be seen against a historical backdrop of economic and (geo)political inequalities, as well as contemporary global-level economic and political disparities, which are enormous, persistent, and deepening, and are a result of disproportionally distributed wealth.

According to the UN's (2005, 1) "Report on the World Social Situation 2005: The Inequality Predicament," one billion people living in the "developed" countries own 80% of gross domestic product (GDP), while the remainder (over 5 billion people) have the remaining 20%. Moreover, in its similar report "Inequality Matters," the UN (2013) mentioned that the absolute gap in mean per capita income between these two categories had increased from $18,525 in 1980 to $32,000 in 2010. This report also showed that in 2010, the high-income countries, which have only 16% of the global population, produced around 55% of global income. However, low-income countries containing 72% of the world's population produced only 1% of global income (ibid.). Likewise, in its recent report of 2020, "Inequality in a Rapidly Changing World," the UN mentions that "Income inequality among countries has declined in relative terms but is still higher than inequality within most countries. Absolute income differences between countries continue to grow" (UN 2020, 20). These two reports paint a sharp and distinctive picture of world inequalities.

In addition to this magnitude of disparities among countries, there are significant forms of institutionalized inequalities prevailing among individuals within each country. Consequently, low-income countries such as Pakistan are struggling in terms of economic self-sufficiency and political stability. For achieving both these states, they are overwhelmingly dependent on foreign aid, primarily from the International Monetary Fund (IMF) and the World Bank. During general elections, Pakistan's current ruling political party, called Pakistan *Tehrīk-i-Insāf* (PTI), proclaimed that the party would not "knock at the door" of the IMF and would build on the country's own resources. Nonetheless, once in power in 2018, the new government moved toward the IMF for a bailout package to run the country due to its precarious macroeconomic situation. Pakistan's 2019 request to the IMF was the 13th such request since 1988, in which the government received US$6 billion for three years.

These rescue packages for the country's faltering economy come with strict terms and conditions, such as the government's promise of specific "structural adjustments" programs. Under such stringent conditions, the government no longer controls the value of the American dollar against the Pakistan Rupee (PKR). The inflation rate continues to increase, and the country cannot even set the price of bread. The terms also encourage several adjustments, such as privatizing state assets and liberalizing the conditions of trade and subsidy cuts. The country stands in an awkward position, as without the IMF, it would have greater challenges in meeting the needs of its citizens. With this organization, the given instructions make it hard for the state to run its economy and prioritize problems. It is arguable that if the IMF's aid had produced a positive impact, then the country would need no more assistance in the present, because it has been receiving this assistance for the last three decades. This constant dependence on aid raises critical questions about the effectiveness of these packages, as it has created the "dependence syndrome" at a country level. This dependence syndrome fosters reliant attitudes and behaviors without thinking about self-dignity, constantly seeking foreign aid and attributing higher value to it than exploring and building on the country's own efforts.[3]

Concerning aid, Daron Acemoglu and James Robinson (2012)—one a famous economist and the other a political scientist—argue in their book *Why Nations Fail* that aid is not the most effective way to improve the situation of low-income countries and break the vicious cycle of poverty. Additionally, Joseph Stiglitz (2000)—a Nobel Prize laureate and former chief economist at the World Bank—has criticized the IMF due to its "cookie-cutter" approach to conditional lending and structural reform. These structural adjustment programs reveal an ongoing "struggle, engagement, and resistance" (Pfeiffer and Chapman 2010, 159).

Needless to say, global stakeholders such as the IMF have not succeeded in helping the country to become self-sufficient (Gera 2007; Z.A. Bhutta 2001; S.R. Khan 2002). Yet it is equally plausible to critically evaluate how effectively the country has been governed at the national level. After over 70 years of independence, Pakistan's governments have neither been in a favorable position nor made significant efforts to build the country (e.g., T. Ali 1983; Nasr 1992). For almost half of its existence, the country has been ruled by army dictators (see Samad 1994; Rizvi 1989). Further impacting an already overwhelming situation, many of the resources have been allocated to the defense sector, and the remaining resources are permeated with massive corruption (Noor 2009; Farooq et al. 2013; Chêne 2008; Javaid 2010; F. Khan 2007). The politicians have "hunted and gathered" resources, built their own small economies, and shifted resources abroad (see O'Donovan, Wagner, and Zeume 2019). I call this *local colonization*. The media have regularly broadcast about their money-laundering and their offshore bank accounts in other countries (see e.g., Sehgal 2017).

Such structures and webs of local and global inequalities take differing forms. The national and global policies and preferences have significantly impeded the creation of a competent and self-sufficient country, which should have appropriately established institutions: for example, an adequate and accessible healthcare system; a viable infrastructure, including the construction of drivable roads; and the provision of affordable public transport to reach healthcare facilities. These policies have hindered the development of educational institutions for raising mental capacity and awareness among the masses, who are instead blamed for clinging to "faulty" beliefs about measles.

The repeated measles outbreaks owe much to such disparities. For understanding this argument, we should inquire about *why* local people hold the view that measles is a sacred illness. It is a fact that most illnesses require some measures to deal with them. The local people do not—and cannot—simply watch their children suffer. They make the best possible efforts according to their belief system—performing rituals for making sense of that suffering and for alleviating it, thereby fulfilling a primary healthcare need. Irrespective of their religion yet with similar economic and political situations, Muslims and Hindus in Sindh province perform a *Chando* ritual based on their association of measles with the goddess *Mātā*, in which a local woman—a healer—recites specific chants and pours drops of milk on to the face of a child who has contracted measles (see Chapter 9). This ritual saves money and time simultaneously, as compared to seeking help from biomedical doctors. However, if fever and pain increase, people still avoid biomedical doctors in favor of local healers, such as a local older woman with specialized knowledge or a Hindu *Hakīm* (a local herbalist who follows *Ayurvedā* or *Unānī-Tib*).[4] These healers, according to those who utilize them, deal with *Mātā* reverently. Since (both Muslim and Hindu) people believe that measles is a manifestation of *Mātā*, they prefer to bring a child who has contracted measles to a Hindu with the belief that this meeting pleases *Mātā*. Thus, bringing a child to a Hindu *Hakīm* serves two purposes—meeting with a Hindu expert and receiving an instant cure (see Chapter 8).

This preference, I argue, may also be seen against limited economic resources to afford private hospitalization or effective healthcare that is unavailable, inaccessible, or unaffordable; therefore, these local people have limited choices beyond observing specific rituals. An entirely different realm stands behind the "sociocultural factors" that are referred to in contemporary media accounts. This domain contains broader and stronger elements—political, economic, and historical—that make populations or regions vulnerable to contracting specific diseases, measles included. These factors significantly shape sociocultural practices by producing particular circumstances to create vulnerabilities in poor, rural populations. These circumstances encourage and facilitate people to hold specific views and compel them to adopt affordable coping strategies. The people of Sindh province understandably utilize the techniques available to them, which also make cultural sense to them. The biomedical realm seemingly exists far away from their everyday realities.

As I have argued above, the measles outbreaks have a strong relationship with structured inequalities that occur in diverse forms and at various levels—local, national, and global. The roots of the problem of the prevalence of measles lie in numerous areas: in the disparities in economic resources for building or visiting a hospital; inequalities in providing facilities and services; a dearth of opportunities to access adequate facilities or receive the best education to learn critical thinking; a lack of awareness of biomedical causes and consequences of a phenomenon such as measles; and the limited power to decide what is good or bad. These institutionalized disparities are a result of *structural power*, in which specific structures are subtly and skillfully built to serve some and to do disservices to others, in what Farmer and colleagues (2013) call "structural violence." Along with Farmer, I argue that people with limited economic resources and political power are subject to such violence—they usually cannot escape these forms of violence. Since these inequalities are structured both overtly and subtly, society offers them options and a vocabulary to rationalize systematic inequalities.

For instance, in Pakistan, many justify their suffering via the cultural concept of "fatalism," or are culturally compelled not to discuss this suffering. Interestingly, Adelson (2008) claims that the same is true in the case of Canadian women, who are also culturally compelled to hide their suffering. Kleinman and colleagues (1997) term this phenomenon "social suffering": the notion that the suffering has been structured in such a way that people construct narratives about being subjected to suffering and justify that subjection as a result of their actions; they do not see their suffering as structurally produced by influential stakeholders. Social suffering refers to ways of suffering that are socially shared and that concern whole social groups rather than merely individuals.

This social suffering prevails across the globe because of the unequal distribution of resources. Frequently inflicting substantial harm on individuals and communities, there is a cause-and-effect relationship among inequalities. For example, due to the lack of resources and then misallocation of these limited resources, it becomes impossible to build proper facilities where people could receive the treatments and education that are necessary for maintaining health. Furthermore, unequal resources impact the distribution of effort, which then affect the extent of the required awareness for the prevention of diseases, including measles, and expenditure on therapeutic measures.

At a household level, particularly in rural areas, inequality of resources and awareness result in gender disparities. The difference begins soon after the birth of a female baby. Baby boys are preferred over baby girls, and women in Sindh receive less education than men due to unequal opportunities.

According to the Pakistani government's (2019b, 161) "Economic Survey of Pakistan," the country stands at 150th out of 189 for its education rate worldwide. The overall rate—for those who are formally educated and are over ten years of age—is around 62%. Of that, approximately 52% of the women of the country have formal education, as compared to 73% of the male population. This rate of education further differs in terms of rural and urban areas, as well as in the provincial divisions of the country. In rural areas, approximately 53% of the population have formal education, and out of a total rural population, the education rate for women is around 40%, in contrast to 66% of men (ibid.). This difference in formal education has resulted in women being less aware and entirely dependent on their male counterparts for sociocultural, economic, and political decisions. Those men and—especially—women who resist the biomedical treatment of measles during outbreaks can be seen against the backdrop of a lack of formal education (see Chapters 10 and 11).

In other words, an individual—who owns enough economic resources, or is formally educated, or male, or lives in an urban area—receives more adequate opportunities and services for health and education. For instance, in urban as compared to rural areas, the formal education level is better; health facilities are more appropriate and effective; access to such facilities is adequate and easier; and electricity is available (to maintain the cold chain of vaccines) (Government of Pakistan 2019b).

Furthermore, I argue that the magnitude of specific economic resources makes some stakeholders more influential than others; therefore, their ideas and practices matter more. For example, the UN has a *de facto* veto over the national government in terms of giving guidelines and benchmarks to be achieved. As Pakistan's media reported in 2013–2014, the WHO mandated vaccination for Pakistanis to travel abroad (Dawn 2014a; A.Z. Bhutta 2013). The central government is more powerful than the provincial governments; the provincial authorities hold more power than the district-level government officials; and the district-level officials hold more power than a vaccinator. All these stated stakeholders are more influential than parents, while a male parent is more powerful than a female parent.

Nevertheless, for exercising power, there is also a reverse order: from bottom to top, the following sphere of influence exists—parent to vaccinator; vaccinator to subdistrict health officials; subdistrict to district officials; provincial government to federal government; and from the federal government to the UN. For instance, a parent exercises power through refusing to vaccinate their child or feeling resentment toward vaccination to express the persistent sociocultural, political, and economic inequalities caused by inappropriate policies of the government and global stakeholders, of which many parents, even in rural areas, are aware. The combination of multiple such refusals challenges the power structures to revise vaccination programs, implement them again, and (re-)arrange additional vaccination campaigns, called "supplementary immunization activities" (SIAs).

People who lack economic resources may suffer the most and use their power of refusal as a form of protest against the government. Similarly, the government may show its power by not correctly implementing the UN recommended protocols. For instance, the WHO mandated vaccination for traveling abroad in 2014, and I received a vaccine and vaccination card to go to Austria. However, the government authorities, despite putting in place the necessary measures, did not check the card neither at the Pakistani nor Vienna airports.

According to Foucault (1982, 789):

> In itself the exercise of power is not violence; nor is it a consent which, implicitly, is renewable. It is a total structure of actions brought to bear upon possible actions; it incites, it induces, it seduces, it makes easier or more difficult; in the extreme it constrains or forbids absolutely; it is nevertheless always a way of acting upon an acting subject or acting subjects by virtue of their acting or being capable of action.

These ways of acting occur at multiple levels—such spheres of power flow from top to bottom and vice versa. The engaged stakeholders consciously or unconsciously use their power to bargain for their products—vaccine, services, and aid—in order to gain more power. Drawing on a Foucauldian view, my argument is that a stakeholder is concurrently powerful and powerless. Yet those who hold greater economic and political power are in a stronger position to influence an action. Stakeholders choose to manifest their power as they negotiate measles and vaccination programs; each of them manifests both potential and helplessness through the ways in which they address measles.

For instance, a vaccinator receives a salary of around US$1 a day despite working in harsh conditions that include a tropical environment, lack of proper transport, and being subject to hunger. In contrast, district officials work in their well-maintained and temperature-controlled offices or visit the field sites in their air-conditioned vehicles. A vaccinator may choose to manifest/protest against such inequalities in multiple ways. Common ways may involve making minimal effort to perform assigned duties, inappropriate ways of following the protocols for vaccination, taking more holidays than allowed, arriving late for work, and fictionalizing facts and figures about vaccinated and unvaccinated children.

This manifestation of inequalities is analogous to Biruk's (2018) study of different HIV/AIDS surveys led by US researchers in Malawi between 2005 and 2008, in which she found that the surveyors, especially the young Malawians recruited by the Americans to conduct surveys, fabricated the data in what Biruk called "cooking" the data. Closser (2010) also made analogous observations based on her work on polio in Pakistan, in which she calls this "negotiation" or ways of "resisting office politics."

These negotiation processes exhibit and manifest the power asymmetries that prevail in Pakistan. Each stakeholder communicates and experiences inequality and distress differently. Such idiographic expressions, which Nichter (1981) terms "idioms of distress," reflect social tensions.

A vaccinator tries to mobilize parents not only to vaccinate their children but to save his/her job and obtain the reputation of a good worker. Analogously, a district-level officer negotiates with the provincial head, and the provincial chief negotiates with the national government, and the latter bargains with international organizations such as the WHO. Larger-scale negotiations occur among these organizations and major donors such as the Bill and Melinda Gates Foundation. These multilevel negotiations demonstrate the hierarchy of positions, which are significantly rooted in economic and political resources. Most often, significant influence and these resources are directly related. Nonetheless, as argued earlier, those who own lesser amounts of resources may also show their influence and (consciously or unconsciously) express the effects of structured inequalities, such as a parent's refusal of a vaccine or a vaccinator's improper way of performing his/her assigned duties. The stakeholders negotiate under specific terms and conditions, such as aid cutbacks or salary reductions. A single stakeholder may concurrently engage in parallel negotiations with others. For example, a vaccinator may be simultaneously negotiating with parents and with higher authorities.

Vaccine refusal on the part of local people is an essential factor for bringing to light sociocultural, economic, and political inequalities. The refusal is concurrently an expression and an effect of a concealed cause or a result of an imbalance existing in the areas mentioned above, meaning that different politics about vaccination prevail in Pakistan as compared to other countries. Vaccination is an essential, yet contested, endeavor that represents a critical context for the concerned stakeholders. Consequently, it has attracted considerable attention from various quarters at both local and global levels. People in Pakistan, especially those in rural areas, question the contents of the vaccine and the intentions of the vaccination advocates. The national and international media have been writing about such suspicions.

For example, on 23 April 2019, the newspaper *Dawn* reported that a man in the city of Peshawar in the Khyber Pakhtunkhwa (KPK) province spread misinformation about the polio vaccine, asserting that it caused children to faint and die. Moreover, the media reported in 2019 that a mob attacked and torched a government health facility and murdered a woman polio worker in the city of *Chaman* in the *Baluchistān* province. These assaults compelled the government to halt the scheduled polio vaccination drive across the country due to safety concerns about the 270,000 polio vaccinators (Dawn 2019). Such news reports, especially in the English dailies of Pakistan, also involve virtual discussions (see Chapter 12).

The media have continually reported on the issue of using vaccination as an apparatus of (geo)politics in Pakistan. The most prominent example of this is the discussion around the "fake" vaccination drive to locate Osama bin Laden, who was the "mastermind" of the 9/11 attacks on the World Trade Center in New York. A Pakistani security analyst termed this fake vaccination campaign "vaccination suicide," because it made people suspicious of vaccination campaigns in general (AlJazeera 2013)—as with the perceived "Western plot" to "sterilize" Muslims (see e.g., Closser and Jooma 2013). Consequently, the vaccination teams became targets of violent assaults by local people who believed that the vaccinators were also "agents" of a nefarious international agenda. Since 2012, over 100 such attacks have been reported in the country by the media, killing over 120 vaccinators, their escorting security personnel, and other citizens (Closser and Jooma 2013; Mansoor 2016).

As previously noted, different stakeholders negotiate, express, and perpetuate inequalities in differing ways. Measles is, hence, more than a bodily condition: it is a window on a world where disparities prevail and where stakeholders negotiate them. I argue that those whose power counts more, that is, the government and global stakeholders, are significantly accountable for the prevalence of measles in rural areas. Indeed, blaming local people and saying that measles is a result of their "outdated" beliefs gives space to the stated stakeholders to conceal their inflicted inequalities and inefficiencies. These influential stakeholders view local people as a significant cause of the problem of measles, while in fact, their created structures play a decisive role in causing such crises.

An Overview of the Chapters in This Book

This book is organized into 11 chapters with a Prologue, this Introduction, and Conclusions. Chapter 1, "Many Anthropologies: Reflections on Theoretical Threads and the Medical Anthropology of Pakistan," describes the body of anthropological literature in which this book is mainly grounded: (1) interpretive anthropology or a "meaning-centered" approach; (2) critical medical anthropology; and (3) the anthropology of global health. Seeing these approaches as complementary to each other, I reflect upon various challenges that one can face while employing them, specifically critical medical anthropology. Along with explaining these theoretical approaches, I also revisit the medical anthropology of Pakistan, in which I describe what thematic areas have been explored and according to which theoretical perspective(s). Here, I not only focus on Pakistani anthropologists but also on international anthropologists who conducted research in Pakistan.

Chapter 2, "Researchlogue: Design, Methodology, and the Circumstances of Data Collection" is a methodological chapter—which I call a *researchlogue*—that illustrates my points of departure and the challenges and circumstances under which I gathered the data for this book, and with what methods, strategies, and approaches. Additionally, in this chapter I provide anecdotes from my fieldnotes, and detail the new qualitative research method I developed, which I call *Kachaharī*, and which has sociocultural roots and significance in Sindh. *Kachaharī* is a voluntary and informal social gathering in which, during the evening, people sit, share, discuss, and talk about life. Using *Kachaharī* prevented me from inventing the answers myself, because local people were leading the discussions. In the latter part of this chapter, I discuss the ethical considerations and potential limitations of my study.

In Chapter 3, "The Settings: The Ethnographic Features of the Two Villages" I describe the primary locales in which I conducted this research. After drawing a vivid ethnographic sketch of Sindh province, I describe the selected districts, *Sakhar* and *Tharpārkar*, and the two villages, *Rahīmpur* and *Rāmpur*. I provide a short history and depiction of their present sociocultural, economic, religious, and political characteristics, as well as of the available governmental health facilities in these districts and villages, because this background and context are necessary to contextualize measles and vaccination in these regions. I show that in both villages and districts, there is a dearth of necessary facilities—for instance, concerning health and education—and of infrastructure, which are a result of various forms of organized inequalities, and which facilitate measles outbreaks.

Chapter 4, "Competing Healthcare Systems: Revisiting Medical Pluralism in Pakistan," offers an overview of medical pluralism in Pakistan. Based on the literature, it briefly describes each existing system, including its historical roots of practices and knowledge, and aims to provide contextual information on people's treatment choices. Each system holds a specific, sometimes overlapping, body of knowledge and practices around questions of conceptualizing, restoring, and sustaining good health. Dealing with an "illness," "sickness," or "disease" differs in the form and content of the related etiology, diagnostics, and therapeutic practices. The apparent intention of all the mentioned systems, nonetheless, is the same: alleviating illness-related suffering and restoring people's health. This brief overview is necessary to illustrate the similarities and dissimilarities among these various medical systems, in order to situate measles and its varying etiologies and treatments, which differ considerably among these systems. Without this context, I would be hard-pressed to explain the contrasts in the cultural view of measles as a necessary sacred illness and the biomedical view of measles as a dangerous infectious disease that should be avoided.

In this chapter, I also address the country's efforts to legalize parts of the pluralistic medical system. For example, *Unānī-Tib*, homeopathy, and *Ayurvedā* have been legally incorporated and there are official schools that teach these healing systems. Nevertheless, the biomedical healthcare system has evolved and received much more attention and funding from the government than *Ayurvedā* and *Unānī Tib*. Yet the resources allocated to biomedicine are insufficient when compared to other governmental sectors, for example, defense. From 2000 to 2020, the country's average budget allocated to healthcare never rose above 1% of the total GDP. Consequently, the biomedical healthcare sector remains overwhelmed: in 2018, according to *Pakistan's Economic Survey*, the doctor–patient ratio was around one doctor for 970 people, one dentist for around 9,540 persons, and one hospital bed for around 1,610 people. These differences in terms of healthcare services and providers further intensify what is known as the "rural/urban divide," in which rural areas have much less biomedical availability than urban areas— thereby demonstrating some of the prevailing inequalities and their substantial implications. I show these differences while turning attention back to the selected villages: *Rahīmpur* and *Rāmpur*, which, again, have no biomedical facilities.

Chapter 5, "Health and Illness: Sociocultural Understandings," focuses on understanding how medical culture and its context in Pakistan are vital to deciphering its dealings with measles and tracing their roots. Focusing on *Rahīmpur* and *Rāmpur* villages where there is no biomedical health facility, this chapter describes the sociocultural understandings of health and illness: how do people make sense of health and illness, and how do they define and maintain health? How do they deal with an illness in terms of their perceptions of its causes or etiology, and how do they decide whether to ignore an illness or consult a specific medical system? What preventive measures are taken to maintain health or to take any further actions(s) to reinstate impaired health? How do people seek health measures by consulting a specific medical system such as *Ayurvedā*, *Unānī-Tib*, or biomedicine, and how do factors—such as beliefs, perceptions, economic situation, education, gender, and geographical area—shape these health-seeking measures? This chapter addresses those guidelines and orientations that culture provides to regulate and give meaning to daily living; these are learned, shared, and passed on from one generation to another. These specific cultural norms can be a source of health when they encourage adopting and avoiding specific behaviors related to daily life activities: for example, food, dress, actions, sleep, hygiene, and dealing with supernatural beings. Not following these cultural norms is often considered to result in ill-health. I describe: (a) how local people conceptualize and work to maintain good health; and (b) how they deal with illness to recover the lost state of health.

In Chapter 6, "Local Rituals of Containment: Emic Perceptions and Practices around Measles," I focus on measles in Sindh province. I present details on the positions, ideas, and practices of local people and *Hakīm* (herbalists), and on government officials involved with efforts to eradicate measles, and ask, what measures do they take? Yet primarily, this chapter devotes full attention to dealings with measles at the local level: it explains why the local people view measles as a necessary sacred illness bestowed by the Goddess *Mātā*, and describes the ritual of *Chando*, which is designed to honor *Mātā*, and in which a child who has contracted measles is quarantined and their treatment is ritually prescribed. In the latter part of this chapter, I draw on print media to describe how government officials view local perceptions and practices about measles. I also elucidate local *rituals of containment* to deal with measles that are designed to facilitate a transition from an unimmunized state to an immunized state via a transitional process that contains the same quality of liminality as other rites of passage (Turner 1974). After focusing on how local people conceptualize and deal with measles and the measures relevant stakeholders take to deal with it, the chapter illustrates measles as a process of transition mediated by these rituals of containment. Through analysis of print media content, I elaborate on how government officials and doctors blame the meanings the local people give to measles and their treatments of it for these outbreaks.

Employing Victor Turner's (1974) concept of "social drama," in Chapter 7, "Social Dramas: Two Measles Outbreaks and Multiple Narratives in Pakistan," I demonstrate how two consecutive measles outbreaks revealed social conflicts in Pakistan. I describe how several stakeholders, ranging from the *Rahīmpur* village of district *Sakhar* to the WHO, interpreted and dealt with the measles outbreaks of 2012 and 2013. This chapter not only presents the perspectives of local people about the outbreak, but also offers the standpoints of government officials and institutions, such as the Aga Khan University; the National Institute of Health (NIH); the Pakistan Medical Research Council (PMRC); the Ministry of Inter-Provincial Coordination (IPC)/Federal Expanded Programme on Immunization (EPI) Cell; the Accountant General of Pakistan Revenues (AGPR); and of international NGOs—WHO, the United Nations International Children's Emergency Fund (UNICEF), and the United States Agency for International Development (USAID). Supplying the comprehensive standpoints of these stakeholders regarding the outbreaks, this chapter highlights the negotiation processes around them.

Profiting from the concepts of "critical events" (Das 1995) and "global assemblages" (Collier and Ong 2005), Chapter 8, "The Critical Geopolitical Events: Making Sense of Anti-Vaccination Sentiment" focuses on how geopolitical regimes have generated favorable circumstances for the development and spread of rumors, conspiracy theories, and resistance, while also causing socioeconomic and political disparities that eventually result in various crises, including health problems. The chapter deals explicitly with how geopolitics have impacted immunization programs in the country and how they have significantly contributed to a set of obstacles to eliminating infectious diseases. I show that the immunization programs have received resistance from some "extremist" segments, for example, some religious leaders and *Tālibān*, and from the society, which relates vaccination to the ongoing geopolitics. Government officials and global stakeholders hold extremists accountable for the low vaccination uptake and the killings of the vaccinators and their security guards, stating that the opinions and actions of these extremists are partially responsible for the spread of the infectious disease.

However, broader geopolitical and economic factors have germinated the seeds of extremism in the country; thus, I show how these lie behind these specific perceptions.

This chapter also offers a historical account of Pakistan–Afghan relations; the USSR invasion; Pakistan's dictator-president Zia-ul-Haq's *Jihād*; and the promotion of the *Mujāhidīn* as villains. The chapter then follows their intricate interconnections with anti-American, anti-Western, and anti-vaccination sentiments. Significantly impacting the country, the critical events related to (geo)politics that I specify have shaped the general perceptions and practices that people in Pakistan hold and perform, including around vaccination. Consequently, they maintain their historically rooted intransigent hostilities and positions against it.

Chapter 9, "National and Global Rituals of Containment: Controversies, Contestations, and Mistrust Surrounding Vaccination in Pakistan," provides general perspectives on immunization in Pakistan. Being a signatory of the United Nations, Pakistan is bound to vaccinate each child to eliminate infectious diseases in order to reduce the disease burden; however, Pakistan's EPI faces multiple challenges. This chapter deals with why vaccination uptake is low in the country, why local people refuse vaccines and show anti-vaccination sentiments, and why they believe that vaccination is a "Western plot" or a "conspiracy against Muslims" that is meant to sterilize Muslim women. Focusing on these issues, the chapter situates controversies around vaccination within broader key events related to geo-bio-politics and explicates the local ideas, rumors, and conspiracy theories woven around vaccination. In short, this chapter deals with how and why a lifesaving scientific advancement—vaccination—has been interpreted differently in Pakistan and often refused.

In this chapter, I also deal with how local suspicions of and resistance to vaccines in general also apply to the Covid-19 vaccine, which is now available in Pakistan, yet only around 31% of the population have received two doses. This problem has been exacerbated by the fact that many rural people in the country do not even believe that Covid-19 is real; instead, they tend to think that it is a governmental scheme to gain more foreign aid (Ali 2020). Thus, as was to be expected, in rural areas, Covid-19 vaccine uptake has been low.

In this chapter, I additionally and importantly demonstrate that vaccine resistance and refusals are not a cause of the prevalence of infectious diseases in Pakistan, but instead are the effects of the aforementioned structural inequities and vulnerabilities. Implementers of vaccination campaigns seem highly focused on dealing with the effects, but not the root causes, which are the factors that are ultimately cultivating the environment of anti-vaccination sentiment, as this chapter will describe.

Having explicated vaccination as a general endeavor in Chapter 9, Chapter 10, "Measles Vaccine: From General to Particular," elucidates the historical development of the measles vaccine and then traces its usage in Pakistan.

Drawing on the information on suspected side effects, and on the rumors and conspiracy theories related to measles vaccination in the country, this chapter inquires: how has measles vaccination been linked to reactions in children that have included the deaths of some, and how have news reports of side effects been discussed and contested online on the websites of some English-language Pakistani newspapers? This chapter highlights various perspectives and rationales woven around measles vaccination in Pakistan, which reveal scales and types of mistrust. As previously argued, these explanations can be better understood against the backdrop of an ongoing interplay between and among sociocultural and politico-economic factors. People suspect both the ingredients of the vaccine and those who advocate for and administer the vaccine. This suspicion is deeply interlinked with the general perception of vaccination as a "Western plot." In this chapter, I also demonstrate how urban "netizens" negotiated the measles vaccine during an online dialogue on media websites. Based on different orientations, standpoints, and experiences, they brought differing claims and counterarguments about the safety or non-safety of the vaccine. These netizens criticized the media, the government, the vaccine, and global stakeholders, and these online sites have emerged as vibrant platforms to contextualize the phenomena of infectious diseases and vaccination.

Drawing on my fieldwork and media content analysis, Chapter 11, "Creating the Anthropology of Vaccination," illuminates some of the international controversies surrounding vaccination via discussion of large "anti-vaxx" movements, and shows what roles anthropology can play in comprehending the reasons behind vaccine refusal and why vaccination is a crucial subject matter for anthropology. To highlight international vaccine contestations, this chapter presents the cases of vaccination refusals in Italy and the USA, the underlying reasons for which differ significantly from those in Pakistan, and which I will address. Owing to the importance of vaccination for preventing outbreaks of infectious diseases such as measles, polio, and now Covid-19—which has brought the issue of vaccination back onto the global stage—I propose the creation of a new anthropological field: "the anthropology of vaccination." I argue that the fields of vaccination and anthropology have much to offer each other, and that anthropologists can play significant roles in reducing vaccine refusals via culturally savvy and appropriate culturally informed educational programs.

In the Conclusions, I summarize the primary issues involved and my findings. I reiterate that in this book, I have substantially profited from various theoretical concepts, including "structural violence" (Farmer 1996), "critical events" (Das 1995), and "global assemblage" (Collier and Ong 2005). I have also benefited from critical medical anthropology and interpretive anthropology. These concepts have helped me to examine measles from two perspectives—as a disease and as an analytical window to the world. As I will explain in these Conclusions, from the first perspective, I have demonstrated that the occurrence of measles outbreaks in Pakistan and elsewhere is related to structured disparities that are, in turn, related to sociocultural, political, and economic factors at local, national, and global levels. From the second perspective, measles as an analytical window has substantially helped me to understand the interplays among these factors. Understanding forms of institutionalized vulnerabilities and inequalities has assisted me in reaching that macro-level where policies are formulated and decisions are taken, which afterward can produce certain top-down forms of structural violence and social suffering from national to local levels. I elucidate that measles offer a platform to observe and analyze the links between micro and macro levels, local and global scales, and the particular and the general. In the preceding chapters, I have shown how these different worlds are interconnected. Peering through the lens of measles outbreaks has made it possible for me—and I hope for my readers—to study and understand various forms of social negotiations, tensions, and contestations, to perceive their underlying currents of mistrust, and to identify their root causes.

I have shown that measles outbreaks in Pakistan are not simply the results of individual behaviors as they are in Italy or the USA. Rather, their root causes include structured inequities and vulnerabilities, lack of effective education for the rural poor, and cultural or religious beliefs that include deep governmental mistrust and that stem from critical events, such as colonization, wars, and a fake vaccination campaign; these critical events are encoded in societal memory and feed into vaccination refusals. Hence, these outbreaks can best be understood against a broader and historical spectrum of economic and (geo)political inequalities, which are enormous, persistent, and deepening. I argue in Conclusions that the Pakistani government will never reach 70% vaccination uptake in rural regions until these issues, and others, are resolved.

In the Appendix to this book, I offer practical suggestions and solutions to the problems with vaccination both in Pakistan and globally.

Notes

1 The names of the villages and interlocutors have been anonymized.
2 *Dawn* is a long-standing newspaper in the country that is considered as particularly credible for two main reasons: its launching by the founder of Pakistan, Quaid-i-Azam Muhammad Ali Jinnah; and its attention to highly important issues and impartiality—its Editorials are written solely about worthy issues.
3 The WHO (2020b) has used this term to define "a cluster of physiological, behavioral, and cognitive phenomena in which the use of a substance or a class of substances takes on a much higher priority for a given individual than other behaviors that once had greater value (…) [it] is the desire (often strong, sometimes overpowering) to take the psychoactive drugs (which may or not have

been medically prescribed), alcohol, or tobacco. There may be evidence that return to substance use after a period of abstinence leads to a more rapid reappearance of other features of the syndrome than occurs with nondependent individuals."

4 *Unānī-Tib* is believed to be an Arabic translation of Greek medicine of the ancient world that reached India through the spread of Islamic civilizations and culture (see Leslie 1963).

1 Many Anthropologies

Reflections on Theoretical Threads and the Medical Anthropology of Pakistan

The Interpretive Approach Revisited

Interpretive or "meaning-centered anthropology," previously termed "symbolic anthropology," provides a foundation for my understanding of meanings and their interpretation. Interpretive medical anthropology entails "symbolizing, conceptualizing, meaning-seeking." Medical anthropologists seek to "make sense out of the experience, to give it form and order" (Geertz 1975, 140). New questions were formulated for questioning and understanding how culture shapes people's patterns of behaviors related to health and illness: what are the relationships among culture, health, and illness? Since interpretive anthropology has placed significant emphasis on the meanings that human beings weave around a phenomenon, this interpretive approach has become well known as the "meaning-centered paradigm" in medical anthropology. This "explanatory model" (Kleinman 1980) approach challenged and influenced the existing epistemological foundations of "disease."

Allowing to understand measles as a state of a body, an illness or infectious disease, this "meaning-centered" approach provides a constructivist argument that public bodies of knowledge are social constructs, and that a body's state is constituted and becomes visible and understandable with the help of anthropological interpretations. According to this model, a body's state can be declared as an illness or a disease; illness is an interpretation in a given local culture and disease is defined by scientific principles in the specialized culture of biomedicine (Kleinman 1978). Through giving meaning to human experience, these explanations shape actions to be taken in the future. Based on their interpretations, individuals decide how challenging the new state of the body is and then choose a response of whether to ignore or treat it (Ali 2011). Hence, these explanatory models play significant roles in analyzing the understanding of patients about their own experiences and help other stakeholders, such as local healers, to deal with these health conditions.

According to Kleinman (1977, 1988, 14–15), considering "disease" as a natural phenomenon and something beyond culture is nothing but a "category fallacy." Kleinman explains: "The reification of one culture's diagnostic categories and their projection onto patients in another culture, where those

DOI: 10.4324/9781003253716-2

categories lack coherence, and their validity has not been established, is a category fallacy" (ibid., 14–15). This constructivist argument (Good 1994) is especially important, viewing disease as ontologically rooted in a human-made system of meanings (Young 1976), and in specific interpretations in particular historical backgrounds, which constitute a critical standpoint for analyzing how these interpretations are contested and negotiated in particular contexts and power relations (Kuipers 1989; Good and Kleinman 1985; Good 1994).

Interpretive anthropology significantly focuses on the construction of therapeutic practices as medical knowledge, and on the interactions of cultural explanations with biology, psychophysiology, and the social relations that influence the diagnosis of the illness and its treatment (Good 1994). We can consider that if diseases are biomedical constructs, biology is also a construct. These studies attended to variations in defining and dealing with an illness while considering that cultural "idioms of distress"—which are "socially and culturally resonant means of experiencing and expressing distress in local worlds" (Nichter 1981, 405)—play a substantial role in those dealings, ultimately making the course of a disease distinct in various societies. Bringing culture to center stage, studies have claimed that it not only shapes the course of a disease (Carr and Vitaliano 1985; Ali 2011), but also may construct specific disorders that another culture might not perceive as a disorder (Good 1994). Attention has been paid to how distinct forms of illness and related trajectories are produced as a result of ongoing interplays between sociocultural and psychophysiological processes.

The meaning-centered paradigm helped me to search for the culturally attached meanings of measles and to discover how a diverse set of stakeholders, which range from a local to a global scale, make sense of measles. This approach provides a framework to collect narratives about experiences, explanations, etiology, and treatment options about measles required for understanding and answering essential questions: which meanings do measles carry, and how do such meanings function in negotiation processes among stakeholders? Why is the etiology of measles expressed in Hindu mythology as a necessary sacred illness? Why do local people observe the ritual of *Chando* and give preference to *Hakīm* (herbalists) over biomedical doctors? Only culturally detailed and "thick" descriptions[1] such as those I provide in this book can answer such questions. Without understanding these multiple interpretations and responses within a sociocultural context, comprehending the reasons behind the occurrence of measles in Pakistan and vaccine refusals would be misleading and hard to relate to within their broader backgrounds.

As Geertz (1975, 28) rightly pointed out, the interpretive approach draws "large conclusions from small" or vast inferences from specific, but thickly structured, cases to generalize extensive statements about a culture's role in constructing collective life. However, critical questions remained unanswered: for instance, how have these specific contexts—in which local people explain measles as a necessary sacred illness—been shaped by their broader context? How is this specific perception and practice connected to the past, especially to the "critical events" (Das 1995) that have significantly shaped the current South-Asian region and the field of global health? These issues will be discussed later on in this chapter.

The interpretive paradigm lacks the rigor to go beyond the phenomena of measles and vaccination. Through this paradigm, meanings can be identified and interpreted in ways that make sense of a given phenomenon, or many. Yet this paradigm pays little or no attention to the circumstances that produce these specific meanings and explanations. The interpretive approach did help me to explain what is happening in the case of measles in Pakistan. However, it did not supply answers to the second level of questions to go beyond the usual sociocultural perceptions and practices of measles as a necessary sacred illness. It was equally important to me to know *why* people hold specific opinions that measles is a necessary and a sacred illness, and what are the underlying reasons, especially for those phenomena that directly result in death or save someone from dying? Describing measles as a necessary sacred illness and interpreting the ritual of *Chando* via thick description are necessary, but so is the question of why these local people hold on to such beliefs and perform specific practices related to measles. Why do formally educated people perceive measles as a disease that can be prevented via vaccination and cured through medication, while less-educated people do not? Or why do specific people consider vaccination as a "Western plot," and why and how did this perception originate?

Despite its limitations, the interpretive paradigm has significantly shaped my views to explain what is happening in the arena of measles and vaccination in Pakistan as well as globally, and has also motivated me to move beyond what is visibly happening, although when and why it is happening remained unanswerable. The "meaning-centered" approach emphasizes discovering meanings in human behavior and places less focus on the broader contexts. It thereby exposes itself to cautious criticism based on the revision of the old as well as the presentation of the new ethnographic data. Severe criticism surrounded it for being "too 'clinical,'" too aligned with medicine's interests, yet lacking sufficient attention to biology and the "scientific rigor of epidemiology or cognitive studies" (B. Good 1994, 55).

In addition to the broader context mentioned above, according to Good (1994) the meaning-centered approach paid insufficient attention to how exactly cultural representations of the illness are produced and reproduced. Individual behavior is significantly shaped by external forces—local, regional, global. Roger Kessing (1987, 161) rightly argued that culture also constitutes specific ideologies that often disguise political and economic realities. Lorna Rhodes' (1990) criticism holds importance as she notes that although critical perspectives tend to emanate from the cultural analysis of biomedicine, the interpretive approach could not draw on these standpoints. Thus, I turn to critical medical anthropology.

Critical Medical Anthropology

My research project also builds on relevant literature from critical medical anthropology for highlighting the broader economic and (geo)political contexts that produce and reproduce specific webs of inequalities, because this body of literature helps to identify causal factors—the hegemonic ideologies and structures of power—that lie behind the outbreaks of measles and particular ways of dealing with the disease.

The term "critical" as used in critical medical anthropology (CMA) denotes an approach that takes it for granted that there is a material reality, and that power is important in the course of events. Rather, it deeply explores often otherwise invisible causal factors. This political economic school of thought draws heavily upon the Marxist concepts of "exploitation" and "false consciousness," and Gramsci's (1971) "hegemony." Due to these roots, the critical perspective helped me to explore connections among broader determinants, such as economic and political factors that directly cause disease, indirectly create circumstances conducive to contracting a disease, and generate explanatory narratives through which people rationalize the reasons for the disease without always understanding these broader factors. These circumstances expose people to precariousness—conditions under which they are more structurally vulnerable to contracting infectious pathogens. The CMA literature has paid significant attention to these broader and influencing circumstances (e.g., Rylko-Bauer and Farmer 2016; Baer, Singer, and Susser 2003; Kleinman, Das, and Lock 1997; Farmer 1996a).

Structural Violence and Social Suffering

Structural violence refers to those social structures, cultural patterns, and political elements that become a system that affects people in an adverse way as that system produces and perpetuates disparities. Paul Farmer (1996a) adopted the notion of "structural violence" from Norwegian sociologist Johan Galtung (1969) in order to explore the institutionalized forms of inequalities and their impact on health and illness. Using the concept of structural violence, multiple studies have explored the overt or subtle ways in which violence is perpetrated, subverted, contested, and appropriated (Rylko-Bauer and Farmer 2016; Qureshi 2013; Massé 2007; Farmer 2006; Farmer et al. 2006; Ellison 2003; Farmer 1996a). Systematic disparities cause "social suffering," in which people bear and justify the critical outcomes of that ongoing interplay among social, cultural, and political systems (Kleinman, Das, and Lock 1997; Kleinman 2000).

Both concepts—social suffering and structural violence—critically discuss the impacts and interplay of institutionalized forms and webs of inequalities that cause suffering and violence. Some stakeholders appear to be overtly constructing such structures in ways that turn them into unnoticed parts of people's daily lives, rendering them culturally normative. Powerful stakeholders are influential and their ideas are given credence and acted upon within society. They aim to control the powerless. On the one hand, suffering is exerted on people in the form of problems and crises. On the other hand, stories of suffering are normalized, and people are either unaware of it or again compelled in a specific way to rationalize it.

This means that lay people's vision is blurred; they cannot hold responsible those who cause suffering; they instead find explanations of suffering in socially constructed narratives. This allows the powerless to live within and according to those realities. For instance, the notion of measles as a necessary sacred illness and the concept of Qismat (literally: "fatalism") exist in Pakistani society as attempts people make to accept their powerless realities. It will be helpful to elucidate this latter concept. Qismat is a concept that Pakistanis, especially the rural population, use in almost all everyday activities. Whenever something happens—such as the death of someone by accident, murder, inappropriate treatment by a doctor—the most frequent sentence one hears is, [in *Sindhī*] *"Jaiko* Qismat *Main Likhayal Huyo"* ("it was written in the fate of that person, so this had to be the way it happened").

This idea of Qismat perhaps trickled down from ancient philosophy in various places and was embraced by the masses in those places as an explanatory framework for their suffering—its roots are thousands of years old. The current powerful stakeholders, such as politicians, elites, and governments, did not create this concept, but they are benefiting from this construction of suffering as inevitable, as part of people's supernaturally determined "destinies." The issue is people sense they have little control over unfortunate events, and they embrace a way of explaining harm. Hence, I argue that rural laypeople appear not to see that equal access to appropriate and adequate healthcare facilities is a prime responsibility of the government. If it is not put in place where needed, then the government should be held accountable. Yet, in Pakistan, usually most of the injustice, violence, pain, and even deaths seem justified in the name of Qismat, attributing them to the supernatural rather than placing blame where blame belongs and taking action, such as protesting against government policies in order to improve their lives.[2]

Fatalism has received plenty of attention in philosophy. The origins of this attention can be traced to Aristotle's work *On Interpretation* (most recently published in 1984), in which he argues against it in the famous "Sea Battle Argument" to draw a relation between logic and necessity in the world around us.[3] Robert Kane (2005, 19) argues that fatalism is "the view that whatever is going to happen is going to happen, no matter what we do." This concept implies a necessitation—events will happen "no matter what," which contains the idea of us being too powerless to do anything about what happens. It ignores the agency behind our actions and how our thoughts and behaviors impact the outcome of an event. Similar to most philosophers, I argue against this idea, mainly due to the ethical grounds that are required for moral responsibility. If a person believes in fatalism, it becomes near-impossible for that person to generate an ethical system in which people can be held responsible for their actions (see Chapter 6).

Kleinman and colleagues (1997) rightly proposed that anthropological analyses should move beyond the visible problems and crises that cause social suffering and study the mechanisms of social suffering. This perspective is vital in order to comprehend the making of social suffering. In the case of measles, although children and their families suffer, they do not see it as suffering, because a strong narrative exists in Sindh province. The story explains that measles is a necessary sacred illness, blessed by the Goddess Mātā, that everyone must contract: "It can occur to you in the grave if you missed it during life," stated one of my interlocutors in his late 40s from *Rāmpur* village.

In this way, suffering and violence are appropriated by powerful stakeholders through structured webs. Both take the form of related words, given that language constructs realities by influencing human beliefs, actions, and behaviors. For example, if the terminology of "sacredness" was changed, or people's perception of viewing measles as a necessary illness was replaced with an understanding that measles can be avoided entirely through proper vaccination, then people certainly would consider measles as suffering, and perhaps even see it as a result of a set of inequalities. But it is also a reality that not all people resist vaccination for measles as they significantly believe in "Western" biomedicine and they consider not opting for it as demonstrating "Stone Age" beliefs.

Moreover, sometimes social suffering can also be categorized in terms of its impact: bearable and unbearable. The influential stakeholders most often exert unbearable suffering, which compels people not to view the bearable suffering as suffering. For example, people often view poverty to be a result of poor governance that exerts suffering on the whole family. Family members worry about the resources to buy food. On the other hand, measles seems to be viewed as bearable suffering that they believe would go away by observing certain rituals for five to seven days. However, hunger cannot go away without the provision of food, even after performing rituals. Measles also does not always go away with ritual; but since people cannot see their children suffering, they observe rituals. They are not aware of the relationship among measles, pneumonia, seizures, and brain damage, which can even lead to death.

Therefore, we should be vigilant in observing the categories of social suffering in terms of its impact. This yardstick, on the one hand, would help to capture all forms of social suffering, and on the other hand, it would prevent those inflicting suffering through intentionally poor governance from disappearing as causal agents.

Therefore, critical endeavors raise questions about the creation of social realities—under what circumstances do they emerge and whom do they serve? (see Baer, Singer, and Susser 2003). The real beneficiaries may be the government, a social class, a gender or ethnic group, and/or stakeholders in such particular cultural conceptions. The CMA theorists question the relationships among external hegemonic ideologies and social patterns, as well as the dominant ideology of biomedicine that permeates almost all countries' healthcare systems (Baer, Singer, and Susser 2003, 37).

For example, Singer and colleagues (1992) have asked, "Why does Juan Garcia have a drinking problem?" The biomedical answer would be that he is addicted to alcohol, that the problem inheres in him, and that he is responsible for getting treatment. In contrast, the CMA answer is much more complex. Juan was born in Puerto Rico into a society in which drinking was a manly thing to do. Because his family was poor (due to colonization), he received no higher education. Once he married and had children, he moved his family to New York City to have a chance at a better life. There he got a well-paying factory job that enabled him to support his family. He was a loving husband and father with no drinking problem at all, until the factory closed and, now in his 50s, he could not find another job. He became depressed and felt unmanly because he could no longer support his family. Hence, he turned to the only manly thing he could do—he started hanging out at a bar and developed a severe drinking problem. So, did this problem inhere in Juan, or in the cultural and socio-structural forces that left him with no other recourse that he could perceive? This is the value of CMA—it allows the researcher to probe beyond the individual and into the deeper structural forces that both heavily influence and severely limit their choices, thereby rendering visible what was formerly invisible.

Accordingly, my research supports the argument of the CMA paradigm that the production of disease and its treatment happen within the broader setting of the world system and within embedded systems of social stratification and structural violence that flow along the lines of social stratification. It is crucial to consider the global context while studying Pakistan's healthcare system. This is because, as Elling (1981) argued, such healthcare systems include international health agencies, corporations, national bilateral aid programs, multinationals (especially drug companies, medical technology manufacturers and suppliers, industrial companies, agribusiness, commercial suppliers of baby food, suppliers of chemical fertilizers and pesticides, and sellers of population-control devices), and the biomedical cultural hegemony that justifies the interventions of such stakeholders on the world stage, particularly in low-resource locations.

Baer and colleagues (2003, 40) contend that the dominant healthcare systems of capitalist countries reproduce class structures worldwide. Their profit orientation has driven biomedicine into a capital-intensive endeavor that depends upon the latest technologies, the extensive use of drugs, and the concentration of services. The State legitimizes and strengthens corporate involvement by supporting medical training and research in the reductionist biomedical framework. I give as an example the World Bank, which has become an active international player in formulating health-related policies and granting financial loans for healthcare endeavors. The Bank influences health policy by cofinancing international and bilateral agencies and matching the funds of recipient governments. The Bank then performs country-specific health sector analyses to propose reforms that are highly compatible with market-driven economies (ibid., 40). The Bank's influence is visible in vaccination programs worldwide, including in Pakistan. Low-income countries, such as Pakistan, have become laboratories where large corporations test their products or "dump" the ones deemed unsuitable for high-resource countries.

There are various specific companies that are involved in the construction, development, and equipping of hospitals, the provision of medical, surgical, and diagnostic equipment, and numerous auxiliary products and services (Doyal 1979). These companies become allies with the elites of low-income countries and then influence health policies by offering incentives: jobs, favors, and outright bribery (Baer, Singer, and Susser 2003, 41).

Moreover, macro-level structures feature highly concentrated power to shape the microlevel structures. The CMA approach is a prime lens for examining the occurrence of measles beyond the illness and concerning economic and political factors. The etiology of illness can be "scientifically" correct, that is, a virus that causes measles can be prevented through a vaccine. Nonetheless, other factors may significantly contribute to providing an environment conducive to the production, distribution, and course of that illness, including measles, especially its outbreaks.

This CMA approach supports questioning the repetitive occurrence of measles in Pakistan: why does measles prevail and how is it negotiated? Through this perspective, this book investigates measles in both local and broader perspectives of political and economic forces, and at the national and global level. According to Singer (1990a, 181), these shape interpersonal relations, determine social behavior, yield social meanings, and form collective experience.

This standpoint offered essential insights that helped to unveil and understand the factors behind the frequent occurrence of measles in Pakistan, which otherwise remained neglected, avoided, and diligently and cleverly diverted. This approach helps to elucidate the factors responsible for people's avoidance of bringing their children to modern hospitals. Why do people refuse and resent vaccination? At the superficial level, people are seemingly the culprits for failure in the elimination of measles, just as Juan Garcia can be viewed as the culprit for his drinking problem. However, behind the scenes, there are structural and eco-political factors that make these people into the culprits, "blaming the victims." The CMA contextualization unpacks these factors by shining a light on several forms of inequalities. As Baer and colleagues (2003) argued, the CMA perspective situates health issues within political and economic contexts (at any scale). These contexts effectively formulate human relationships, shape social behaviors, create collective experiences, rearrange local ecologies, and influence their cultural meanings (ibid., 4).

Agreeing with Good (1994), I note that illness (measles in the current case) can be a "misrepresentation" if it is defined in a particular perspective to ultimately serve the interests of influential segments of society, such as elites, beneficiaries of dominant economic arrangements, the medical profession, or an empowered gender. It is, therefore, necessary to study the interactions among several levels: macro, national, institutional, community, and micro—to look at measles from both emic and etic perspectives. This entails examining the intersections of broader economic patterns, the national economic and political structures, the healthcare system, the popular and folk beliefs and actions, the experiences of illness, behavior and meaning, human physiology, and environmental factors (see Young 1980; Frankenberg 1980; Morgan 1987; Ong 1988; Morsy 1990). This study connects explanations of measles with the underlying causes of those interpretations. The CMA perspective provided a conceptual framework to question perennial measles outbreaks and helped me to analyze the connections between macro- and microstructures. I have significantly benefited from this conceptual framework in understanding how dominant systems produce meanings through the social and institutional rules and practices that shape and influence our lifeworlds (e.g., Foucault 1980).

Building on CMA, I unpack the underlying circumstances that compel many Pakistanis to consider measles to be a necessary illness or vaccination as a "Western plot." These works have offered a relevant set of terminologies of inequalities and significantly made me (like many others) aware of the forms of suffering that many people have been witnessing and experiencing. My awareness has also been formed in the crucible of the inequities that I myself, an anthropologist from the Global South, have faced, along with my family and my community, as I describe below. The following "critical reflections" concern research practicability, research ethics, and the personal and political dangers of telling the truth.[4]

Critical Reflections on the CMA Paradigm: Practicability, Ethics, and Dangers

Critical dispositions are paramount skills that enable one to explore deep meanings. Yet conducting studies with a critical lens is a daunting task as it requires a researcher's vigilance and poses several challenges and problems. Critical studies often need to involve quantitative and qualitative research methods and to adjust them to complement each other. Thus, the first problem that I faced was the suitability of research methods to obtain both qualitative and quantitative data, because quantified data are also essential for critical ethnographies. Quantitative data offer a vital understanding of the economic and demographic state of an individual, a family, or a community. The data help to comprehend inequalities. I developed a survey to learn about people's socioeconomic situations—such as demographics and income patterns—to situate into this context the occurrence of measles, while arguing that such factors compel people to hold specific views about the disease.

The second challenge with this approach is related to the application of those methods. In some geographical locations, especially those that have experienced colonization, people have widespread suspicions about surveys; thus, carrying out quantitative research is a challenging task.

The third problem concerns academic freedom and autonomy. Criticality can pose precariousness—sociocultural, economic, and political—for a researcher, and especially for some researchers and in some specific geographical settings. The CMA literature has rarely discussed how this approach can propel a researcher into a state of precariousness. The critical approach aims to uncover the powerful sociocultural and politico-economic forces—hegemonic institutions and ideologies—or "culprit" factors at work that construct the underlying circumstances to silence and marginalize some people, ultimately restricting human freedom and affecting human dignity. Yet these factors largely stay subtly complex, at least from nonacademic eyes. Aiming to explore and expose such subtle but crucial factors, a critical paradigm intends to seek how "truths" are being socially constructed temporally and spatially. It unveils the interests of influential stakeholders, which then can be used against a particular researcher if they do not like what the researcher finds.

For the current project on measles, employing the critical paradigm to deeply describe the interplay between internal and external factors was a somewhat frightening task. This is because, in Pakistan, this lens could result in severe implications for me personally due to the involved stakeholders, who—zooming in and out—are the USA, the CIA; Pakistan's politicians, its army, and the Inter-Services Intelligence (ISI); and "Big Pharma." These stakeholders are influential and hold specific interests, and their policies and practices have adversely impacted the country. This is because the extremists, who now are called *Tālibān*, were deliberately produced in the name of the "greater good," and because the country spends a considerable amount of its budget on the army (due to constant fear and threat of wars with India) at the expense of sectors like education and healthcare. As a result, the country suffers severe consequences of *Tālibān* production and has been unable to develop its nonmilitary institutions, which should fulfill people's basic needs.

I often thought that the safe way to proceed would be to refrain from applying critical theories in order to keep myself out of trouble. Yet as a scholar, I could not in good conscience take this approach. Thus, I chose to apply the critical approach to do accurate and comprehensive analyses while drawing on credible sources and observations, and then take the position of challenging hegemonic and hidden power structures, such as capitalism, neoliberalism, "Western" domination, colonization, political corruption—for the greater good. Finally, fighting a great "battle" with myself in which fears, anxieties, ethics, and obligations participated, the latter two won to compel me to employ criticality.

Criticality is not dangerous for every researcher. Being a critical and conscious thinker and working with a critical standpoint is usually nonproblematic for those researchers who mainly belong to the Global North to conduct their research, perform their analyses, and return to their own countries. Undoubtedly, they do face other challenges, such as having to learn a new language or "going native," but they rarely have to fear for their lives; however, sometimes they do have to fear for their jobs. For instance, in Pakistan, Svea Closser (2010) conducted her work on polio and mentioned the "politics" behind the "failure" of a mega polio program. Although she exposed critical factors, it is less threatening for her to live in her own country and conduct her work in Pakistan or other countries because she holds US citizenship. The latter identity appears a privilege, as on 27 January 2011, Raymond Davis—a US soldier who was working for the CIA—was believed to have killed two men in *Lāhore*, Pakistan, and despite that, was set free after deep negotiations.[5] This appears a promising case of how different identities can give some advantages or disadvantages to (not) ward off dangers.

Thus, I argue that using a critical lens is extremely important, but not applicable to all endeavors nor suitable for every researcher to employ. The anthropologists coming from former colonies and low-income countries need extra vigilance while conducting "anthropology at home." This conclusion favors classical anthropological fieldwork patterns, in which anthropologists always researched a society that was not their own. The challenges of conducting fieldwork in one's own country were not apparent to the first generations of anthropologists. In contrast, doing anthropology at home features other advantages that I call "plug and play," because the anthropologist is already familiar with the emic perspective—the widely held views—from the inside. This familiarity offers the researcher an edge, since s/he has already completed the *rites de passage* that are often required to be an ethnographer.

The fourth limitation concerns the consequences of such studies for the interlocutors. Our studies can be dangerous for them in at least two ways: we may change their views to make them more conscious of the systemic disparities they are suffering from, and ultimately, they can challenge the hegemonic ideologies and structures of power that inflict the suffering. We can change the views of our interlocutors during and after our fieldwork. When we participate in their lives, we learn from them, and they from us. Our continuous conversations, especially the critical ones, compel them to think differently. We convey another worldview to them, which perhaps the interlocutors never thought of before. I do not claim that they are "unconscious," but what we do adds a new perspective to that consciousness and makes them more aware. Because they want to know, we often tell them about the problem we are studying, which earlier they may never have considered a problem.

Moreover, if we feed back to them with theses or articles, some of them—if not all—can read the stories we have created from their views. Our analyses can further convey to them that what is "normal" to them is "abnormal" in the wider world. Informing our interlocutors about our work based on their accounts and maintaining trust relationships have long been considered as our obligation (e.g., Caplan 2004; Jorgensen 1971).

Therefore, simply by sensitizing them about the root causes of their suffering, we indirectly pit our interlocutors against the people inflicting the suffering. The inflictors can proactively exert further suffering as a punishment for speaking the truth because those suffering are now aware of the problem, which ultimately can make the inflictors have to defend themselves.

That means that although we may leave our fields, our impressions and perspectives remain, and we may still cause problems and suffering for our interlocutors and ourselves. We set off ripples of change at our respective field sites. This precariousness-related puzzle raises questions about research ethics and limitations, especially regarding using critical lenses. Anthropologists should also conduct research to identify whatever new suffering we may leave behind. This way, we can reflexively study the critical problems of the critical paradigm. Therefore, I maintain that how to protect both researchers and their interlocutors after applying the critical approach should emerge as a new and important theme in CMA.

Anthropology and Global Health

Global health has received ample anthropological attention (e.g., Biehl 2016; W. Anderson 2014; Farmer et al. 2013; Singer and Erickson 2013; Fassin 2011; Escobar 2011; Kleinman 2010; Collier and Lakoff 2008; Baer, Singer, and Susser 2003; Farmer 1996a).[6] These researchers have paid attention to how and why health has become a global project and research obligation. History shows us that specific key political and historical processes, which Veena Das (1995) called "critical events," are behind this development. Critical events, according to Das, can be viewed as those events that carry profound, broad, and long-lasting impacts and consequences. Prior to global health policies, there were different endeavors such as "international health." The focus of "international health" was to control epidemics across the boundaries between nations (Brown, Cueto, and Fee 2006).

The internationalization of health and illness goes back to the era of colonization, invasion, and missionaries, who both faced the new diseases they encountered and brought their own diseases with them, including measles, thereby killing many of the people whom they intended to serve. As an example, measles and other infectious diseases brought by the early missionaries and sailors to Hawaii killed off one-quarter of the Indigenous population. Thus, the presence and prevalence of measles in colonized countries may be a direct result of colonization.

For some, the roots of international health are found in the eighteenth and nineteenth centuries when the missionaries established clinics and the colonizers organized large-scale campaigns against infectious diseases in their respective colonies for their own sake, to protect themselves from the infections and keep their colonized populations healthy so that they could work for the colonizers (Lane and Rubinstein 1990; Leng 1982; El-Mehairy 1984; Asad 1995). Briefly, this interaction provided the foundations of today's international healthcare systems. The attitudes of the colonizers toward the "natives" and their measures for protecting themselves and coping with the novel settings shaped the world differently. It was an interaction between them and the settings, and between different medical systems—the one the colonizers practiced and the "other" one that native communities believed in and practiced.

Thereafter, the health arena took another turn, in which it was reconceived in light of "technical" parameters of the concept of "development" while labeling diseases as signs of "underdevelopment." Escobar (1984, 2011) argued that "underdevelopment" was formulated as a technical issue, which needed the technical expertise of the "developed" nations to be solved. This new conception provided high-income countries with the authority to intervene in low-income countries because the colonizing countries regarded development and modernization as part of their primary agenda, which also included the massive exploitation of the natural resources and workers of the colonized countries.

However, "international health" changed into "global health" over time, in which health is no longer viewed only as an individual concern or a national responsibility. Health and healthcare have become perceived as a global problem as well as an obligation, especially when health is disturbed by microorganisms: viruses and bacteria. The promotion of health has turned into a global endeavor due to human-made alterations such as population growth, unequal distribution of resources, and international travel (Singer 2015), as recently evidenced by the coronavirus pandemic. What is more, the weaker national healthcare systems are believed to be significant threats to other countries due to the spread of infectious diseases such as measles, Ebola, avian flu, and now Covid-19 and its variants. As mentioned earlier, Pakistan has remained under the spotlight due to the ongoing prevalence of measles and polio. (Although polio has been eradicated in most of the world, it still exists as a serious threat in Pakistan and neighboring Afghanistan, as I will discuss further in Chapter 10.) Due to this prevalence, vaccination was made mandatory for Pakistanis to travel abroad.

Owing to the rapid spread of diseases, global stakeholders have become more interested in global health, realigning and repositioning themselves to that focus (Hafner and Shiffman 2012) as the WHO has been continuously adjusting its interests and expertise in the field of global health (Brown et al. 2006). Similar observations have been made by Closser (2010, 46), who observes that this international organization has been practicing the "culture of optimism" and has been rewarded by receiving funds from its donors to continue its worldwide projects.

Considering improving health as a global challenge opened new avenues of intervention: humanitarian and business. This new packaging of health as a global problem now appears to need global solutions, most especially as a result of the coronavirus pandemic, which affected—and continues to affect—both low- and high-resource countries. Yet, as has become abundantly clear, high-resource nations are far better equipped to deal with this global pandemic than low-resource nations. Adams (2016b, 187) argues that, ideologically, the solutions to global health problems should be cost-effective, practical, technologically sophisticated—affordable, but also profitable—and accountable to the public. This ideation attracted a wide range of stakeholders such as academics, scientists, experts, administrators, and business personnel.

To address the multitude of burning global health problems, new economic and technological forms have emerged. A new range of professions has materialized from conceiving an idea to making it real in a laboratory, and from laboratory to the delivery level. Brown and colleagues (2006) argue that moving away from the older conceptualizations—such as colonial era "tropical medicine" and postwar "international health"—has gathered diverse actors and interests situated in diverse places, which has made the field of global health into a "big business."

In his article "Bureaucratic Aspects of International Health Agencies," George Foster (1987) identifies four types of bureaucratic organizations involved in tackling health crises: international (multilateral) organizations, governmental (bilateral) organizations, nongovernmental organizations (NGOs), and philanthropic foundations. Biehl (2016) claims that such changes in the ways of engagement for conceiving of and dealing with health have significantly changed ideas, practices, and the political capacities of state and non-state actors, which currently are more visible.

Farmer and colleagues (2013) view global health as an "assemblage of problems." The problems, in the case of measles in Pakistan, have emerged in the form of mistrust, suspicions, rumors, conspiracy theories, and ultimately suffering embodied by diseases and deaths. These "hidden agendas" in Pakistan have fueled massive resistance against population control and vaccination programs. For example, a "fake" vaccination drive was used as a cover in 2011 by the American CIA in the northern areas of Pakistan, especially in Abbottabad city, to discover the location of Osama bin Laden. This misuse of the hepatitis vaccine, an example of hidden interests, was declared by a Pakistani security analyst to be a "vaccination suicide" (Al Jazeera 2013), and indeed it most definitely heightened people's fears of and mistrust in the country's vaccination program, as described in Chapter 11.

Andrew Lakoff (2010, 59) divides contemporary global health into two regimes: global health security and humanitarian biomedicine. According to him, the former regime focuses on diseases that still might occur or reoccur, such as virulent influenza and smallpox. Although these diseases may not cause outbreaks, numerous stakeholders, including multilateral health agencies, national disease control departments, and laboratories, are engaged to provide "early warning" systems while considering the probable political, economic, and health-devastating consequences. The latter regime deals with those diseases that are presently infecting people in low-income countries such as malaria, HIV/AIDs, Ebola, and Covid-19. Both these regimes, according to Lakoff (2010), are "global" because they cross the boundaries set by the national governance of public health. The engaged stakeholders in these regimes make a global space that results in sites of knowledge and intervention.

Medical anthropology has significantly focused on the concept of "the global." In his book chapter "That Obscure Object of Global Health," Didier Fassin (2012, 96) interrogates the concept of "the global" to "unveil the dialectic of spatial expansion and moral normalization" and "health" to highlight the "tension between the worth of lives and the value of life." He claims, "Global health has become an effective signifier. Independent of the object to which it refers, it transmits an idea of change, of worldliness, of postmodernity. This dimension—which makes it a keyword of our time—should not be understrated" (ibid., 101). Fassin further wonders about the functions of global health; he wonders whether this concept is more about "Western" power to define and transform the world or about the practical matter of dealing with the world's health problems.

These diverse perspectives allow the researcher to particularly focus on global health for documenting and analyzing the power relations and people's requirements in tension with various national and global stakeholders. In the case of this project, they include laypeople (*Hakīm*), biomedical doctors, politicians, federal and provincial governments, national institutions, and global organizations, for example, the WHO and United States Agency for International Development (USAID). The global stakeholders issue protocols to the Pakistani government to conduct various programs to deal with measles and other infectious diseases and to measure their progress. For following these guidelines, the government receives aid not only for dealing with infectious diseases, but also for developing the fragile economy. Thus, global funding plays a pivotal role in global health.

Funding and Metrics in Global Health

The funds, from an economic perspective, involve the processes of production, (re-)distribution, and consumption. Over time, these processes of funding have become the subject matter of several disciplines of the social sciences. To investigate the mechanisms of funding, McCoy and colleagues (2009, 413), while considering them as a "fragmented, complicated, messy and inadequately tracked" phenomena, divide these mechanisms into three phases: provision, management, and spending. This "chaotic" state of funding requires critical study to track the real beneficiaries (ibid., 407). The studies should specifically be critical about the funding that goes to the low- to middle-income countries (LMICs) with an apparent aim to upgrade their healthcare sectors. At the same time, the other realms—such as poverty, food insecurity, malnutrition, inaccessible clean water, hygiene and education, humanitarian and emergency aid—that affect health are less prioritized (ibid.). These realms are far more critical and relevant to health because of their considerable influence on it. As discussed in Chapters 9–12, many laypeople refer to a lack of economic resources, clean water, food, and medicine. Due to the unfulfillment of these needs, they perceive the danger of no food to be higher than that of contracting measles, and thus are reluctant to skip even one day's work to take their children to be vaccinated or to take a child with measles to a medical facility.

Moreover, quantification has emerged as an objective determinant of science (Porter 1995), and one can observe the "critical turn" in anthropology and sociology to study the quantification of a phenomenon, as profoundly as possible, because some stakeholders use it as a tool to construct realities that allow them to exploit or justify their interventions in megaprojects (Adams 2016a; Espeland and Stevens 2008). Weightage is given to high or low numbers according to a requirement for creating a specific impression as is visible in the cases of infectious diseases and vaccination. There is always that "culture of optimism" (Closser 2010, 46) or what I call an *optimism bias*: "good numbers" are relative phenomena.

Furthermore, global health programs produce specific models of formulating a problem and then designing strategies to deal with it. These models incorporate the differences embedded in belief, behavior, and context to give background information, but do not necessarily value them in designing interventions. Pinto (2008) terms global health as a "black box" because of its discriminatory approach to suppressing the local contexts and specificities (regional, cultural, and national) in interventions or research. Counting is a vital part of such programs, as in the programs focusing on the elimination of infectious diseases, where there is considerable reliance on statistics.

Moreover, strategies and ways of dealing with infectious diseases are linked to the concept of modernization: vaccination can also be seen as a tool for differentiating the "traditional" and "modern." The people who are against vaccination are labeled as "traditional" due to holding old beliefs, and those who accept vaccination are the "modern" ones with innovative ideas.

Global Health as a Global Assemblage of Problems

Furthermore, global health can be seen in Collier and Ong's (2005) phrase as a "global assemblage": the site of formation and reformation of individual and collective lifeworlds. I see that our contemporary lifeworlds are connected in such extremely sensitive and inextricably intricate ways that if something happens in one place, it leaves a significant impact on the other places as well—in the well-known "butterfly effect." By employing this metaphor, I note the fact that, due to intricate interconnections, there is always a causal relationship between two close or distant occurrences: (in-)significant effects of a happening anywhere can be felt in the rest of the world. The causal factors can relate to temporal or spatial contexts, which can further be interrelated with past or contemporary events. In the "butterfly effect," my study illustrates the links between vaccine refusals and geopolitics. Vaccine refusals, in Pakistan and elsewhere, are intricately rooted in temporal, spatial, current, and past critical events. These refusals, via halting the elimination of infectious diseases, including measles, cause further micro and macro effects across the world. For instance, considering measles as a "threat," at a microlevel, the respective province organizes supplementary immunization activities (SIAs); or at the macro level, the WHO offers further guidance, and "resources" to Pakistan; or the organization makes the "yellow" (vaccine) card mandatory to travel abroad. In this way, as microlevel refusals are the effects of other (in)visible causes, they become a cause of several other effects, such as a largely unvaccinated population, which results in disease spread, which in turn results in illnesses and deaths. This chain of cause–effect–cause continues.

To consider global health as a mix of numerous determinants, not just biological, Farmer and colleagues (2013) propose a "biosocial" approach. Digging deeper to understand the factors that structure the problems, they raise a salient question about the ways in which history and political economy can help to comprehend the twisted distributions of wealth and illness around the globe (ibid., 2–3). This approach seems an extended version of the "structural violence" concept that Farmer (1999, 2003b, 1996b) developed in the late 1990s while arguing that improper distribution of wealth has impacts on the poor, and these impacts have not been significantly investigated. He, with Campos (2004), called for a "resocializing" of ethics—especially bioethics—to investigate the asymmetrical distribution of powers and positions. Apart from legal responsibilities, practices of global health projects should be right, just, and fair.

I argue that anthropologists should work more on making visible the invisible structures in global programs, and make efforts to analyze and explain the "butterfly effects" of every policy and practice. For example, the butterfly effect will help to understand and explore how a fake vaccination drive in Abbottabad district affected vaccination uptake in other regions of Pakistan, and at an international level too. Also, how did that fake drive affect other areas in which foreign stakeholders are involved? Such studies could help to improve programs, decrease human suffering, and extend our knowledge. Anthropology should unveil nonmedical determinants by gathering and analyzing the broader power constellations, institutions, processes, and ideologies that structure disease and health. Such analyses should be empirical, historically rooted, and not limited to one part of the world. Inquiries, as Biehl (2016, 135) suggests, must focus on places affected by global inequalities and neo-ideologies, such as neocolonialism, neoliberalism, governmentality, and humanitarian reasoning. Farmer and colleagues (2013, 9) propose that emphasis should also be placed on the role of non-state institutions such as NGOs and private philanthropists.

Anthropologists have studied the global in the local and not so much the local in the global, especially in relation to health and illness. I argue that we should reverse the direction of our analysis or move our inquiries toward the latter. For instance, my research has explored how an ordinary person perceives the measles vaccine, and how a simple vaccine refusal compels the policymakers at diverse levels to redesign the vaccination programs and protocols, as I will further demonstrate later on.

The Medical Anthropology of Pakistan: A Long Way to Go

Thus far, anthropologists have not fully explored the medical landscape of Pakistan, although some works inside and outside the discipline have been conducted, mainly by "non-native" researchers (e.g., Mull 1991, 1997; Mull et al. 1994; Closser 2010, 2012). At the country level, some graduate-level theses have been produced, especially at its public university, named Quaid-i-Azam University, which have mainly emphasized health-seeking behavior (e.g., Anjum 2000); sanitation and health (e.g., Maqsood 2001); environment and health (e.g., Iram 2003); maternal health (e.g., Shah 1999); local perception of health (e.g., Shahzadi 1999); ethnomedicine (e.g., Ashraf 1994); and the relationship between culture, health, and illness (e.g., Ali 2011).[7] Such theses have employed what William Sax called "five-decades-old anthropological approaches" (personal communication, Heidelberg 2018). Furthermore, a few studies have focused on infectious diseases in Pakistan like measles (Mull 1991, 1997), polio (Closser 2010, 2012), and HIV/AIDS (Qureshi 2015, 2013).

Dorothy Mull (1997) collected data on measles in Sindh province. In a household study on childhood diarrhea and malnutrition with 150 mothers of malnourished children, she encountered a measles outbreak and obtained data on measles. With only three detailed case histories, Mull's work, *The Sitālā Syndrome: The Cultural Context of Measles Mortality in Pakistan*, is the only anthropological research that has focused on measles in the country and the province. Yet this study has weaknesses: it was conducted more than two decades ago and since then, the sociocultural, economic, and political situation of the area has changed significantly. In addition, Mull's work was concentrated in an urban area. In Pakistan, especially in Sindh province, rural and urban areas differ substantially in terms of facilities, such as education and health (see Government of Pakistan 2017b, 2017a, 2019b). These differences result in a distinguishable perception and practices toward life, including health and illness, between rural and urban people.

Moreover, the Covid-19 pandemic has opened a new horizon for medical anthropological work. Although some work has been done during the pandemic (see Ali 2020a, b, c, d; Ali and Ali 2020; Ali and Davis-Floyd 2020; Ali, Sadique, and Ali 2020, 2021; and Ali et al. 2021), much needs to be done in the post-pandemic phase.

More specifically, studies need to focus on infectious and noninfectious diseases in relation to sociocultural, historical, economic, (geo)political, and biopolitical factors. These perspectives will help stakeholders to better understand the production, distribution, and course of illnesses. It is important to shift our focus from "five-decades-old-anthropology" to the current turns in the discipline. For instance, not a single study in Pakistan has employed the syndemics approach proposed and led by Merrill Singer beginning in the 1990s and which is ongoing.[8]

These thematic and theoretical gaps demand anthropological investigations into "biosocial" aspects of health and ill-health. These anthropological works will contribute practically and theoretically by providing information about the roots of sociocultural practices. New studies should move the debate to the next level to ask why, for example, people view measles as a necessary sacred illness; or why diabetes has become endemic in the country; or why some theoretical threads are less dangerous to employ in Pakistan than others?

There are many anthropological studies concerned with various forms of sociocultural, economic, and political inequalities at the global level. Yet, studies from this perspective that have focused on Pakistan are scant. The medical anthropology of Pakistan holds great theoretical, applied, and methodological importance. It can use different entry points such as what I identify and introduce as "societal memory" and "local colonization," which can help study health problems, interconnections, and interplays between several factors, competing narratives, and stakeholders that significantly affect health. Methodologically, I introduce a new qualitative method that I call *Kachaharī* (Ali, 2022), which can be an intriguing method to conduct further studies. This method is socioculturally rooted in South Asia, including Pakistan. *Kachahār* is a local word that means discussions; ethnographically, it "is an adaptation of the 'focus group' discussion, with the difference that the discussion is driven not by a researcher but by participants; it builds on an existing culturally recognized local social process for discussing and solving a particular problem" (Ali, Sadique, and Ali 2021).

Concluding Remarks

This chapter has described the various concepts and approaches I have built upon and profited from to conduct my research and to analyze my data. Interpretive and critical approaches are center stage. I combined these theoretical approaches, which throw light from different angles on one and the same problem about human imaginaries and practices related to health and illness. These approaches, therefore, work in a complementary fashion.

To further address my topics, I refer to Ortner (2016, 49), who states that the "culturalist" approach—the notion that culture takes central importance as an organizing force in human affairs—helps us to learn about how culture offers people meanings in their lives, and how anthropologists decipher those meanings in their thick descriptions. The critical perspective investigates how economic and political forces—locally and globally—shape people's lives as much as or more than culture.

Both of these approaches—the culturalist/interpretive and the critical perspectives—view and understand the world differently, and their proponents often criticize one another for their limitations. The interpretive culturalist approach criticizes the "reductionism" in the work of the critical paradigm—for example, that it considers people's lives as reflexes of mechanical forces. The critical theorists critique the interpretive theorists for overvaluing culture while ignoring the harsh realities of power (ibid., 49). The critical theorist goes one step further in insisting that culture also constitutes the ideologies, such as fatalism, that disguise political and economic realities that keep people in poverty (Keesing 1987, 161).

I see the criticisms of both paradigms against each other as valid. I also perceive the weakness of each paradigm as its strength. The importance of the meaning-centered—interpretive, culturalist approach—consists of valuing culture and weighing culture's influence in the lives of its participants. In contrast, as Ortner (2016, 49) put it, the value of the critical "political economy" approach lies in its focus on "the power, inequality, domination, and exploitation" that may create specific cultural patterns. I see these approaches not as contradictory but as complementary, because both shed light on differing yet equally important phenomena: culture does have extremely potent effects on people's beliefs and behaviors, while hegemonic powers do exist and do generate top-down influences on culture and belief.

With its emphasis on interpretations of illness, the interpretive approach supported me in understanding and explaining what measles is to a diverse set of stakeholders—how do they define it and what effects does that definition have on how they deal with it? In contrast, maintaining that the origin of an illness resides in configurations and disparities that occur at several levels, the critical approach guided me to understand the underlying causes of outbreaks and why stakeholders hold specific explanations for the occurrence of measles. It provided the key to understanding how geopolitical and economic regimes have rather cleverly and subtly carved out diverse local and global inequalities, which then result in various crises, as well as in benefits for these regimes, such as ongoing funding. The existence and specific shape of measles in Sindh province are a result of this unequal distribution of resources, lack of healthcare institutions, and a dearth of adequate facilities and lack of public awareness, in particular, about vaccination.

These aforementioned perspectives support the formulation of essential questions about the links between global geopolitics and local anti-vaccination sentiments and outbreaks of infectious diseases. Why did Juan Garcia have a drinking problem, and how did the critical event of a fake vaccination campaign to locate Osama bin Laden fuel anti-vaccination sentiments, including the killing of vaccinators in Pakistan? (see Chapter 11). In addition, the "anthropology of infectious diseases" (e.g., Singer 2015)[9] and the "anthropology of global health" have informed my analytical approaches. Having explicated the primary theoretical frameworks that inform this book, I turn now to the following chapter, "Researchlogue: Design, Methodology, and Circumstances of Data Collection."

Notes

1 Clifford Geertz (1973) was the first anthropologist to distinguish between "thin" and "thick" descriptions. "Thin" descriptions are straightforward accounts of an event; "thick" descriptions layer in the meanings of that event.
2 One can easily point toward the 1968 Movement in Pakistan, mainly in Sindh province, which was about the dictatorial regime of Ayub Khan. It may be a good entry point for anthropologists to explore how the entanglement of sociocultural, (geo)political and economic factors occur.
3 In *On Interpretation*, Aristotle argues, "Hence, if in the whole of time the state of things was such that one or the other was true, it was necessary for this to happen and the state of things always to be such that everything that happens of necessity. For what anyone has truly said would be the case cannot not happen; and of what happens it was always true to say that it would be the case."
4 Due to space limitations, I do not go into the details of the 1990s debates between meaning-centered and CMA.
5 Some anthropological work has started to highlight the vulnerabilities of the researcher (e.g., Biner 2017). Now, the British Academy runs a "Researchers at Risk" scheme. In cooperation with the Institute of Social Anthropology, the *PrecAnthro Group* and the Swiss Anthropological Association, EASA's Annual General Meeting (AGM) Symposium, *On Politics and Precarities in Academia: Anthropological Perspectives,* was organized in November 2020 at the University of Bern. During this symposium, I gave a talk on precarity in being an anthropologist in Pakistan and a Pakistani anthropologist abroad.
6 Merrill Singer and Pamela Erickson. *Global Health: An Anthropological Perspective.* Long Grove, Il: Waveland Press, 2013.
7 These are some of the theses. My sense is that there are around 70 theses in the domain of medical anthropology at Quaid-i-Azam University. I cannot mention all of them here due to unavailability of online records; and due to space constraints in this book. There is a need to research and write about the work in medical anthropology in and of Pakistan.
8 Following this approach, we are leading the following volume: Ali, I., Merrill, S., and Bulled, N., eds. *COVID-19 Syndemics and the Global South.* London: Routledge, 2023.
9 Singer, Merrill, *The Anthropology of Infectious Disease.* Walnut Creek, CA: Left Coast Press, 2014.

2 Researchlogue

Design, Methodology, and Circumstances of Data Collection

In the Introduction and Chapter 1, I described the subject matter of this book and the theoretical concepts and frameworks that I employed to thoroughly study measles outbreaks and vaccination. In this chapter, I describe the research designs and methodologies that I have used for conducting the research on which this book is based. For this chapter, I attempted to write what I call a "researchlogue" to show how I approached the field; described the challenges and circumstances under which I gathered my data; and outlined the methods, strategies, and approaches used. I present several anecdotes from my field diary that demonstrate my research journey. As part of my researchlogue, I begin with an anecdote from my field diary:

> It is a summer day in May 2014. The temperature is rising steadily from morning to noon since Sindh province is situated in a subtropical region, where the temperature in the summer frequently rises above 46°C (115°F). Despite the rising temperatures, the routine activities of life never stop. Similarly, for reaching and vaccinating every child, the government's 12-day supplementary immunization activities (SIAs) against measles are underway throughout the province from May 19th to 30th, 2014. These activities may be seen against the background of the measles outbreaks in 2012 and 2013. Thousands of vaccinators and social mobilizers are engaged in the form of teams. There are fixed-site teams, which sit at one place, such as a hospital or a bus station, to vaccinate children, and there are mobile or outreach teams that are continually moving from one house to another for immunizing the targeted children.
>
> To observe these immunization activities, we are at the *Sakhar* district's control room that is governing the vaccination campaign in the district. My today's task is to observe the vaccination campaign in rural areas. Its exact location is unknown, except that it will take place in the cluster that was severely affected in the outbreaks of 2012–13. The village *Rahīmpur* lies here.
>
> My research assistant and I have a motorbike (a Honda 70—a small four-stroke-motorcycle, which some vaccinators get from the government). It is essential to mention that this small bike is not comfortable,

DOI: 10.4324/9781003253716-3

especially for the long rides and during hot weather, as we are covering our heads and faces with scarves and wearing sunglasses. Yet the hot wind and sunlight are burning our bodies, particularly our uncovered body parts, e.g., hands and feet.

In contrast, the officials—of the government and WHO—have an air-conditioned vehicle followed by an escorting police jeep in black. The officials generously offer a ride in their car that I politely refuse in order to experience the hardships that vaccinators (particularly those who are engaged in outreach teams) face to cover scattered areas on a bike, especially during the hot and humid summer.

We start our journey on a small, paved road, locally called a "link" road, which contains many ditches. In terms of width, it is so small that two trucks or buses can hardly pass or cross each other. The temperature is around 30°C at the beginning of the journey, and in the afternoon, it crosses 40°C. The vehicle of these officials is leading, followed by a police vehicle and then our bike. We head toward a village that has no road but a *Sarrak* [an unpaved passage or road] within the agricultural fields. The *Sarrak* continues for almost 10 km, and the mentioned vehicles leave a cloud of dust behind. Now the small dunes to cross appear. The vehicles of officials crossed them with no effort while our bike is unable to cross the dunes, despite our enormous efforts.

Therefore, there are two apparent solutions: to leave the bike there or carry it in our hands to cross. The second option is more convenient and appropriate because we still have to reach the village. Without switching it off, I become able to cross the dunes with the help of acceleration. The sand that is coming from the empty spaces of the sandals is burning my feet because of its heat. Although the dunes are approximately 1 km long and 300 km wide, this small journey to cross them makes me and my assistant sweat immensely and gather dust on our hair and clothes. I am feeling burning on my body due to perspiration and dust. This small act of participation offered indispensable and profound insights about the circumstances under which vaccinators perform their duties.

After taking the *Sarrak*, we finally reach the village. The vehicles of the officials are already there. The vaccinator is making announcements on a small, mobile loudspeaker to inform the villagers about the vaccination and the location of an *Otāq* [a guest room for the male members of the village and also for male guests] where the team is staying. Gradually, people start to gather. The event turns into a gathering. Villagers begin bringing their children to get vaccinated. Children are panicked: their cries are dominant, as many of them are crying even before vaccination. Simultaneously, officials are keeping records, discussions are underway, and the district health officials and the WHO person are inspecting the entire event. Their clothing is different from the inhabitants of the village, not merely in terms of quality and cleanliness, but also in terms of patterns, as the WHO person is wearing pants and a shirt and two of the officials have baseball caps. Whilst the people of the village are in *Shalwār-Qamīs* (loose trousers and shirts) or *Lungī* or *Goadd* (a type of sarong that is wrapped around the waist and worn in place of trousers, especially by men from South Asia), *Sindhī Topī* (caps) and *Patko* (turbans). Policemen[1] in their uniforms (light black pants and shirts) are holding handguns, such as AK47 Kalashnikov rifles and revolvers. Although vaccinators are busy vaccinating the children, they seem under tremendous pressure as well, due to being continuously monitored by the district and the WHO officials.

This vignette paints a valuable picture of how SIAs are organized, and particularly of how the mobile vaccination teams perform their duties. Also, the vignette offers an understanding of the experiences and circumstances under which I gathered the data for this book. Without quoting any literature, in what follows I directly and candidly elaborate on the ways in which I gathered my data and pieced it all together.

My Strategy

I write this section in the present tense, in order to convey to the reader a sense of my fieldwork experiences as they occurred in the moment. Fieldwork is always challenging. It requires essential preliminary planning, patience, and tolerance. Although I belong to Pakistan and am thoroughly familiar with almost everything there, planning my fieldwork is still necessary. The first thing I plan is to send an email to the Federal Minister of Health to get an appointment with him so that I can introduce the project, seek permission, and conduct an unstructured interview. Unfortunately, the Minister's response never arrived. Although I kept wondering whether or not to commence my fieldwork, I nevertheless organized the fieldwork at the beginning of 2014 with an inductive approach to keep my options open. The broader locale is in view: selecting two villages from two districts of Sindh. I do not decide in advance which specific villages and districts to study, preferring to gather more information first. My preliminary design is to collect information about the outbreak from the District Headquarters (DHQ) hospitals, *Talukā* (subdistrict) Headquarters (THQ) hospitals, and Basic Health Units (BHUs). My plan for where to start is initially vague. Yet I can see that the significant sites of data collection should include the national office of the Expanded Programme on Immunization (EPI), the health ministry, district health offices, and district offices for the EPI. Nonetheless, after arriving in the field, it became clear that neither DHQs, THQs, nor BHUs could provide sufficient data about the measles outbreak, but the federal EPI center could. Thus, I plan to commence my fieldwork at the federal level.

In January 2014, I enter my field at the stated level. The underlying reasons for initiating fieldwork in *Islāmābād* are not only gathering the required data on the outbreak in order to select the villages to study, but also informing the national EPI officials about my research project and visiting the WHO office. Therefore, my research journey starts at the federal level: I first wander around the National Institute of Health (NIH). I already know the location of the NIH, as I lived in *Islāmābād* from 2005 to 2013 until my arrival in Austria to pursue my PhD studies. I had also accompanied some allergic patients from my native [in *Sindhī*] *Taluko* (subdistrict)[2] to the NIH during that stay of eight years, as there is one of the best biomedical centers of the country to deal with allergic patients.

Accordingly, my fieldwork begins with multiple visits to the NIH, as the EPI and the WHO country offices are at the same location. During this time, luckily, I arrive at a laboratory where the samples of suspected measles arrive from across the country for tests to be conducted to confirm whether or not measles is present. I had not come across that type of laboratory in the country before. Thus, it is a great beginning to "thrust my nose" like Malinowski (1922, 6) into all measles-related information and institutions. Upon my arrival there, I approach a man who is around his 50s and wearing a white overall. After he is informed about my visit, he brings me to the person-in-charge, his boss, where a brief informal meeting occurs. The person-in-charge of the laboratory then directs me to his assistant (the same person I met earlier) who is responsible for conducting the experiments and for record-keeping. The meeting with the assistant continues for two to three hours and proves to be a significant source to learn of the procedures and protocols for declaring whether (or not) there is an outbreak. He nevertheless shows diffidence in sharing the records of cases reported during the outbreak, considering it confidential. He shares what he considers permissible during our discussion.

Eagerly awaiting the Minister's response, in order to gain access, I make as many efforts as possible to get to know acquaintances and friends who are perhaps working at the NIH or the WHO headquarters. This strategy for finding someone is often practiced in the country and exemplifies the expression "When in Rome, do as the Romans do." Nonetheless, during the implementation phase to commence my fieldwork, I am very concerned because the fieldwork is continuously changing into zigzag patterns. To deal with this anxiety, I keep myself engaged in collecting news reports related to measles and vaccination.

Since nothing significant is coming up, one day I decide to visit the WHO office to check the protocols required to get an appointment. The WHO office gives the impression of a fortress. Foolproof security is provided by a wall containing a barbed wire fence and big cement blocks at the main entrance to stop an unwanted vehicle's attack (as on 20th September 2008, a truck filled with explosives entered and detonated in the Marriot Hotel in *Islāmābād*). At the same location as this office, there is a check-point containing alert security guards, who are ready to fight as and when needed. This fortress-like outlook frightens me. Maintaining my composure, I talk to the security guards, who inform me that only officially invited visitors are allowed. I return with the hope that I would receive that invitation after finding a relevant person who could help me to obtain it.

Meanwhile, I reach the health academy, where, by chance, I meet a professor of public health. We have a brief conversation during which I share my anxieties. He encourages me and comments that this is what fieldwork is about, and that a researcher must take into account all experiences of difficulties in accessing people and initiating fieldwork in the design of a project.

Visiting the WHO without an invitation does not work. My efforts to establish acquaintances continue. After almost ten days, my unceasing efforts finally pay off, as one of my friends introduces me to a person named Shabīr (a pseudonym), who is working in the federal EPI office, responsible for training, capacity building, and vaccine maintenance (cold chain, record-keeping). My friend gives me his cell number. That day, I am profoundly happy. I feel like Sherlock Holmes, as a clue to a riddle has been found. The very next day, I call Shabīr on my mobile phone, and introduce myself while referring to my friend. Shabīr responds positively, as my friend had already informed him about me, and invites me to his office. I accept the offer with no further delay because time is passing quickly. According to my initial study design, this expedition was supposed to take place in three months, and I have to travel far and wide to visit the districts and the villages. On the next day, I arrive at his office. Shabīr, in his forties, welcomes me. After hugging each other and shaking hands, we enter his well-furnished office, containing a comfortable couch, the country's flag, and a picture of the country's founder.[3] Shabīr is also from Sindh province, so we speak the same language. We start a discussion that offers me a preliminary understanding of the making of vaccination programs in Pakistan. He orders his assistant to bring Chānh (black tea with milk) and biscuits. He shares his information about outbreaks and vaccination programs, and his acquaintances in the office of the WHO. He informs the national EPI manager—his boss—about me and arranges a meeting with him. To do so, he goes there and secures an appointment for me. "Tomorrow, the EPI manager has some spare time to meet," he states. Now, finally, things are going in a more desired way as clues are leading to other clues.

As decided, I arrive at Shabīr's office the next day to meet the manager. Shabīr accompanies me to the manager's office, which is superbly furnished. The manager welcomes me with a smile and shakes my hand. He has limited time, so it is important for me to inform him about everything as briefly as possible. In that brief meeting, I introduce myself and, most importantly, the project. He finds the project "intriguing" and "indispensable." Although the meeting goes well, he demands the project proposal and an approval letter from the university. This demand puzzles me. I am profoundly reluctant to share the proposal due to fears of "copyright" and "misuse," as many people use submitted proposals, even theses, for their purposes with their own names. In some cases, people actually sell the project proposals. Being aware of this potential danger, I face an awkward situation. It is like standing at the edge of ethics, where a researcher tries to ward off any danger or trouble and needs to decide what to do next. With anxiety, I hesitate to provide him with the proposal. Yet the second demand is fulfilled by providing a letter from the scientific committee of the University of Vienna, describing my project and its approval.[4]

One important point needs to be mentioned here. In these offices, a dress code is crucial because the clothing, including shoes, is used to judge a person's personality and worth. Consequently, at the federal level, I am highly conscious of dress patterns. I wear smart Western trousers and a shirt because most people working here dress like that. My reputation is compounded by my knowledge of English: good English is considered a sign of knowledge. People who dressed in native patterns, such as the turban, were humiliated by the British, who forced their "servants" to wear them, especially the doormen who used to stand at the entrance of their houses and hotels. Using dress patterns and English as parameters to measure the worth of a person is what I call "debris" from the British colonization. Both phenomena work as identifications of "rational" and "irrational" people. English is still an official language of Pakistan, although the country's parliament has been discussing making Urdu an official language for several years.

These meetings and discussions paved the way for me to gather insights about Sindh's affected districts and the EPI district offices; for example, their location and structure, which were utterly unknown to me earlier. To get there quickly, I continue searching for EPI locations and asking some friends in the province. This information helps me to choose both the districts and the villages, as I will further describe below.

The journey now begins toward the south-eastern part of the country: Sindh province. To continue the data "hunting and gathering," I plan to travel to the province from *Islāmābād* to reach the district EPI centers and to choose the villages in February 2014. There are three options to get there: by air (two cities, *Sakhar* and *Karāchī*, have airports), by road, and by train. Traveling by air is more expensive than the other two options. Trains are noisy if one is not in what is locally called a six-person lower air-conditioned cabin, or a single-person air-conditioned parlor compartment, and are always confronted with delays. Thus, both options are inexpedient, except for a bus. Therefore, I book a bus ticket and depart from the country's capital in the late afternoon. I reach *Sakhar* district the next morning after an 18-hour journey.

After entering the province, a new world begins for me, geographically and ethnographically (see Chapter 5). There are hot summers, as although it is February, the outside temperature is rising and my body is sweating.

Ethnographically, one can observe shrine behaviors, a different *Shalwār-Qamīs* (trousers and shirt) clothing pattern with a unique *Sindhī* cap, turban, language, and historical buildings. The influence of Hinduism remains visible in meeting patterns, rituals, and architecture. *Sakhar* district also contains historical Hindu temples and sacred places such as *Sadhbelo,* which is on a small island in the *Sindhu Daryā* (Indus River), and *Satyan-jo-Āstān* (literally: a residence of women who threw themselves onto their husbands' funeral pyres).

After reaching the district, my next task is to locate the district EPI office. By taking a taxi, I reach the *Sakhar* EPI office, which has a big signboard at the main entrance declaring that it is a governmental building. The first impression of the building is that it is in a dilapidated condition, as the cement of the walls is falling off. After entering the building, I meet a person and ask him who the officer in charge is and where s/he is. He says, "In charge's office is a few doors down the hall." I reach a room with an open wooden door. The person in charge, Mr. *Rānno* (a pseudonym), is facing the door, and four other persons are sitting facing each other. To my *"Aslam-o-Alikum,"* I receive a response of *"Wa'alikum-a-slam."*[5] Everyone stands up to show respect and meet me (it is a norm in the province to show deep respect). We hug each other and shake hands. After that, I introduce myself and my research endeavor. *Rānno* is highly obliging, even in our first meeting. He shares that other researchers also visit him, so I am not the first one. He is quite welcoming, encouraging, and helpful. A *Kachaharī* starts, led by *Rānno,* as the other four persons are also participating. To reiterate, a *Kachaharī* is a small informal discussion that has roots in the local socio-cultural norms. He introduces the four people to me as vaccine supervisors. What luck! *Rānno* orders *Chānh* (again, black tea with milk)—a *Kachaharī* without tea is incomplete. Our *Kachaharī* continues for one hour, during which he willingly provides the required data and introduces me to his staff. During several *Kahchārīon* (plural of *Kachaharī*) with him and others, I gather sufficient data regarding the number of cases in the outbreak, the names of the affected villages, the local responses, the design of the vaccination program, weak areas in vaccination, and local politics. He shares a list of cases that occurred in the outbreak, broken down into *Talukā* and villages. He never asks me about a permission letter for the research and continually encourages me in my work, which he considers a significant contribution to the province and the country. However, he does want me to meet the Executive District Officer (EDO) health—the government's district official responsible for the health department. The EDO is in charge of the entire office as well as of the district.

Hence, it is necessary to seek the EDO's consent by informing him about the project. I make an appointment. When I go to meet him, around seven people are already standing and waiting in the corridor. The door to his office is closed. The assistant inquires if I am there to meet *Sāhib* (literally: boss).[6] I nod my head to indicate yes, I have come to meet the EDO *Sāhib.*

He asks me to write my name on a piece of paper, which I do (my name and the university's name), and give it to him. He takes the slip inside, and surprisingly I am called in prior to anyone else. After entering, following the local norms, we shake hands. He asks me, "Yes, son! What can I do for you?" As many people are waiting outside to meet him, I briefly introduce myself and the project. "Excellent! Please meet Mr. Rānno. He can give you all that required data," he suggests politely. He then briefly shares his views on the outbreak and the workings of the EPI. The meeting lasts for around half an hour. Thereafter, we say *Khudā Hāfiz* ("May God protect you") to each other.[7]

This visit to the district office sets my next course of action, in which I select the village of *Rahīmpur*, the district EPI cell, and generate interactions with the vaccinators and supervisors. This visit solves the puzzling parts of my study, and ultimately proves to be an essential step for the continuation of the project. According to the given list of cases in the district, the village of *Rahīmpur* reported the highest cases, that is, 50 during the outbreak. Now my task is to find this village. The information on the *Taluko* is available, but not the exact location. I have a partial understanding of the area, as when I was a teenager, I once went there. There is no proper public transport available in that area, except at hourly intervals to catch a van. It is possible to reach the general area by van, but not a village. Therefore, to reach the village, the sole option is to take a motorbike. I take a 70cc motorbike with my research assistant. After putting a bottle of water, a note pad, and a camera in our bags, we begin the search in the morning. This area falls into the Thar Desert and is called *Nārā* Desert, but it now has irrigation water available. Agriculture has significantly evolved in the last two decades or so. It is also home to various social groups, locally called *Zāt* (caste) such as *Shanbānnī* (a Baloch caste), *Bhanbharā* (not Baloch and locally called *Hur*)[8] (see Chapter 5). Finally, we reach the village of *Rahīmpur* at noon with aching bodies, and after interactions with several people to ask how to find this village.

Working in my "own" area or doing "anthropology at home" have advantages and disadvantages, which have been highly discussed and debated in anthropology (see Peirano 1998; Van Dongen and Fainzang 1998; Greenhouse 1985; Strathern 1987; Edward 2014). The utmost and distinct advantages, in my case, are knowing the language, the area, the dress pattern, and what Malinowski (1922, 23) calls "the imponderabilia of actual life." In order to follow the customs of that *Sindhī* society, finding an *Otāq* (again, a guest house and meeting room for male members) in the village is the utmost priority. After following the broken link road that led to the village, I observe its physical layout: small white dunes, *Pakā* houses, and *Katchā* houses (see Chapter 5). Interestingly, the endpoint of the road is a place containing a *Masjid* (mosque), a school, and the *Otāq*. With no hesitation, I proceed to the *Otāq*, where Mr. Sāhil, the *Waddairo* (chief) of the village, is available. Following cultural norms, he stands up to meet after my *Salam*.[9] He begins our interactions with a question of how I am, as per his cultural training.[10]

My responses to this question lead to a full introduction of myself, my project, and its purpose.

In the afternoon, the schoolteacher joins us after closing the school, and I need to introduce myself again. After that, a *Kachaharī* begins. We find common ground in Shia Islam, by discussing the brochures of *Zayārāt* (see Chapter 5 for an elaboration on shrine behavior) and the *Alam* (flag).[11] I begin the discussion on these topics, which stimulates them, and they start talking continuously about the *Mojza* (miracles), *Karam* (blessings), and the experiences of their *Zayārāt* (see Chapter 3). They love to talk about such things. Meanwhile, it is lunchtime; thus, they offer *Mānī*, which includes vegetable curry and *Chapāti*, despite my insistence otherwise.[12–13] The *Kachaharī* continues till evening. This first meeting proves a significant entry while creating a base for further work. Afterward, the *Kahchārīon* (again, the plural of *Kachaharī*), in which they share the accounts of the outbreak, continue.

Moving to the Thar Desert

Without going into minute details of the village of *Rahīmpur* here (but see Chapter 10), I now provide a brief introduction to the south of Sindh province: the *Tharpārkar* district.

No direct public transport runs between *Sakhar* and *Tharpārkar* districts.[14] However, connecting transport options include by train, bus, or van to reach *Hyderābād* (the second largest city of the province) and then take a bus to *Mithī*—the headquarters of the *Tharpārkar* district. Alternatively, a van can be taken to *Mīrpurkhās* (another provincial city) and then a direct bus to *Mithī*.

During the summer season, traveling by public transport, especially in a non-air-conditioned train or even an excellent air-conditioned bus, is not easy. Public transport, particularly vans and buses, is always overloaded. Vans, for instance, accommodate four persons on a three-person seat. Trains are mostly unpunctual and also overloaded. And the well air-conditioned buses that depart from the northern areas, for example, Gilgit-Baltistan, Khyber Pakhtunkhwa (KPK) province, or from *Islāmābād* are always full or do not stop.

Consequently, on the suggestion of a friend, I take a van from the *Nārā* Desert to *Mīrpurkhās* and then a bus to *Mithī*. I hadn't known about that route before, as the road was newly constructed. My wish was to arrive on the same day. Traveling via *Hyderābād* was undoubtedly time consuming, as vans or local buses take more than five hours to reach there and four to five hours to reach *Mithī*.

Moreover, there is an interval between the departures of two public transport vehicles. Hence, in a new city, I wanted to arrive as early as possible in the evening so that I could find accommodation. According to a friend's suggestion, traveling via *Mīrpurkhās* takes less time than traveling via *Hyderābād*. However, this too does not work because the van is slow due to regular stops to drop off and pick up passengers. Also, at one point during the journey, the driver decides to stop and load all the passengers onto another van. It is irritating, but only patience helps. Owing to the heat, all passengers, including me, are sweating. The summer season in this province never spares anyone from perspiration. It is already evening when we reach *Mīrpurkhās*; hence, I decide not to travel to *Tharpārkar* and instead to stay that night in a hotel in *Mīrpurkhās*. Staying there is not a pleasant experience due to its location close to the area where sex workers (male and female) ply their trade. The next morning, I take a bus (non-air-conditioned) and arrive in *Mithī* around 11.00 in the morning. I book a room in a hotel in the center. In front of this hotel, yellow-colored *Ching-chi* (rickshaws) are waiting in a row. This is my first time there—my first-ever encounter to see cows freely roaming intrigues me, so after having lunch at the hotel, I start wandering around the city.

Most of the country's and province's Hindu population live here in *Mithī*. The grey-colored (specific to this region) cows (the majority are cows with a few bulls) with big horns roam.[15] Also, there are Hindu *Mandar* (temples); a *Shamshān Ghāt* (a cremation ground); mosques; neem trees[16]; vendors selling fresh fruit and vegetables; (I)NGO offices; a famous well of sweet-water that belongs to a family who sells the water. On a mound of a dune, there is a picnic spot that offers a panoramic view of the city. The accent completely changes here, as I speak *Utrādī*—a northern accent—and here it is *Lārrī*—a southern accent. The *Lārrī* language is politer and more submissive, contrary to the *Utrādī* language, which is more authoritative and egoistic. In *Uttar* province (north), *Mān* ("I") is used, and in *Lārr* (south), the equivalent is *Āu'n* (that can be translated as "me"). It would be fascinating to further explore these linguistic differences, but I must move forward.[17]

The next morning, my purpose is to go to the district EPI office. To do so, taking a *Ching-chi* is an excellent option. I just ask the *Ching-chi* driver to bring me there and pay him PKR20 (around 15 euro cents). I arrive at the EPI center with my black backpack, where I meet an employee in the corridor. He asks, in Urdu language with a *Sindhī* accent, "*Ha Lālā! Kaisy Ānā Huwā*" (Yes, Lala! why are you here?). Well! It surprises me, and I start pondering over why he is speaking in Urdu, giving me the title of *Lālā*, which is used for *Pathān*, Pashtun, or *Pakthun* from the KPK province.[18]

Nonetheless, my response is in *Sindhī* with an *Utrādī* accent, but he again responds in Urdu. After telling him that I belong to this province, and asking to speak in *Sindhī*, he starts communicating in *Sindhī*. After a brief introduction, he tells me about the office of the person-in-charge of the district EPI—Mr. *Sukhyomal* (a pseudonym). I go to his office, where he is sitting alone. He is a medical doctor and in his late fifties. He welcomes me with a handshake, and we hold a brief meeting. In my first impression, *Sukhyomal* does not seem as open and willing to share the data as *Rānno* of *Sakhar* district. I then return to my hotel.

The room during the day is sweltering. Also, there are constant power-cuts, which locally is called "load-shedding" of electricity. Load-shedding means that electricity is not provided 24/7 or with full voltage. It occurs in intervals, which can be one hour of electricity and one without. The interval can, in some areas, be day and night.

While wandering around, I observe children, girls and boys, adults playing cricket in some sandy grounds with a cemented pitch. The craze for cricket in the subcontinent is comparable to football (soccer) fever in Europe. I play this sport, too, and am not bad at it, as I remained a captain of the departmental cricket team in Pakistan and of the Pakistani cricket team in Vienna. Cricket, I must mention, is also one of the "leftovers" of the British colonizers in addition to the English language and the dress pattern. To my knowledge, cricket exists in most former British colonies.

In the evening, I go to a cricket ground where young boys and some adults are playing, who ask me if I would like to play. Given that anthropologists conducting fieldwork must make every effort to build rapport and mingle with the people under study, my response is a big "YES!" Hence, they put me on a team. Fortunately, I perform according to the expectations of my team, and we win the match. This interaction leads to further interactions. They want to know more about me, [in *Sindhī*] "*Adā! Tawhān Pānn Kair Āhyo? Hin Sheher Main Nawān Āhyo?*" ("Brother! Who are you? Are you new in this city?"). Our interactions offer opportunities to give them a detailed account of my arrival and to mingle with them. This proves to be more of a rapid process than expected as they invite me to join them very early the next morning, as they play cricket regularly before sunrise. I happily accept the offer, and the next morning, I wake at dawn.

On the way to the cricket field, I observe women coming and going, holding small pots in their hands, moving them toward and away from the ground. This intrigues me, so before going to meet the players, I go to see these women, who are giving food—smashed grains of wheat, rice, flour, and pulses—to ants at their burrow. When I ask, they tell me that these are creatures of *Bhaggwān*, and feeding them brings luck, fortune, and averts troubles. They have been practicing this custom since olden times. I had never observed such practices before—first cows just roaming around, and now women feeding ants.

Afterward, I join the players. We play a match and then have a brief *Kachaharī*. Playing cricket and holding post-cricket *Kachaharī* does not cease as long as I am in the city. They become acquaintances, and I am no longer new in the city. This looking around with an open mind is allowing me to directly see things, meet people, and gather data.

For instance, one day, the president of the country was there to visit the area—the media were repeatedly broadcasting about the deaths caused by malnutrition and measles—and security is strict. The police are inspecting every vehicle. Some roads are closed, and police are stopping *Ching-chi* rikshaws on the road leading to the district EPI center. I am also in a *Ching-chi* to go to the center when it stops. There is a barrier preventing people from going in this direction. Suddenly, a policeman comes to me and says, "*Sain* (sir), please, you can go." This policeman and I had played cricket together; I had not known that he was a policeman. Rapport plays its part, and I reach the center.

Contrary to the *Sakhar* district, the district health officials here are less welcoming. My preliminary observations include that they are afraid that I might disclose their "weak" points. There is an invisible resentment to share the "secret," especially with *Sukhyomal*—the person-in-charge of the expanded program on immunization (EPI) in this district. Despite this apparent resentment, they do share some primary data, which help me to meet the vaccination teams and other health staff. More importantly, these visits contribute considerably to my selection of the village of *Rāmpur*.

During that phase, I come to know about one friend of mine who is working in the district with an international non-governmental organizations (INGO). We have a meeting in which I share my project. He offers me accommodation, as he is living in a four-bedroom house, given by the organization, in the city. I accept the offer and leave the hotel. During my stay, the hotel manager informs me that someone inquired about me and checked my identity card—the copy submitted to the manager, because the area is under intense surveillance. After all, (a) the Indian border is quite near; and (b) drought in the Thar Desert has attracted several international as well as national nongovernmental organizations, religious parties, and government officials, including the president. The governmental intelligence agencies are keeping an eye on the area. For the drought, in particular, I observe 4×4 vehicles (especially Pajeros) crossing or moving in the city with green plates that mark them as vehicles of international organizations.

I move to my friend's house. One day he takes me with him to his office in a given vehicle, as he is going for an official visit, and simultaneously wants to show me the Thar Desert. As soon as we leave the city, the red-brown dunes start containing wild plants, and there are some green trees where cattle are wandering and grazing. Also, I observe children holding empty pots, especially pitchers, in their hands as a symbol of the need for water. They are showing them to specific vehicles. As my friend has been working there for a few years, he tells me that they need some aid and they know that the vehicles belong to (I)NGOs. The children with empty pots and innocent, questioning eyes try to stop us by showing us the empty pots, which is a deep reflection of drought.[19–20]

Now having enough knowledge about the area, I decide to visit the village of *Rāmpur*, because that village had also reported various cases of measles in 2012 and 2013. To go there, I need to take a minibus, locally called a "coaster," which goes every hour from the city until 6.00 pm. I walk to the bus stop and wait under a gigantic neem tree. This time, a policeman—who is standing almost 100 m away—calls me by making a "*shhh*" sound and a hand gesture: a gesture that is considered culturally impolite and unacceptable. I, therefore, ignore him completely. He shouts again and asks me to go there. There is no other choice than going to him. He starts communicating in Urdu, addressing me with the same title "*Lālā*" as mentioned earlier. I then inform him that I am not a *Pathānn* (*Pathān* in *Sindhī* language) but live in Sindh. He demands that I show him my identity card. After that, he finally starts communicating in *Sindhī*, and later we find out that we both speak *Serāikī*.[21] Thence, he shares that if I were from KPK, he might have wanted some *Kharachi* (bribery). An ordinary person always fears the police, because the police are strong across the country. However, not all police officers are bad and corrupt.[22]

Finally, the coaster arrives. I get in, and it is highly decorated with locally made, colorful handicrafts on the inside. Its front part is (always) reserved for women, who are dressed in colorful clothes, white bangles, and have covered faces. The men are sitting in the back seats of the coaster with *Shalwār-Qamīs* and turbans. It is like a mobile home, in which people are eating, women are breastfeeding their children, and Bollywood songs are loudly dominating the whole atmosphere. After almost two hours, the village's stop arrives. I get down and follow a link road that is under construction at that time. The road goes in between the brown dunes with wild plants and trees. It takes half an hour's walk to reach the village. I get a panoramic view from a mound of dunes that allows me to see the scattered *Chanworā* (huts). Some of them are newly built, some are old, and some are burnt down. After getting closer to the village, I observe peacocks and peahens roaming around; a donkey working at the well to take water out; and women are filling pitchers of unglazed pottery with water; two men are putting unfired pottery in a simple kiln.

I ask a man about *Patel* (the influential person). He informs me that an old man has died; thus, *Patel* is sitting at the house of the deceased family to share their pain and perform specific offerings such as prayers. On request, he brings me there. Twenty men are present and sitting on the *Rillī* (handmade bedsheet) carpeted on the floor under a *Chanworo* (hut).[23] After inquiring about the deceased, I learn from people that he was a Hindu, and it is the second day after his death. This knowledge puts me into an awkward position, as I know Islamic ways to condole people by reciting some verses from the holy *Qurān* but am unaware of how to condole a Hindu. I utter *Rām Rām* while folding my both hands and inquire as to who has died. I utter some prayers verbally and inside my heart. After that, the *Patel* leads the discussion that turns into a *Kachaharī* on the causes of that person's death.

These sketches from my fieldwork offer a general but distinct impression about the field, the people I have been working with, and how I gained access to the field. The villages were at my best objectively selected. Yet there may be subjectivity involved in that selection.

The Study Design

For my research, I have employed several methods as per the anthropological orientation. The hunting and harvesting of data at the beginning of the project were planned into three phases. The first phase was a preliminary phase to visit the field, introduce the project, make the unfamiliar familiar, build rapport and trust, understand the necessary horizons and boundaries (in terms of difficulties), and set the pace to conduct thorough research. Its time duration was three months, originally scheduled from November 2013 to February 2014. However, due to the prolongation of the Austrian *Visum* (visa)—a requirement to study and live in Austria—that was expiring at the beginning of January 2014, I postponed the first phase to cover the period from the beginning of January 2014 to the end of April 2014. I had planned the second phase to take place from July to December 2014 to gather the detailed data in a place that was now known and familiar. This phase was double the length of phase one, because of its importance in terms of collecting the "raw material" for my research project. The third phase began right from the conceiving of the project and ran to the completion of the project—concatenating the pieces of data together. This phase comprised the translation, transcription, analysis, and writing of first, my PhD dissertation, and now, this book.

Nonetheless, and as often happens, after I started my fieldwork, various unwanted and unexpected problems and emergencies led to a revision of the plan. Most importantly, I learned about the governmental 12-day Supplementary Immunization Activities (SIAs) against measles across Sindh province that I wanted to document. Initially, the campaign was planned from 28 April to 9 May 2014. However, eventually, the government postponed it "over the failure of the department concerned to devise a micro-plan before its launch[ing]" until 19 May 2014 (Pakistan Press International 2014). As a result, I extended the first three-month phase to a ten-month fieldwork phase. I converted the original two-phase design into a single continuous phase to study the vaccination campaign, the occurrence of which was a fortunate coincidence for me. In Pakistan, emergency-based campaigns do not occur frequently. Proving an essential event for my research project, this campaign offered direct insights and inferences about its administration and the local perceptions related to the vaccination campaign. This campaign in Sindh province was accompanied by refusals, resistance, and resentment against the vaccine, based on local and global politics (see Chapters 9–12).

During that phase, I collected data through several methods, including participant observation, *Kachahari*, building rapport, interviewing key interlocutors, socioeconomic survey forms, informal meetings and unstructured interviews, gathering and reviewing secondary materials, and media reports. The primary units of data collection were the local people, local healers, vaccinators, biomedical doctors, Lady Health Workers (LHWs), government officials, and INGO officials. Moreover, I also conducted two follow-up phases in 2015 and 2017, which lasted for a few months each, and through which I complemented and updated my data. It is also important to mention that (similar to most anthropologists), I have not stopped collecting data thus far, as I have been collecting reports and views from the inter-locutors through phone calls. I have incorporated much of this more recent data into this book, and will use the remaining data for future research and publications.

My Approaches

For conducting this long-term ethnographic project, I mainly oriented myself with two anthropological approaches: the Extended Case Method (Burawoy 1998) and Multi-sited Ethnography (Marcus 1995). Selecting appropriate orientations was a challenging task mainly for two reasons. First, the project studies the interlinkages, the interdependencies, and the interconnections among the local, the national, and the global and their impacts on each other. Second, besides the two specific villages I studied, the rest of my research was what George Marcus (1995) terms "multi-sited." By multi-sited, I mean that I conducted this research in multiple locations, and all of them were at vast spatial distances from each other. Both the selected villages were far from each other, the federal capital was farthest, and the "global space" was omni-present. For instance, reaching the village *Rahīmpur* from *Islāmābād* needed around 18 hours by road during 2014 (now one may reach it within 10–11 hours due to improved roadways).

Moreover, in reaching this vast geographical field and building clear rela-tionships among my research sites, the Extended Case Method (ECM) played a significant part. This is because ECM, according to Burawoy (1998), employs reflexive science to ethnography for extracting the general from the particular, moving from one to the other, as well as connecting the present to the past. The ECM approach advocates for an extended stay in the field while employing participant observation and using the critical theoretical framework. Specifically, the Extended Case Method helps to analyze com-plex microsocial events to reveal structural characteristics at a macro level (see Gluckman 1961) or investigate "the interrelation of structural ('univer-sal') regularities, on the one hand, and the actual ('unique') behavior of indi-viduals, on the other" (Van Velsen 1967, 148).

In combination, both of these orientations supported me in using measles as an analytical entry point to comprehend the institutionalized structures that create fertile ground for systemic inequalities to thrive. Both orientations helped me to understand and to distinguish the general or macro (global- and national-level policies and practices) from the particular or microlevel (mea-sles outbreaks and vaccine resentments and refusals), while drawing on past critical events to connect them to present events.

The Villages

Seven districts of Sindh were significantly affected during the measles out-breaks of 2012 and 2013. Covering all of them was impossible due to constraints of time and resources; thus, I chose two villages: *Rahīmpur* from the *Sakhar* district and *Rāmpur* from *Tharpārkar*. There were multiple reasons behind those selections. First, since measles is believed to be a manifestation of *Mātā*, it was necessary to select villages with different geographical locations and religious practices. *Rahīmpur* village is in the northern part of Sindh province with many more Muslims than Hindus, while *Rāmpur* lies in a southern district of the province with a higher number of Hindus than Muslims. First, via these selections, I wanted to compare the perceptions of and dealings with measles to understand differences and similarities in terms of religion. Second, both the villages differ from each other in several ways besides religion, most importantly regarding the modes of production, infrastructure, political systems, healthcare services, and social organizations. The third reason is slightly related to the second. *Rahīmpur* was at the epicenter of the outbreaks of 2012 and 2013, while *Rāmpur* village lies in an area that is severely affected by malnutrition, where over 100 children died during those years, and the deaths were associated with measles. The government and the politicians continuously contested the deaths that occurred in both villages and their districts.

Methodological Orientations

Again, this book is based on long-term ethnographic fieldwork that I mainly conducted from January to October 2014 in Sindh province of Pakistan, followed up with two short field trips in 2015 and 2017. The primary methodological orientation that guided this fieldwork was "multi-sited ethnography" (Marcus 1995). This orientation was used against a backdrop of the dispersed, multicentered, and multifaceted nature of the topics of measles and vaccination, which are characterized by an entanglement of a multitude of actors, localities, rationales, and practices. I wanted to include as many such "sites" as possible. The interlocutors I worked with included local people, *Hakīm* (*Unānī* and Ayurvedic medical practitioners), vaccinators, biomedical doctors, government officials, politicians, and representatives from the WHO, the Global Alliance for Vaccines and Immunization (GAVI), the United Nations Children's Fund (UNICEF), and the United States Agency for International Development (USAID). I also analyzed the situations concerning vaccination and local, national, and international media content in other countries.

For this ethnographic project, I employed several methods: participant observation, informal discussions, interviews with key informants, a socioeconomic survey, theoretical sampling (a well-known method in grounded theory studies to seek additional data based on concepts developed from initial data analysis), and a new qualitative method that I developed, which is called *Kachaharī* in the *Sindhī* language. *Kachaharī* can be defined as an informal, voluntary, and socioculturally obligatory gathering, which usually takes place in the evening at an *Otāq* (a guest house used for male members

Table 2.1 Mapping basic features of the selected villages

Rahīmpur Village	*Rāmpur Village*
Greater number of Muslims	Greater number of Hindus
Mātā—do not know the specific name	*Sitālā-Mātā*
Kālkā Devī Mandar (Hindu temple)	*Mandar* (Hindu temple)
Mosque present	No mosque present
Worship of *Allāh*	Worship of *Mātā* every Monday
"*Uttar*" (Northern) Sindh	"*Lārr*" (Southern) Sindh
Agriculture (semi-desert)	Rain cropping (desert) (relying on rain to produce crops)
Less number of cattle	Cattle as a source of income and food
Pakā houses (bricked houses)	*Chanwaro* or *Jhuggi* (huts)
Waddairo (political organization)	*Patel* (political organization)
Handpump/electric motor	Well
Clean drinking water	Unclean and stagnant drinking water
Joint families	Joint families
Endogamy/exogamy	Exogamy/endogamy
Small town nearby	Small town nearby
Transportation: mainly private by jeep, motorbike	Transportation: mainly public by bus and private truck
Close to the Indian border	Close to the Indian border
Hindu *Hakīm* (herbalists)	Bhopa "Hindu *Hakīm*"
Women healers	Women healers
No modern healthcare facility nearby	No modern healthcare facility nearby
Sindhī	*Mārwarrī* (mother tongue), *Sindhī*
High literacy rate	Low literacy rate
A primary school in the village	A primary school nearby

only). *Kachaharī* is similar to a Focus Group Discussion (FGD) because it often involves many people. Nonetheless, it differs from an FGD because local people have the authority to run it. In *Kachaharī*, the participants lead, and the researcher attends as a participant. I have discussed these differences and similarities elsewhere (Ali 2022). This qualitative method has its roots in the sociocultural settings in which I conducted fieldwork. Besides using primary field data, I also used official documents and media news reports as secondary sources of information.

Ethical Considerations

Analogous to other studies, the research I conducted also has a few ethical considerations that are worth mentioning. The involvement of multiple stakeholders made the project sensitive because it contains, collects, and communicates the geopolitical and biopolitical links and interests of those visible and invisible stakeholders located at various places. I was often engulfed by thoughts and anxieties about how this work should be conducted, processed, and presented. During a presentation of the project at a symposium, one commentator posed a thought-provoking question: for whom will this work be used? Another professor asked how this work would be perceived, given that it shows the connections of Hindu mythology in modern-day practices while considering the Indo-Pak partition; one of the central reasons for this partition was religion: Hindus and Muslims have vastly different belief systems, which made them want to separate into two different nations (see Hoodbhoy and Nayyar 1985).

Whom my research will serve and how it will be perceived largely depends on its readership. This research might serve two purposes—knowledge creation and transformative values—(a) the anthropological literature on measles and vaccination, mainly from Pakistan, has been scant; and (b) my data might be used by the government, policymakers, and global stakeholders to increase vaccination uptake by using the information—the emic perspective—that I provide about the sociocultural and religious reasons for vaccine refusals and working with that information to try to change people's beliefs, for better or for worse.

Another aspect of limitation related to ethics is the trustworthiness of the research—that is, how to respond to the interlocutors in terms of revisiting the information they have given. Providing this book and the research articles that accompany it and asking for feedback would be one way to get back to the interlocutors. However, then the question is, who should be given this chance: all the interlocutors or only a few? The stakeholders involved range from the local to the global level: for example, laypeople, local healers, government officials, and the (I)NGO personnel (to mention a few). Offering a chance to them to read their standpoints and revise this book, if they wanted to, would raise further issues concerning the complexities of power, reporting, privilege, and would certainly be costly in terms of time and resources.

More importantly, the project raises critical issues of "truth" and "honesty": whose truth should be presented and to what extent? This is because every "truth" has a different entry point and is valid under certain circumstances. Should it be told metaphorically or detailed comprehensively? What consequences would it entail, not merely for interlocutors, but also for the researcher as well? The topic involves numerous ethical points, for example, the ethics of "true" research, the ethics of protecting interlocutors, the ethics of refraining from aiding someone else's hidden and vested interests.

To deal with such ethical challenges, as previously noted, I adopted the critical paradigm to describe and analyze the situation as clearly as possible, primarily through narratives of my fieldwork experiences that I have transformed into data (see, e.g., Stoller 1989). Moreover, to protect the interlocutors, I have anonymized their names, except those that have been reported in the media.

Limitations of the Study

In addition to its ethical concerns, this research has some limitations. The first limitation is related to the "anthropology at home" debate. Working "at home" was simultaneously an advantage and a disadvantage. To recap from above, researching at home is like what I call "plug and play," because it needs no extra time to build rapport with the interlocutors, learn their language, "go native" (I already am a native) and describe the view from inside. Such work also helps to avoid full reliance on translators. Over a century ago, Rivers (1906, 9) hinted that translators share their "own version" of hearing and comprehending because they do not have the same level of language proficiency in the second language when translating from their primary language. Simultaneously, neither the researcher nor the translator is proficient in each other's language. This can result in partial truths. Researching at home where you already speak the local language(s) instead is relatively easy in this regard, since the researcher is already attuned to the culture in advance through the process of enculturation. The researcher does not merely work as a researcher but also as a member of society.

On the contrary, the disadvantages include that while working at home, researchers might avoid or miss some aspects and connections related to a topic. They may unintentionally and subjectively take things for granted that they ought to be noticing. One of the limitations of this study lies in this disadvantage.[24]

The second limitation is linked to this first one, which is related to a prior local understanding of measles that also seems to concurrently be helpful and a hindrance. Being a member of Pakistani society and belonging to one of the districts that was subjected to the measles outbreak, I have witnessed how measles is locally dealt with, and I hold some subjective experiences and judgments. Family members always shared stories concerning "*Wadi-Mātā* or *Māī*" (a great deity used for supplications against smallpox) and "*Mātā* or *Māī*," (the goddess believed to be responsible for measles). My family members received inoculations against smallpox, and my father has marks of smallpox on his face. Also, my grandfather's mother was a local healer, who was invited by the inhabitants of our village in Sindh and nearby villages to diagnose and deal with measles. If *Mātā* (measles) is present, the ritual of *Chillo*, including numerous "dos" and "don'ts," must be observed (see Chapters 9 and 10). To observe the ritual of *Chando*, my father's grandmother often visited a house where *Mātā* had manifested in a child. I have observed occurrences of measles and entire ways of dealing with it. I contracted measles when I was an infant, and my mother's brother's son died due to it; we were treated according to local measures that were further shaped by the economic situation of our family (see Prologue). Thus my childhood orientation has helped me significantly to comprehend the phenomenon of measles at a local level. Simultaneously, this orientation might have made me biased in some ways, making me more sympathetic to people who observe such rituals and romanticizing the rituals themselves due to their cultural meanings to me and to my family. This might have blurred my research lens. On the one hand, I am looking at measles from a critical perspective in terms of why people hold such views, and on the other hand, I may not see measles as a genuine problem because I have witnessed countless people recovering from it, apparently through this ritual.

The third limitation is a gap in the present research that is related to children's voices. Children are the center of dealing with measles by all stakeholders, and an indirect focus of my research. Yet their perspective is missing: how do children feel after contracting measles or being vaccinated; what are their fears, emotions, and views? The question of why I could not include children requires a brief explanation. First, the key reasons include constraints related to time and resources, since working with children necessitates extra time and different research methodologies (e.g., Clark 1999, 2011). Second, children were not the main focus of this research, even though measles and vaccination are directly related to them. Due to these reasons, bringing children's voices into research demands and deserves further careful anthropological inquiries. Children have received less attention from researchers in terms of valuing and comprehending their standpoints. The voices of children and their experiences about vaccination are missing in measles research and in research on other infectious diseases.

The fourth limitation is geographical. Since this study was conducted in Sindh, I see potential limits in relation to other provinces and areas of the country, because Pakistan is a country where subcultures prevail. Owing to these distinguishable subcultures, other provinces may have a different interpretation of measles and vaccination. In KPK province, the anti-vaccination sentiment is intense as compared to the rural parts of Sindh. And in almost all Pashtun-settled areas, resistance to vaccination and anti-Western, especially anti-American, perceptions are more robust than in areas of *Sindhī, Punjabī,* and *Baloch* settlements. Due to strong religious views in some parts of the country, one may also find local views that considering measles as a manifestation of *Mātā* is un-Islamic.

The fifth limitation is related to sampling. The study employed a nonprobability sampling methods such as theoretical and convenience sampling, which always carry specific limitations. In this sense, the results of this research cannot be generalized.

The sixth limitation is about my inability to meet with all involved stakeholders. I could not manage—due to several constraints related to time and resources—to hold interviews with the officials of the UN or the WHO (for instance), who were living in Geneva or New York.

The final limitation concerns time. The fieldwork on which this book draws was conducted primarily in 2014. Since then, several new things have happened in the country in general and in the arena of infectious diseases and vaccination in particular. For instance, Pakistan has a new government; and mobile technology and the internet have widely spread in the country. And the ongoing Covid-19 pandemic has overwhelmed the entire world, including Pakistan (I. Ali 2020a, b, c, d; Ali and Davis-Floyd 2020; Manderson and Levine 2020). Changes like these might have influenced local perceptions of infectious diseases, including measles and vaccination. Moreover, the data about measles from the WHO have continuously been updated, and measles cases significantly increased in 2018. Although I have revised my data in the light of these new developments, it was not possible for me to revisit the selected districts and villages in order to check on any new developments there.

Conclusion

In this chapter, in what I have called a "researchlogue," I have described my methodologies to show my points of departure and to illustrate the circumstances and challenges under which the data were gathered and with what methods, strategies, and approaches. I have noted that at the beginning of this research project, I had planned to conduct my fieldwork in three phases: (a) a preliminary phase to visit and become acquainted with the field; (b) a secondary phase to gather the detailed data; and (c) the data analysis to compose first my PhD dissertation, and now this book. Nonetheless, as so often happens during ethnographic research, after I started my fieldwork, various unexpected problems led me to revise my initial plans. Most importantly, I learned about the governmental 12-day SIAs against measles across Sindh province that I wanted to document in any case. As a result, I extended the first three-month phase to a ten-month fieldwork phase in 2014. In addition, I undertook two short field trips in 2015 and 2017 to update myself on more recent events.

As I have explained in detail above, I selected two villages—*Rāmpur* and *Rahīmpur*—from two different districts, that is, *Sakhar* and *Tharpārkar* of Pakistan's Sindh province. Several criteria guided my selection: (1) different geographical locations and religious practices; (2) distinguishable modes of production, infrastructure, political systems, healthcare facilities, and social organization; and (3) one of these villages—*Rahīmpur*—was the "epicenter" of the measles outbreaks of 2012 and 2013. Moreover, I introduced and explained a new qualitative research method: *Kachaharī*. Using *Kachaharī* allowed me not to ask leading questions or guide the discussion because it was led by a local person. In the latter part of this chapter, I have discussed the ethical considerations and the potential limitations of this study. I turn now to Chapter 3, in which I discuss local perceptions and practices of measles in Sindh.

Notes

1 All of them were men; thus, I use the term "policemen."
2 In the Sindhi language, a subdistrict is called *Taluko* and its plural form is *Talukā*.

3 In the governmental offices, you would always see a picture of Quaid-i-Azam Muhmmad Ali Jinnah—the founder of the country.

4 My anxiety can also be seen in the broader context of Pakistan in terms of how different structures have affected the country and culminated in types of mistrust and corruption, which further impede the country's economic growth.

5 The common greetings to wish safety upon each other. The literal meaning of these phrases is "peace be upon you."

6 *Sahib* is a common word used for bosses or government officials. It can also be used as a suffix to names to show respect.

7 This is one of the popular expressions to utter at the time of parting. It can also be *Allāh Hāfiz*. The other expressions used in Sindh include *Sadain Gadd* (together forever); *Sāth Salāmat* (our relations should stay safe); *Sik Salāmat* (our curiosity to see each other may stay safe).

8 They are *Murīd* (followers) of *Pīr Pāggārā*—who is a spiritual leader and also president of a political party: Pakistan Muslim League Functional. Presently, it is the *Pīr Pāggārā* VII. To learn about who *Pīr Pāggārā* is and what the *Hur* movement is called, please read Sodhar and Shaikh (2015).

9 Shorter version of *Aslam-o-Alikum* that means peace.

10 This is a frequently asked question, in which the person who asks the question actually wants to know the social group ("caste") of the other person. The expected answer is to tell the "caste." There is no visible hierarchy, but it exists invisibly. People treat others accordingly. People start to infer from the references who you are, as there are certain prejudices related to each social group. The inferences can bring you rapidly closer or put you at a distance. I deliberately started my response with my name and the university, because this makes a great difference in terms of mingling with people and obtaining data. During my fieldwork in Sindh province, I wore the same clothes as the interlocutors. Whilst following Malinowski's recommendations to "go native," I struggled significantly in the beginning. I used to wear simple *Shalwār-Qamīs* (loose trousers and shirt). One of the seniors—who had his master's in anthropology—suggested to me to change my dress. I hesitantly wore trousers and a shirt the next day, and the villagers who had been ignoring me suddenly welcomed me. Drawing on my previous fieldwork experiences as well as experiences whilst living in the province, I put the PhD in the first sentence of my introductions.

11 A religious flag that is associated with *Ahl-e-Bait* (family of the Holy Prophet Muhammad), worshipped and esteemed significantly.

12 It is used for chapati as well as a general term for a whole meal, which may contain rice, chapati, curry, and so forth.

13 I was treated as a *Mehmān* (guest) and if your guest goes hungry, thence, it is considered as against *Mehmānnawāzī* (treating guests). There is a common belief that guests are like food—in other words, *Allāh* sends the food of a guest to the host. A guest is considered as a blessing, sent by *Allāh* to the ones dear to Him.

14 At least at the time of my fieldwork, there was none.

15 In the past, it used to be like that (free animals) across the Sindh, as my grandfather tells, but this is now no longer the case.

16 To understand what this tree offers in a place where water is scant, please read this poem written by Elsa Qazi—a German girl married to a Sindhi:

> *My lovely Neem*
> *That intercepts sun's scorching beam,*
> *Yet bears the heat all day*
> *Without the rain's refreshing spray,*
> *Thou charm'st the wanderer's woe away*

With soothing shade
How strong you are, how unafraid,
How green thy leaves in spite of all
The mid-day flames that burning fall
Upon thy unprotected head …
Could man be both as thou and rise
Above the earth, with the sheltering arm
To save the suffering ones from harm,
From sorrows, poverty and vice
Through sacrifice
Could man be steadfast, and like thee
Face every fate, would it not be
Fulfilment of life's loftiest dream
My lovely Neem!

Elsa Qazi (2017)

17 There is a popular perception that inhabitants of the *Utar* are more arrogant, egoistic, and clever than the people from *Lārr* who are expected to be the other way around.

18 Perhaps my skin color is brighter than most Sindh inhabitants, i.e., whitish, especially compared to those living in the rural areas. This incident was not the first time that I happened to be perceived as non-*Sindhī*. Though such a title was given to me before in my province after spending my eight years in Islamabad, I have been addressed as Lala. There can be several underlying reasons of addressing me as a Pashtun: origin, dress pattern, orientations, lifestyle, and habits that I received whilst studying in the capital, or in the Afghan refugees' settlement in the province after the USSR invasion. Although my family has been living in the Sindh province for many generations, my grandfather shares that our fore generations migrated from somewhere in the Middle East, settled in Baluchistan province in the beginning, and thence migrated to Sindh. We abandoned Baluchi and adopted *Serāikī* as our mother tongue.

19 Sometimes, some of these children get scared by the people in these cars. They cry, scream, and run away if you try to communicate or approach them. For instance, one day, we (my research assistant and I) were walking back from the village at a time when the fruit of a local tree—*Khabar*—was ripe. Three children around seven to ten years of age—two girls and one boy—were on the tree picking the fruit. They started screaming and crying as soon as we talked to them.

20 This also signifies the "dependency syndrome" resulting from the activities of the NGOs. People of the area are now "expert" enough to differentiate a private vehicle from a public one. Most of them look for some aid. There are number of NGOs—local, national, and international—working here.

21 Some linguists classify it as a separate language, and some consider it as a dialect of Sindhi. It is a mother tongue of some social groups in Sindh and, particularly, it is spoken in the southern parts of *Punjāb* province. It is said that the *Baloach* social group, who left *Baloachī*, speak *Serāikī* now as their mother tongue.

22 One needs to be highly obedient; otherwise, you may end up in jail. A simple sepoy is more potent than a professor. Mistaken or not, if one is caught, then one is caught. The only possibility is to pay some *Kharchī* and go away. Corruption is quite prominent in all the country's institutions, and bribery is just one form of it. In religion, *Rishwat* (literally bribery) is *Harām* (literally "forbidden") but, despite that, it does exist. The value is not to be corrupt; the fact is that corruption exists. There are undoubtedly various concomitant and confounding factors related to it. The poor are even further vulnerable.

23 The plural of *Chanworo* is *Chanwarā* in Sindhi.
24 It is important to reiterate that objectivity is no longer sought for in anthropology, as we long ago concluded that it is impossible and unnecessary to achieve—all anthropologists interpret their fieldwork experiences through their personal and cultural lenses.

3 The Settings
The Ethnographic Features of the Two Villages

An Overview of Sindh Province

This region, where the Indus Valley civilization prevailed, witnessed several invasions that left prominent and permanent impressions on people's lives. These included the invasions of the Achaemenid Empire (Persian Empire— under Darius I in the sixth century BCE) and Alexander the Great's invasion (in 326 and 325 BCE with an army led by Macedonian Greeks). After Alexander's death, the rule of Seleucus I Nicator and the Mauryan Empire led by Chandragupta Maurya began in Sindh in 305 BCE, followed by the rule of Indo-Greeks and Parthians in the third to second century BCE. Then the rule of Scythians and the *Kushāns* started, which continued from 200 BCE to 100 BCE. Under the rule of the *Kushāns*, Buddhism spread in the region. After that, Persian *Sāsānids* ruled from the third to the fourth century CE.

Afterward, Islam was introduced in the Indian subcontinent, when Muhammad bin Qasim—a Syrian Arab commander of the Umayyad caliphate—invaded Sindh in 711 CE. That invasion gave Sindh the title of *Bābul-Islam* (literally: the door of Islam). The Umayyad and Abbāsid caliphate (712–900) included Sindh in Al-Sind, which was the administrative province of *Al-Mansūrah*—the empire's capital. From the tenth to sixteenth centuries, Arab governors established their own dynastic rule due to weakening caliphate strongholds. After that, the Mughals invaded and ruled the region from 1591 to 1700. The *Soomrā* took the reins from the Mughals and were defeated by the *Kalhorrā*. The *Tālpurs* replaced the *Kalhorrā* and ruled until the British arrived for trade. The British invaded in 1843 and made Sindh part of the Bombay presidency. In 1937, Sindh became a separate province. The British divided it into different administrative units—*Talukā*— to collect tax through chosen *Zamindars* (landlords). According to a report, "Pakistan Emergency Situational Analysis: A Profile of District Tharpārkar," of the United States Agency for International Development (USAID) (2014b), the British developed such areas into urban centers and provided roads and schools. This development attracted people from rural areas and other provinces. After the British departure and Indo–Pak partition in August 1947, Sindh became part of West Pakistan until the separation of Bangladesh in 1971.

DOI: 10.4324/9781003253716-4

These invasions left significant impacts on Sindh, which can be seen in the sociocultural, economic, and political landscape of the province. Briefly, subsequent changes occurred in health-related ideas and practices, such as the practice of *Unānī-Tib* (a holistic traditional medical system) and the introduction of the biomedical healthcare system—all are related to the described invasions in one way or another (see Chapters 6 and 7).

Although the current government is a parliamentary system of government that was borrowed from British colonizers, several clans have entirely dominated the political and economic patterns of the country, including Sindh province. The style and forms of domination are similar to British colonization; hence, I call it *local colonization*. The clans include the Mahar family; the Syed or Shah families; the Bhuttā family (Zulifqār Ali and her daughter Benazīr served as Prime Ministers of the country); the Wassān family; the Zardārī family (Asif Ali Zardārī served as the 11th president of Pakistan from 2008 to 2013); the Soomoro family (Muhammad Mian was the president and Prime Minister of the country); the Magsi family; the Jatoi family; the Jāmoot family; the Jjām family, and so forth. These families have created their *Jāgīr* (fields or zones) in which everything is under their control, and they have been hereditary rulers of Sindh province; hence, feudalism still prevails not only in the province but across the country. In their zones, nothing goes against their will, including the governmental institutions. They are the new dominant chiefs. They influence the provision of facilities as well as the induction of staff. They are well-equipped to dominate and resist any potential threats to their power.

Among other key factors, their vested interests and corruption considerably affect the establishment of necessary institutions and infrastructure, such as healthcare facilities and services. They not only influence the building of facilities but also intervene in the hiring of health staff. For their own healthcare, they consult the competent biomedical doctors, the properly established private health facilities, and also go abroad—most often to the UK and the USA—for their treatment. Specifically, the village of *Rahīmpur* is under the premises of one of the stated political families. The village has a half-constructed and dilapidated paved road, electricity with low voltage that is often turned off, and a healthcare facility at around 10 km. In contrast, in the same geographical location, the zone of the new political chief enjoys a properly constructed paved road, 24 hours high-voltage electricity, and adequate and effective healthcare facilities.

Rahīmpur Village

Geography: *Rahīmpur* is located in *Sakhar* district; it is almost 40 km away from *Rohrrī* and *Sakhar* city. The village is on the northern side of the province, situated in the alluvial plain and desert, close to the Indian border, which is approximately 200 km away (see Figure 3.1). As mentioned earlier,

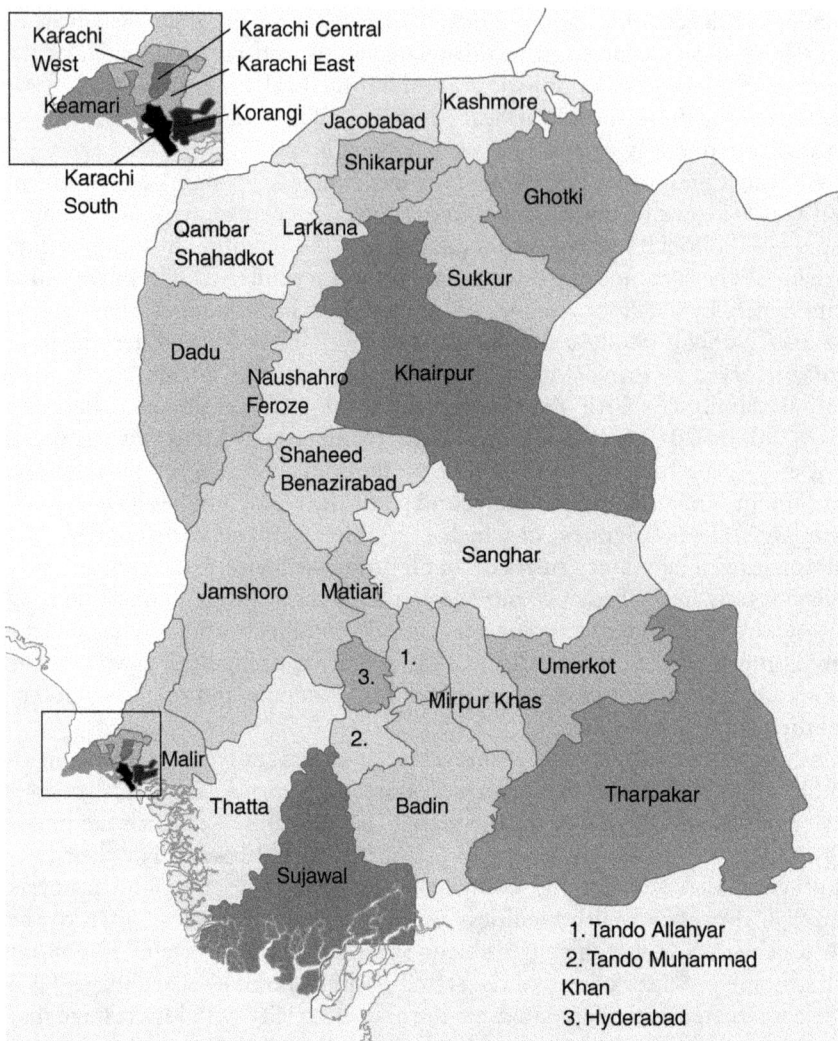

Figure 3.1 Map of Sindh.
Source: Government of Sindh (2020)

this village attracted media and political attention due to the intensity of the measles outbreak with high morbidity and mortality rates.

Social Groups and their Sociocultural Patterns: Three social groups, *Bhanbharā*, *Mallāh*, and *Mārraichā*, are settled here. According to the Socioeconomic Census (SEC), the village has 72 households: 40 *Bhanbharā*, 20 *Mārraichā*, and 12 *Mallāh*. The total population comprises approximately

500 individuals. A joint family system comprises 10–15 members. Although there are a few nuclear families consisting of four to five members, the biggest extended family includes 30 members. The head of a household is always a male member, which demonstrates that males (elders, especially while keeping male gender as a point of reference) enjoy power and position; take decisions (sometimes elder women, especially mothers, influence these decisions); and are responsible for earning money. Female counterparts do the home work: the child-rearing and caring duties, cooking, washing, and cleaning.

In terms of marriage patterns, although monogamy and endogamy are the preferred practices and choices for Muslims, there are a few cases of exogamy and polygamy. Parents make the nuptial decisions. The first option is to marry a cousin (father's or mother's sibling's child), and in the case of unavailability, the next choice is to find a partner from among relatives, and thus the same social group. No one marries outside of the social group; they are endogamous. In contrast, the *Mārraichā* do not opt for endogamy, but exogamy. To them, all girls and boys of a family and relatives are siblings; therefore, they search for a marriage partner entirely out of family and relatives. For them, unknowns are the only choices.

Purdah or locally called *Parrdo* (female seclusion) is strongly observed in *Bhanbharā* and *Mallāh*, as compared to *Mārraichā*. Women stay inside the houses and interaction with *Nāmehram* (an outsider, and religiously forbidden to meet and talk with) is predominantly forbidden. The purpose of this is to observe *Parrdo* and reduce the chances of illegitimate relations and *Zana* (adultery), which are great in Islamic teachings. A woman's body, it is believed, has several attraction points to enchant the opposite sex and some supernatural beings such as Jinn. Therefore, the women of Muslim social groups are advised to stay inside the boundary walls of their houses and cover their whole body either with a headscarf or a black Burqa in case they need to go out (for healthcare, for instance). These values are determined by religious teachings, yet sometimes one can observe women breaching such values. In contrast, the women of the *Mārraichā* social group can go outside without any restriction, but they have a paradoxical type of *Parrdo* system. The females always keep their faces covered with a headscarf, especially from their husband's father and brothers, but social mobility is quite flexible, as, again, they can go outside.

Religion: This village has a predominantly Shia-Islam population with a smaller number of Hindu. Almost in the center, the village has a *Masjid* (literally: mosque) that is used to call *Āzān* (Arabic: Adhan) and perform *Namāz* (literally: prayers) three times a day, though only male members can observe *Namāz* there.[1] During the month of *Ramazān* (Ramadhan, the month of fasting), the villagers are expected to perform communal prayers. They also communally hire a *Maulvī* (a religious person), who plays a preponderant role in leading *Namāz*, calling *Āzān*, teaching the Holy *Qurān*, especially to children, and inculcating Islamic knowledge (on purity and danger, for example). Every evening, almost all male members come to the mosque to observe *Namāz* and end the fast with food such as dates, apples, *Pakorry* (fried snacks made up of several ingredients such as onions, tomatoes, green chilies, red chilies, salt) and *Sharbat* (handmade syrup). During the other months, the number of people observing *Namāz* decreases, but someone from the village calls *Āzān* regularly. Moreover, *Mārraichā* being *Ādivāsī* and practitioners of Hinduism have sacred pictures or statues of gods and goddesses for worshipping on altars reserved for this inside their houses.

Moreover, all social groups believe in saints and visit their shrines for seeking help, including the miraculous healing of any illness. There is a shrine of a saint nearby in the village and a sacred place called *Qalmī Qurān* (handwritten Holy *Qurān*). They also visit other shrines in the province, such as *Shahbaz Qalandar* and *Shah Abdul Latif Bhittaī*.[2] Moreover, *Bhanbharā* and *Mallāh* go for *Zayārāt* to visit the shrines of *Hazrat* Ali, Imam Hussain, and their families in Iran, Iraq, and Syria.[3] The visitors are titled *Zawār* (for male) and *Zawārann* (for female), which becomes a prefix to their names. When they return, they are always warmly welcomed by the villagers and the relatives, who garland them and give them some cash. They make vows for anything such as health, children, good fortune, and economic sustainability. According to them, only the luckiest people are called by the Imams to go there. People keep saving money and sing particular songs to show respect, attachment, and beg for invitation from the Imams. In one of the *Otāq* (again, a guest and meeting room for male members), there was a banner (20×15 meters) on the wall concerning the communal visit to these places under a person ordinarily called *Aggwānn* (literally: the leader). It is like a company of travel agents who advertise trips with a fixed amount to pay to mobilize people, since paying visits to such places is always considered both a blessing and the culmination of a dream. Everyone hopes to visit at least once in a lifetime.

In contrast, *Mārraichā* only visit shrines in the province. The *Bhanbharā* and the *Mallāh* do not worship at *Kālkā Devī Mandar* (a Hindu temple) that is at a distance of around 60 km. Yet during the days of the outbreak, the *Mārraichā* either took their children to this shrine or brought them water from it (see Chapter 6).

Language: *Sindhī* is the primary language (see details on the province and districts), which is used for communication, taught in schools, and is the language of the newspapers. This is the mother tongue of all Muslim social groups. Even the *Mārraichā*, whose mother tongue is *Mārwarrī*, speak *Sindhī* proficiently as they learn it from childhood.

Housing Patterns: The village has *Pakā* houses—made of fired bricks, cement, or mud with a roof of bricks with the support of iron girders— and semi-*Pakā* houses—built with bricks (fired and unfired), mud, and roofs made with wood from bushes obtained from the nearby sand dunes and their agricultural fields. Yet there is a third type of housing called *Katchā*, in which the *Mārraichā* live, constructed with mud, wood, and bushes. The first two types have a boundary wall (mostly made of clay) for protection from thieves and to observe *Parrdo* (women's seclusion and as a boundary of the property). The *Katchā* house does have a boundary, but it is made of plants and branches of trees like *Bbabbur* (botanical name: *Acacia nilotica*) and *Bbair* (botanical name: *Ziziphus vulagaris*) that have thorns. All houses are single story and have a big courtyard with a kitchen built of semi-*Katchā* (in *Pakā* and semi-*Pakā* houses). Almost every house has a hand pump in the corner and a place for animals that can be semi-*Katchā* or completely *Katchā*. Animals, however, are also tied outside their houses under trees during the summer season in the daytime.

Sleeping Patterns: The day begins at dawn when people wake and give fodder to their animals. After that, male members head toward the agriculture fields for excretion purposes with a ewer in their hands to clean their lower body parts afterward or use water from a watercourse. Some of them, thereafter, return to their houses to drink *Chānh* (tea) and get tools to go into the fields, though most of them already carry tools with them for gathering fodder for animals—cows, buffalos, goats, and sheep. They visit their fields to tend the crops, pick weeds, and harvest the crops (depending on the season).

On the contrary, women do have reserved space or a latrine inside their houses to meet their excretion requirements. Some fold the bedsheets used during the night, bring the *Khat*[4] (literally: charpoy) inside (depending on the season); clean the house; prepare *Lassī*, food; and some join their male counterparts in the fields to help with gathering fodder and crop harvesting. However, a few of them who work in the nearby town or as teachers get ready early in the morning and do other chores in the evening. During the summer season, the afternoon is for resting if it is not a wheat-harvesting season, while in the winter season they continue working at intervals.

Subsistence Patterns: As previously noted, most inhabitants are engaged in the agriculture sector, more than half of them have land, and the rest of them work as farmers on someone else's land. However, the *Mārraichā* are entirely landless as they migrated to Sindh province only a decade ago. Even their residential space, which consists of white dunes with no agricultural use, belongs to the *Bhanbharā*. In the past, this whole area encompassed white dunes that have been transformed into fields for agriculture over the last two decades with the building of canals and migration. Yet there are still many dunes of white sand (this area is semi-desert).

As mentioned above, many male inhabitants are farmers and day laborers, and women are mostly homeworkers. Only two men from the village are teachers; one works in print media as a reporter.[5] Those who are engaged in farming have a seasonal income, while teachers have a monthly income. Laborers, however, have a daily or weekly income. The average income of the villagers is USD50–100 per month, depending on occupation and profession.

Food Patterns: Their means of subsistence significantly shape their food choices, though religion plays a fundamental role in determining food patterns in terms of *Halāl* and *Harām* categories (yet these are not limited to food). The *Bhanbharā* and *Mallāh* social groups keep their own produced wheat—an essential ingredient of their food—for an entire year in round tin barrels. The *Mārraichā*, however, receive three to six pounds of wheat as a labor per acre that hardly is sufficient for six months. Therefore, they buy wheat flour or wheat from the market on a weekly or monthly basis.

The essential food items include *Mānī*,[6] or rice, and curry. *Mānī* is cooked using wheat flour, while curry varies and may include chicken, beef, fish, eggs, vegetables, pulses (a type of legume), chickpeas, and importantly *Sāgg*[7] (green leaves of specific plants, especially mustard leaves gathered from the fields). Some of these are homegrown such as eggs and vegetables. There are three primary mealtimes for food intake. The first is *Nairan* (breakfast), which starts early in the morning around 8.00 am, and comprises *Mānī*, butter, *Lassī*, and maybe curry—all homemade and homegrown. Some also drink *Chānh* in the mornings, which was uncommon in the past. Second, *Mānjhāndo* (literally: lunch) starts around 2.00 pm and often contains *Mānī* with some curry. The third meal, dinner, begins in the evening around 7.00 pm and includes bread with curry or milk obtained from buffalo or cows. The second and third mealtimes sometimes contain *Bhat* or *Pulāo* (rice with potatoes), *Biryānī* (rice with chicken or meat or beef), and white rice with pulses or *Sāgg*.

The cooking and serving of food are the women's responsibility, and male members are served first, although, in some cases (ideally), children and older people are served first. On the arrival of a guest(s), or a marriage or death events, the food significantly differs in terms of type and quantity. For guests, lunch and dinner must contain chicken or fish[8] or meat or beef, and *Mānī*, though rice or something else is an optional course. *Chānh* is also compulsory in the morning, or during the day. The *Nairan* is, however, the same as previously mentioned. Before sleeping, milk is served to guest(s). During marriage and death ceremonies, cooking *Biryānī* is typical (see the section on marriage and death patterns).[9]

Political Organization: To briefly describe the political organization in *Rahīmpur* village, there is an influential person locally called a *Waddairo* who settles any disputes. The issues can include: (1) familial issues when someone refuses to give or take a girl for marriage or if a marriage does not go well, (2) issues of illegitimate relations, or (3) issues of land distribution and the encroachment of territory. In other words, he settles disputes and blood feuds. The level of intensity determines the participants, solutions, and punishments. Yet some issues are solved by families without publicizing them to avoid shame; some involve politicians, *Pīr*[10] and *Waddairā* (plural of *Waddairo*) of other villages. The following is a scene from the field that gives an example of a dispute.

Nabīl, who is an elder brother, has been seriously sick for a couple of years. He was the breadwinner of his family and reared his younger four siblings—two brothers and two sisters. His parents are dead, and his younger brothers are grown up and dominating the home affairs. In his forties, he returns home, as he is no longer in a physical position to earn money. He is frustrated because he cannot earn money, and his younger siblings are not respecting him. After the constant frustration of some years, he expresses this grudge one day while loudly asking his brothers to pay him the share of building the house a decade ago. Nonetheless, his brothers refused to pay the share, which created a dispute among them.

Without involving a *Waddairo*, all the siblings sit together and listen to his concerns to solve the dispute. He shares his life struggle to feed the entire family even when their father was alive but old enough to earn money, and then their father died. *Nabīl*'s sisters, who are married, together decided that they (sisters) have not acquired their due share of the property, so the younger brothers should obey them and in return look after *Nabīl*, who is in dire need of care. This way, they settled the dispute, which in most cases becomes intense and results in a blood feud. Thereafter, *Nabīl* stays at home, receives a room, and is looked after.

Moreover, another dispute occurred in which a married girl was murdered by her husband's brothers in the name of "honor," considering her relations with another man. To solve this dispute, a *Faislo* (a local justice system) was called in which several *Waddairā*, local politicians, and local people participated. During *Faislo*, both parties shared their concerns, after which the killers were found guilty, and a monetary fine was fixed on them to pay to the deceased woman's parents.

Education: In terms of literacy and education, formal education levels differ according to age and gender. Children receive formal education and religious teachings, including how to recite the Holy *Qurān*. In adults, a small number of people are formally educated. The maximum education is the master's level—only four men hold this degree. A few adults do have a religious education but not formal education. Gender-wise, a smaller number of females have a formal (as well as higher) education compared to males. The younger generation, however, has obtained primary education. The highest education level in females is a secondary school certificate (12th grade). Among adult women, there is only one 18-year-old girl who has reached that level. Nonetheless, the girls and adult women (not all, but a few) do know how to recite the Holy *Qurān* and observe prayers.

Dealing with Health and Illness: Local people do not merely consult a single health sector, but most often seek multiple, pluralistic consultations: they consult a *Hakīm*, visit shrines, go to religious leaders or a person who knows the Holy *Qurān* for verbal healing and visit a biomedical healthcare facility. This consultation nevertheless depends upon the given etiology of the illness and their economic situation.

For *Sāyā* or what is called "spirit possession"—in which someone is believed to be possessed by a specific spirit or spirits, the voice and agency of the possessed are associated with the spirits (Boddy 1994)—a suitable option is to visit a shrine and a faith healer for chanting specific verses. For orthopedic problems, they visit a bonesetter who is famous in the area. They visit a *Hakīm* for illnesses, such as fever, cough, and measles. Although in the village there is no *Hakīm*, there are two Hindu *Hakīm* in a nearby small town at 10 km distance away, where a BHU, private clinics, and a school are available. These *Hakīm* have been practicing *Hikmat* (literally: wisdom) for the last few generations. One *Hakīm* is almost 70 years old, and the other one is around 50 years old. It was highly thought-provoking to observe in their clinics that they do not merely refer and use their homemade herbal medicines such as *Phakī, Kakh,* and a *Sharbat* prepared from several plants, gold, or pearls, but that they also use aspects of biomedicine such as paracetamol, syrup, injections, and drips. The following description from the field highlights that coexistence of medical knowledge and practices at one of the *Hakīm*'s clinics:

> It is an afternoon in winter. Although it is not too cold, one still needs a sweater or a shawl to keep warm. The small bazaar of various shops—with groceries, clothes—is full of people and motorbikes. A police vehicle is beeping a horn or has switched on a siren, which usually declares a state of "emergency," but it was not like that. Over time, this sounding of a siren has emerged as a practice that police vehicles and also some private vehicles of "affluent and politically backed" people do often to show off or to have "fun." My RA and I turn our bike into a small street, which is around six to eight feet wide, and find the clinic after approximately 20 meters. We take the stairs. The *Hakīm* is sitting in his rolling chair. As we enter, people present there, including the *Hakīm*, look at us. We meet the *Hakīm* and introduce ourselves. He offers us chairs to sit. He quickly inquires about our purpose for visiting him. He is quite busy in dealing with the patients. He warmly welcomes us and offers tea. Following is the brief scene of the clinic.
>
> An older man is on an oxygen machine. One medical representative—of a pharmaceutical company—wearing trousers and a shirt with a tie is sitting in a nearby chair facing the *Hakīm*. Some boxes of medicine, which he brought as a sample, are placed on the glass top table. The wall behind the *Hakīm*'s chair displays pictures of *Mātā*, other Hindu gods and goddesses, verses from the Holy *Qurān*, and modern biomedicine brochures, e.g., with tables, injections with smiling faces of white-skinned and golden-haired children and women, as well as brochures for prevention of infectious diseases, made by the INGO, World Vision. The *Hakīm* quite often goes into the women's patient room, where otherwise only women are allowed.

This stated setting of one of the *Hakīm*'s clinics certainly shows many aspects of health-seeking behavior in the area. The boundary-crossing coexistence of religious and modern biomedicine there—which has been created and put in place for many purposes—is highly significant. During the onset of measles (or an outbreak), the *Hakīm* are consulted for healing.

As noted earlier, people of the village strongly believe in the power of the saints to miraculously heal any illness. Most often, it is a parallel choice of dealing with an illness. There is a shrine of a saint nearby in the village and a sacred place called *Qalmī Qurān* (handwritten Holy *Qurān*). A *Qurān*, which is quite old and put in a glass box, is believed to have flown to this place. Not only people of this village but from the whole area and other districts visit and make vows. However, these are not the only choices; as previously noted, they also visit other shrines in the province, such as Shahbaz Qalandar, Shah Abdul Latif Bhittaī, Sachal Sarmast, and Ubhan Shah. In the whole province, one can observe several *Muqbrā* (shrines), which are believed to be the embodiments of saints. Most people respect them, and certain saints are famous for specific illnesses. The *Bhanbharā* and the *Mallāh* also pay a visit to shrines of Hazrat Ali (the cousin of the Prophet Muhammad and husband of his daughter Fatima), Imam Hussain, and their families in Iran, Iraq, and Syria. Moreover, the *Bhanbharā* and the *Mallāh* do not worship at the *Kālkā Devī Mandar* (a Hindu temple), yet during the days of the measles outbreak, they, including the *Mārraichā*, either took their children to this shrine or brought them water from it (see Chapter 6) to seek their health.

Moreover, the local people prefer to consult a *Daī* (a traditional midwife and healer) during pregnancy, delivery, and to deal with measles. A *Daī*, who is an old lady of another social group from a nearby village, visits the village often to check and know if somebody is pregnant. She remembers the days and trimesters. These people also, in some cases, go and pick her up, especially to attend births. It is essential to mention that she is not chosen in extreme circumstances. For example, if the situation of a pregnant woman is critical, then local men bring her to a biomedical private or government hospital. A Basic Health Unit (BHU) is consulted for an antenatal check-up or specially to learn the gender of the conceived baby through an ultrasound. However, a woman healer, who observes the rituals for measles, lives in this village. She has memorized the lyrics of the *Bhajjan* (see Chapter 6).

Available Amenities in *Rahīmpur* Village

School: The village, as mentioned earlier, has one primary school, where the total number of enrolled students is 110. There are around 35 little children who go to school but are not yet formally enrolled. There are two teachers—both are male. For further education, students need to attend middle school and college, which are 10 km from the village.

The Biomedical Health Facility: The village has no biomedical health facility. The nearest BHU is around 10 km away; it provides biomedicine for the promotion of health, prevention, cures, and referrals. This facility operates community-based or outreach programs such as vaccination and offers support to the Lady Health Workers (LHWs) in clinical, logistical, and managerial terms. Other available services are treatments for Acute Respiratory Infection (ARI), malaria, tuberculosis (TB) control, and Mother and Child Healthcare Centers (MCHCs). Approximately 85 staff members work there, who comprise physicians, dentists, technicians, vaccinators, and LHWs.

During the fieldwork, this center was under a limbo state to become a Rural Health Centre (RHC). One staff member—whose village is around 100 km away from there—told me that the induction of new staff in this facility had been approved, but a promotion of the unit is still pending. According to him, this limbo state has created a sense of confusion and uncertainty among the staff, and indeed, working at an RHC is better than a BHU due to facilities and benefits available for the staff. This unit has a catchment population for vaccination of around 30,000. Moreover, inhabitants of this village consult this BHU, although the first response for dealing with measles occurs at a household level. Concerning the vaccination routine, inhabitants of the village shared that a vaccination team visits the village every second or third month of a year.

Animal Husbandry and Human–Animal Relationships: People keep their cattle in the courtyard of their houses, and share their own living space with the cattle during the winter season to protect the latter from the cold. The social groups that are economically weak, such as the *Mallāh*, and especially the *Mārraichā*, also share the same space with the cattle, even sleeping there at night. People do not feel cynical about animals or consider the feces of animals as unhygienic or harmful to health. They dry dung and use it as a fuel for cooking food.

Roads: To reach the village, there is a half-constructed paved road, which was in a deteriorated condition at the time of my fieldwork. This passage is linked to another paved road that links to the district and the health facility. Since there is no public transport, the preferred way of transportation is motorbike. In the area, people rent their bikes. Influential people, however, have a car, a jeep, a tractor, and a few motorbikes.

Drinking Water, Sanitary, and Hygienic Patterns: The village has subsoil water—which tastes good—available for drinking. Every household has an installed hand pump, and a few have electric motor-pumps for taking a bath, washing clothes, and sometimes for providing animals with drinking water. The *Mārraichā* people, however, fetch water from hand pumps of the *Bhanbharā*, and their women wash their clothes at a nearby watercourse.

There is no adequately developed sanitary system. Some of the houses do have toilet facilities, and there are self-constructed trenches for drainage, which are open. The low maintenance of this system, hence, invites flies and mosquitoes. The rainwater also flows and sometimes makes difficulties for the pedestrians. Most male members of all social groups and the women of the *Mallāh* and the *Mārraichā* go to agricultural fields for defecation. The timing, usually, is early morning or late evening when it is quite dark.

Electricity and Communication: I discussed earlier that although electricity is available, the voltage is always low with frequent load-shedding.

During summertime, the voltage drops further, and fans run slowly and light bulbs dim. A few people have installed solar plates to produce solar energy, as the sunlight is quite strong in terms of heat and stays longer in the region, especially in the summer. The nearest post office and police station are at a distance of 10 km. To receive a letter, people prefer to give a "care-of" address.

In the olden days, especially before the Internet and mobile phones, the primary sources of information and entertainment were radio, word of mouth (still an active channel of information flow and sharing), and television. At present, a few people have android mobile phones, some of the villagers have simple mobile phones, and a few of the houses have televisions. Educated people, such as teachers, buy newspapers produced in the *Sindhī* language (but not daily).

Rāmpur Village's Ethnographic Characteristics

Geographical Location: This village is around 50 km away from *Mithī*, where the district headquarters (DHQ) hospital lies and many children suffering from measles and malnutrition outbreaks were brought for medication during 2012 and 2013. Located in the Thar Desert, the village is situated in the monotonous mounds of sand. Other villages in its surrounding area include *Godyār, Miyār, Khākīno, Gopatār, Āsār, Gomānā,* and *Dhani*. Most often, and especially for the "outsider," making a village boundary is challenging, as one village encompasses dispersed *Chanworā* (huts). The first mistake an observer may make is to view the scattered buildings as more than one village; this impression can only be corrected by local people.

After entering the village, as noted in Chapter 2, one observes scattered *Chanworā*—new and old constructed—on the dunes. Cattle, peafowl, and children make up part of the first impression. The location of the *Chanworā* indicates the social groups: the *Bhīl* and the *Menghwārr* are on the outskirts (at the entrance of the village) and then the *Thākur* are on both sides of a paved road, and the *Kumbhar* inside. Facing the sunrise, the *Menghwārr* are on the right side at quite a distance away.

According to the Socioeconomic Census (SEC) that was conducted in 2014, this village has over 1,000 inhabitants living in approximately 150 households—around 80 households of *Thākur*, 50 of *Menghwārr*, 15 of *Bhīl*, and 10 of *Kumbhar*.

Religion and Social Groups: The Hindu population is predominant in this district. One might expect there to be no social hierarchies among them, yet these become apparent after living there for a time. Yet the former discrimination against the *Menghwārr* and the *Bhīl* is not as strong as it used to be stated that when a Brahmin sees and meets an *Ādivāsī*, he has to then observe rituals of "purification." Local people themselves do not seem to feel the discrimination against them; nonetheless, the *Thākur* (to my understanding) enjoy the top position, and the next two groups are *Ādivāsī*. Without openly claiming to be superior, the *Thākur* certainly do not consider the *Menghwārr* and the *Bhīl* to be equal to them. The lower social rankings of the *Menghwārr* and the *Bhīl* appear when one sees specific pots kept on walls reserved in the *Chanworā* of the *Thākur*. An *Ādīvāsī* can come inside the homes of the *Chanworā* without any discrimination, yet they would be served from different pots than those used by *Thākur*.

Nonetheless, there was no visible difference or treatment toward the Muslim social group—the *Kumbhar*, whose members prepare unfired earthenware for usage for all groups. A *Thākur* shares pots with a member of the *Kumbhar*. Interestingly, the *Menghwārr* do not consider the *Bhīl* to be equal to them; because the latter group does not merely eat meat, but eats the meat of dead animals that may have died a few days ago due to any other reason and give off odors.

The village has several sacred places, which include *Mandar*, shrines, *Marrhī*, *Thān*, and memorial stones. However, there is a hierarchy among them; in descending order, it goes as follows: the Mandar of *Mālhann*; the shrine of *Hārīo*—who was a devotee of *Mālhann Devī*; *Marrhī* of *Kaisar Purī*; *Māujī Thān*, *Manbhan Thān*, *Gogo Thān*; and the memorial stones (of Sati and heroes) (see Kalhoro 2015). Apart from these sacred places, there are reserved spaces in the houses of the *Thākur*, the *Menghwārr*, and the *Bhīl* for worship, which contain small altars for pictures and statues. The *Kumbhar* observe prayers in their houses as the village is without a Masjid. The languages spoken in this village include *Dhātkī* (linked to *Mārwarrī* and *Sindhī*), and the inhabitants are also proficient in the *Sindhī* language and can communicate effectively.

Political Organization: The village head—usually known as a *Patel*—is an older man who solves problems. The chances of the occurrence of problems are, however, quite minimal. In the Thar Desert, feuds rarely exist, except for some disputes and quarrels. People here live peacefully. As noted earlier, animals are always unchained and unaccompanied by their owner. There is no fear of thieves. Moreover, the *Patel* comes from the *Rājput* social group, and other social groups also have their influential people, called *Mukhī*. For small issues, each social group first consults its influential person.

Family and Marriage Patterns: Joint, as well as nuclear families (less common), prevail in this village. According to the SEC, the largest family has 13 family members, and the smallest has four. A male member is the head of the family; however, in decision-making activities, older women such as mothers and grandmothers of the head also play a significant role: the *Rājput* and the *Kumbhar* practice endogamy. To them, the underlying logic includes being easy to accommodate with a known person, family, and knowing the character of each other, considering their social groups better than others. Owing to exogamy, daughters will go to "outsiders" and will suffer if they are away from sight. In contrast, the *Bhīl* and *Menghwārr* opt for exogamy, considering cousins (from mother or father's side) equal to siblings, as was also observed in *Rahīmpur*. They search for matches in far-flung areas to ensure that there have been no blood ties between the two families for generations. Some mediators also help to search for a proper match.

Housing Patterns: As stated previously, houses are locally called *Chanworo* or *Jhuggī*, built from bushes, branches of trees, wood, mud, and in some cases, unfired bricks. The bushes, branches, and wood come from the trees available in the area. According to local people, *Mātā* recommended some specific trees and bushes that include *Kandī/Khejrī/Jhand/Sangrī* (*Prosopis cineraria*), *Kumbhāt/Kumātiyo* (gum arabic/*Acacia Senegal*), *Bbair* (Indian Iujube/*Ziziphus vulagaris*), *Aku/Aakado/Aakra* (Giant milkweed/*Caliotropis procera*), *Kirarr/Kair/Ker/Kareel* (*Capparis decidua*), *Khabarr/Khāro Jaal/Bada Peelu* (*Salvadora oleoides*), and *Khip/Kheemp* (broom brush/*Leptadenia pyrotechnica*). Both male and female members go to gather the material and bring it on donkeys and camels or also on their heads and shoulders. Family members and some relatives work together to construct the *Chanworo*. Creating its circular shape, they build a wall with mud and unfired bricks or clay, though there are also houses built by fixing the wood in the ground, and they are then covered with mud, or some houses are built only with bushes, branches, and wood. The size of a house varies, but the general size is around 10–12 feet inside. The roof is conical and skillfully thatched with stalks of locally available plants and trees. In the center, there is a pillar of wood— obtained from trees such as *Kandī Khejrī/Jhand/Sangrī* to support the whole *Jhuggī*. The houses also reflect the economic and social position of the people. One may have more than one *Jhuggī* or one built with fired bricks and colorful ropes (e.g., some houses of the *Thākur*). One family may own from one to six *Jhuggion* (plural of *Jhuggī*).

Not only are the materials and trees recommended by *Mālhann Mātā* for constructing a *Chanworo*, but also what and how to construct it. Again, a circular shape with a conical roof using local bushes, branches, and wood is permissible. Materials to be avoided include cement, fired bricks, and rectangular shapes. Failing to follow the codes brings harm. For instance, during my fieldwork, almost 50 houses caught fire and burned down. People were saying that the fires occurred because these people violated the codes as they used some cement and bricks to build walls: the fires were a punishment from *Mātā*. (These houses had wooden roofs.)

Subsistence Patterns: In terms of economic and subsistence patterns, people predominantly depend on the rain because of the unavailability of an irrigation system. The rain helps them to grow crops such as millet, pulses, chilis, tomatoes, and watermelon. Camels are mostly used to plow the land. Chemical fertilizers are used minimally (or not at all). As already mentioned, the primary source of subsistence is animals such as cows, sheep, camels, and donkeys. Cows are treated as sacred animals and are the highest yielder of milk. Sheep are a source of wool, and camels are a primary source of transport. People also work as laborers in nearby cities and prepare handmade crafts. Making embroidery, *Rillī*, is quite popular, especially among women. The *Kumbhar* are engaged in the making of unglazed pottery.

Food Patterns: Staple foods include millet and wheat. People prepare *Mānī* (bread) with the flour obtained from millet or wheat, and serve it with pulses, vegetables, beans, and *Sangrī* (seed pods obtained from local *Kandī/Khejrī*, *Rohirrā/Luar*, and *Kumbhāt/Kumātiyo* trees). During the extreme summer and the days of drought, people extensively rely on *Sangrī*. Animals and people simultaneously depend on these two trees which, despite the extreme temperature, remain green and provide this fruit. Of course, the economic position of a family also considerably shapes food patterns. Consuming vegetables, for instance, is not affordable for all the village inhabitants and they cannot grow them due to the dearth of irrigation water. As in the *Rahīmpur* village, food is eaten three times a day—in the morning, at noon, and in the evening. Yet the type of food eaten at noon and in the evening differs significantly between these two villages. During times of drought, these people only eat *Sangrī* or vegetables (who can afford it) with water. Those who cannot afford depend on wild food such as *Sangrī*. Due to food shortages, the curry contains more water than ingredients. One day I was given *Mānī* at a *Thākur* house, after playing a local game usually called *Shīhan-ain-Bbakrī* (literally: lion and goat) at noon. It included *Chapāti* and Indian baby pumpkin.[11] The bowl contained more water than pumpkin. Similar to *Rahīmpur*, cooking and serving are the responsibilities of women. Men eat first; however, children and elders receive food as soon as possible, or children and fathers eat together while the women eat last.

Education: Many inhabitants have no formal education. *Thākur* have more formal education than other social groups because they are slightly better off economically. Overall, there are around 70 individuals who have formal education, and most of them are children attending school. The highest level of education in the village is the higher secondary school certificate (HSSC). There are two individuals with HSSCs, five with secondary school certificates (SSCs), six with middle school (eighth grade) education, and around ten with primary education. The remainder of the 70 are presently enrolled in the school. For education and school-going enrollment, the male ratio is higher than for females.

Interestingly, the ratio of educated women was higher in the *Menghwārr* social group. Among the adult population, the average literate male is in his 50s, as compared to the average literate female, who is a teenager. Moreover, there is one primary school 1 km from the village, with three teachers. Children do not only come to school from this village but also from nearby villages that have no schools. The college for grades 11 and 12 is around 25 km away.

Patterns of Dress: Gender and religion significantly influence dress patterns. Females wear a *Ghāgharā* (blouse) and a *Pothīo* (a smaller blouse) for the upper part of the body. Married females also wear white bangles up and down their whole arms, covering everything from the shoulder to the hand— and a nose ring. An unmarried female wears bangles from elbow to hand and wears no *Nath* (nose ring that goes from nose to one ear). The male members wear *Dhotī* or *Lungī* (a type of sarong) and *Pothīo*—shirts.

Most importantly, the dress patterns of the Hindus and Muslims vary. *Kumbhar* females wear loose *Shalwār-Qamīs* (loose trousers and blouse) and wear colorful and thinner bangles. The male members also use *Shalwār-Qamīs* and *Dhotī*, but the wearing style is different. Used as a source of identification, dress patterns reveal to which social group an individual belongs.

Available Facilities in *Rāmpur* Village

One private bus, locally called a "coaster," runs as a leading public transport provider between the district headquarters, other cities, and villages. It was old in condition, yet fully decorated with locally produced handicrafts such as handkerchiefs and decorations made from beads. Bollywood music (most of the time), or *Sindhī* songs are regularly played at a high volume during the ride. The front half of the seats is reserved for women and the second half for men. However, if the number of women increases, then men offer seats to women. The conductor of the bus asks men to stand up, or men intentionally do that, as offering a seat is considered a gentleman's act. Men also sit on the roof of the bus if needed. The interval between the two buses is always one to two hours. Besides the bus, a few people have motorbikes. Apart from road transport, people use camels and *Kekrro* (a local name for trucks) to travel across the mounds of sands. Trucks, which are also quite old, have distinct types of tiers and are used for carrying weight and as public transport. There is one truck available in the village that is used for the stated purposes.

Drinking Water: As in the district *Tharpārkar*, since water is scarce, people considerably depend on rainwater, accumulated in the reservoirs in the form of ponds and wells (in the district headquarters, there is a famous well of sweet water owned by a family, who sells and supplies it to the whole city using donkeys and camels). This water is consumed for drinking (by humans and animals) and domestic purposes. Donkeys and camels help fetch water from the wells, and after that, people either take it in earthenware or rubber bags – made up of the inner tubes of tires – which are carried with the help of donkeys and camels. Women can also go to fetch water and bring in on their head or waist. They reserve that water in a small dig in the courtyard of their houses; the dug-well is either made of cement or is a big pot of glazed pottery. As noted earlier, the quality of water has a strange color, taste, and odor. The groundwater is saline to brackish and contains a high concentration of several salts and minerals that are considered harmful to humans and animals. Despite that, people use it for drinking, cooking, washing, and bathing.

Sanitation and Hygienic Patterns: In *Rāmpur* village, the houses are without a bathroom or latrine. For defecation, people go to the open fields and mounds of sand, preferably during darkness either early in the morning or late evening. For the children, however, there is no time limit. The sanitary system is entirely nonexistent. As far as hygienic conditions are concerned, animals also have close abodes to where the humans live. People do not avoid animals such as buffalo, cows, goats, and sheep. Kitchens are mostly open; thus, the wind easily brings particles of sand into the curry or *Mānī*. And house cleanliness is the responsibility of women, who clean their houses daily.

Electricity Supply: The village has a low-voltage electricity supply; some people own simple non-android mobile phones—there are no smartphones at all. To charge them, people have 8–10-inch solar plates. Usually, communication occurs through word of mouth. The news reaches people via radio, or sometimes, people bring Sindh newspapers from the city. Television is nonexistent here. There is no police station nearby, except one in the district headquarters as mentioned above.

Healthcare System: The village of *Rāmpur* has no biomedical healthcare facility. Local people, like many in the desert, use home remedies, especially plants to deal with health and illness. To stay healthy, most people sleep and rise early. For pregnant women, each social group has a *Daī* (a traditional skilled birth attendant) who provides care right from conception. Deliveries of women take place at home, not at hospitals. One local woman administers vaccinations against tetanus to the pregnant women along with her husband. During my fieldwork, this vaccination was organized. Her husband (one of my key interlocutors) hung a banner at his small shop in the village and started vaccination. He had a register containing the names of candidates to receive the vaccination.

Concluding Remarks

In this chapter, I have described the locales where the research was mainly conducted: *Rahīmpur* and *Rāmpur* villages. I provided a short history and depiction of their present sociocultural, economic, and political characteristics because these characteristics are necessary to contextualize my discussions of measles. The chapter not only detailed the ethnographic features of the selected locales, but also described the available governmental facilities, health, education, and roads in particular. This illustrated a dearth of necessary facilities—for instance, concerning health and education—and infrastructure, which are a result of various forms of organized inequalities and that further result in severe consequences, such as outbreaks of measles. In the next chapter, I will describe the cultural conceptualizations of health and illness in both villages.

Notes

1 This is because practitioners of Shia-Islam call *Āzān* three times a day and can perform the five sets of prayers at three times: *Fajir* (morning); *Zuhar* and *Asar* (noon and afternoon); and *Magharib* and *Ishā* (sunset and night).

2 Both are two famous saints of Sindh province where thousands of people go to seek the saints' support for various aspects of their lives, such as seeking health.

3 For the practitioners of Shia-Islam, these shrines hold great importance; thus, every practitioner of this sect tries to pay a visit to these places.

4 Its plural is *Khattun*, which is a wooden frame having four legs woven with ropes hand-made from bushes.

5 During my last follow-up visit in 2017, I came to know that he has left this job of reporter and now manages his land.

6 The term *Mānī* denotes homemade bread as well as being a general term for food. People may inquire if someone has eaten food with '*Mānī Khadhi Aaahy?*' Or '*Mānī Khaibi?*' (Have you taken your meal, or would you like to have a meal?)

7 This food is highly romanticized, especially by the older generation.

8 They buy fish from fish stalls that is obtained from nearby rivers.

9 See Mintz and Du Bois (2002), who have published an extensive review of food to discuss it both as subject matter and an analytical tool to expand the anthropological debates further.

10 Syed and *Pīr* are believed to be the descendants of the Holy Prophet Muhammad, who draw their lineage from the Prophet's daughter Fatima.

11 Two people play with two pieces each on drawn lines on the ground. You first place one piece, then the other player places his/her piece, and then it is your turn and the other player's turn. The central purpose is to block the pieces from moving further.

4 Competing Healthcare Systems
Revisiting Medical Pluralism in Pakistan

Indigenous Systems of Medicine

Analogous to many other places of the world, Indigenous medicinal systems have prevailed in the Indian subcontinent for centuries and sometimes for millennia, such as *Ayurvedā*, *Siddhā*, *Unānī-Tib*, homeopathy, and home-based measures. According to Akbar Zaidi (1988), before several invasions by the Greeks, the Arabs, the Turks, the Khiljis, the Tughlaqs, the Syed and Lodhis, the Mughals, the Portuguese, and the British, *Mohen-jo-Daro* (literally: "Mound of Dead") located in Sindh province, and the Indus Valley civilizations had a medical system with a focus on preventive medicine. Banerji (1974, 1333) considers this emphasis on prevention as a "mature attitude of the society towards the health problems."

Subbarayappa (2001) mentions that *Ayurvedā* started in the first millennium AD with the help of sages and physicians, who recognized various potential herbs that were helpful for health promotion, prevention, and cures. This knowledge laid a theoretical and conceptual foundation for the various Indian medical systems. For Che and colleagues (2017, 21), these systems profoundly reflect the culture—traditions and religion—of the Indian civilization. These authors have categorized Indian medicine into two types of systems: the classical and the traditional. The first comprises *Ayurvedā*, *Siddhā*, *Amchī*, *Unānī-Tib*, yoga, and naturopathy, which are not geographically or linguistically specific but can be found in different countries. These systems are well-codified in Indian scripted treatises. In the past, people studied these systems via apprenticeship with mentors, and at present there are schools in both India and Pakistan to promote these classical systems. The traditional system is specific geographically, linguistically, ethnically, familialy, and individually, and is embedded in "the tribal, folkloristic, local health, and household remedies, as well as bonesetters, practitioners in the treatment of poisonous bites, and birth attendants" (ibid., 21).

With their different cultures, all the invasions, as mentioned above, affected the society and culture of Hindustan (the former name for the Indian subcontinent) at the time. Likewise, they also influenced the existing medical systems by introducing their ideas and methods of healthcare and medicine (Zaidi 1988; Banerji 1974). On the British invasion, Banerji (1974,

DOI: 10.4324/9781003253716-5

1334) argues that "every facet of Indian life including the medical and public health services were subordinated to the commercial, political and administrative interests of the imperial government in London." Imposing Western biomedicine on the local people, the British colonizers significantly impacted the Indigenous medical ideas and practices. Consequently, the preexisting medical systems faced a vicious cycle in terms of neglect; negligence then made it gradually harder for the Indigenous system to compete with the powerful—economically and politically—Western system. This new flourishing system was highly favored among the emerging Indian elites, who received education in the "Western" style. Thus, Banerji (2004, 125) claims that when "Western" biomedicine flourished with spectacular developments, people with limited competence and resources controlled the Indigenous medical systems, which ruined the scientific or empirical basis of local systems.

Advocates of *Ayurveda* started referring to its "Golden Age" before the Islamic invaders introduced *Unānī* medicine (Leslie 1989). And they significantly criticized British-imposed allopathic medicine for "denigrating Hindu medicine" and "promoting an alien system" (ibid., 240). The introduction of an alien system caused disturbances and resentment in society. People continued to use the old medical practices. In my field in Pakistan, two Indigenous medical systems are prominent: *Ayurveda* and *Unānī-Tib*. It is not only people who practice *Tib*, but the government has also taken measures for functioning, acceptance, integration, and incorporation of *Unānī-Tib*, but not for *Ayurveda*. However, India has recognized both systems at the policy level (see upcoming sections).

Ayurvedā: An Overview

Composed of two Sanskrit words—*Ayur* meaning life and *Vedā* meaning science, knowledge, or wisdom—*Ayurvedā* translates as a "science of life" (Che et al. 2017, 21). According to these authors, this science originated around 6000 BCE in the Indian subcontinent. *Ayurveda* is a "comprehensive" and "holistic" healing system that deals with physical, mental, and spiritual well-being (Che et al. 2017; Subbarayappa 2001; Kurup 1983).

The codification of *Ayurveda* in Sanskrit occurred between the second and seventh centuries BCE. According to Hindu mythology, the gods transferred *Ayurveda* to humans (Leslie 1989). Bagde and colleagues (2013) claim that Brahma transferred *Ayurveda* to the God Daksha Prajapati, and then to the twin brothers named Ashvin Kumars.[1] After that, transference continued, and it reached human beings (ibid.). The primary source of *Ayurveda* is *Charaka Samhita*, available in the Vedas, the Hindu sacred texts, written in the Indus Valley around 1000 BCE. Che and colleagues (2017, 21) view *Ayurveda* as "a prevention-oriented holistic science of natural healing" that prescribes diet, medicinal herbs, physical exercise, and meditation. It is appropriately codified and rooted in the culture of the people of India (ibid.). In *Ayurveda*, the human body is an amalgamation of "*Pancha Mahabhutas*" (literally meaning "five humors"): *Prithivi* (earth), *Apas* (water), *Tejas* or *Agni* (fire), *Vayu* (air or wind), and *Akasha* (ether or void) (Ranade 2001). These elements have specific physiological expressions: chyle,[2] blood, flesh, fat, bone, marrow, and semen (Ranade 2001; Leslie 1963).

According to Vedic philosophy, there is an inherent connection between the universe and human beings. Changes in the climate, society, economic patterns, lifestyle, food patterns, emotions, and relationships create an imbalance among the elements mentioned. They can adversely impact an individual's state of mind, body, and soul.

Ayurvedic texts describe three states of the human body based on *Tridosha*, that is, *Kaphā*, *Pittā*, and *Vatā*, which resemble the present concepts of motion, energy, and inertia (Kurup 1983; Che et al. 2017). Synchronization among these states, or *Doshā*, guarantees good health, even if a causative organism is present in the body; but an imbalance among them causes illness, which requires the holistic healing of *Ayurvedā* (Kurup 1983). *Kaphā Doshā* (inertia) synthesizes the cells by maintaining the body's cellular and intracellular structures; *Pittā Doshā* (energy) is responsible for the metabolic and biochemical processes in the body such as producing heat and energy, and *Vatā Doshā* (motion) regulates the energy flow through and among the cellular structures and controls the other two *Doshā* (Che et al. 2017). The elements air and ether are dominant in *Vatā*, making this first state responsible for movement and activity. *Pittā*, the second state, includes fire, producing heat, and helping with appetite and digestion. *Kaphā*, the last state, contains earth and water, and is responsible for water and other bodily fluids (ibid.). There are a further five types of each *Doshā* responsible for distinct functions (Kurup 1983; Ranade 2001), which I do not describe here in detail.

Subbarayappa (2001) has mentioned three major types of Ayurvedic *Cikistsa* (therapy): (a) *Daiva Vyapasrayd* (divine therapy), (b) *Vukti Vyapdsraya* (rational therapy), and (c) *Sattvdvajaya* (psychotherapy). Initial divine therapy is for illnesses caused by an unseen phenomenon, such as *Karmā*. This therapy is done in terms of prayers, incantations, amulets, and propitiation of certain gods and goddesses. In *Vukti Vyapdsraya Cikitsa*, *Tridosha* is analyzed for its etiology, and the treatment is according to the five elements to restore the disturbed balance. *Sattvdvajaya*, according to Sudarshan (2005, 226), is about "mastering the mind" by restraining oneself from excessive or unnecessary sensory functions, which is done through meditation, yoga, chanting, breathing exercises, *Pancha Karmā*, and herbs. The herbs are the heart of this healing. They may be flowers, fruit, roots, stems, and leaves, and require a process for use. Without a proper process, however, they are just herbs: nothing more. The scriptures discuss more than 15,000 herbs. However, approximately 850 are in everyday use. (For its practice in Pakistan, see the next section.)

Unānī-Tib Revisited

Charles Leslie (1963) views *Unānī-Tib* as an Arabic translation of Greek medicine of the ancient world that reached India through the spread of Islamic civilization and culture. Yet, it is debatable who originally founded this form of medicine.[3] This term contains the history in its etymology, that is, *Unānī*, meaning "Greek" (Ionian) and *Tib* (Arabic), meaning "medicine" (Sheehan and Hussain 2002). Its practitioners are called *Hakīm* or *Tabīb*. *Tib* prevails in the subcontinent, Arabian, Central Asian, and Middle Eastern regions, as well as many other countries (Sheehan and Hussain 2002; Rafatullah and Alqasoumi 2008). Nonetheless, according to Husain and colleagues (2010), some variations exist in practice due to differences in culture, history, personal attitudes, and philosophy of a particular region. In Hindustan and Pakistan, for instance, Che and colleagues (2017) view some changes that have occurred by adding different knowledges and practices.

The backbone of this system is the four *Akhlāt* (humors) in the body: *Khun* (blood), *Bulghum* (mucus), *Safra* (yellow bile), and Sauda (black bile). Humors have four essential *Quwāt* (qualities): *Garmī* (heat), *Sardī* (cold), *Rutubāt* (moisture), and *Yabis* (dryness), and any one's dominance makes an individual body distinctive from others—like *Dumwī* (sanguine), *Balghumī* (phlegmatic), *Safravī* (choleric), and *Saudawī* (melancholic) (Israili 1981; Sheehan and Hussain 2002; Khaleefathullah 2001).

Disturbances in humors cause an imbalance in the body, resulting in ill-health. According to Sheehan and Hussain (2002), *Unānī-Tib* defines the human body as being in three states: (a) in a healthy state, the body can potentially perform all usual tasks; (b) during ill-health, the body works improperly and is unable to move, eat, and digest; and (c) in-between state, in which the body works and performs tasks, yet not at the optimum level. The third state indicates that something wrong is disturbing the body's equilibrium.

Sheehan and Hussain (2002) further elucidated that the *Unānī* system provides a six-factor framework to deal with health: (i) the natural air; (ii) food and beverages; (iii) movement and rest; (iv) sleep and wakefulness; (v) eating and evacuation; and (vi) emotions. Health requires an equal proportion of such factors in terms of quantity, quality, time, and sequence. An imbalance causes ill-health.

In *Tib*, mention Sheehan and Hussain (2002), each body has a different temperament, which is determined by age, gender, environment, food intake, sleep, and work. Therefore, a *Hakīm* should have an in-depth understanding of the humors to make a faultless diagnosis because the diagnosis determines "the regimental therapy"[4]—intrusive and nonintrusive. A *Hakīm* needs to match the temperament of the patient and the therapy. The therapy includes avoiding, adapting, and adjusting some personal habits, for example, food, sleep, exercise, routine, and environment, and specific actions causing psychological changes. The *Hakīm* and patient both arrange future appointments to examine the situation and share experience, respectively, especially after the therapy. If the recommended therapy does not work, the *Hakīm* recommends specific "active and intrusive" therapies (Sheehan and Hussain 2002, 126). Guy Attewell (2013, 141) cites Tabatabai (1912), who argues that a *Hakīm* does not recommend "any element which is not found in the human [body] composition [as this element] will be harmful to it because it is 'unnatural' [*Ghair Tab'i*]."[5]

For various diseases such as jaundice/hepatitis, sterility, epilepsy, mental issues, depression, *Unānī* is considered a "superior" and suitable medical system (Sheehan and Hussain 2002; Shaikh and Hatcher 2005).

Ayurvedā and *Unānī-Tib* in Pakistan

According to the WHO (2007a, 32), 70% of Pakistan's population, mainly settled in rural areas, use classical and/or traditional medicines, including *Ayurvedā*, while considering it as "efficacious, safe, and cost-effective."[6] The same report further mentions that around 45,000 traditional healers (the majority in rural areas) and over 52,000 registered *Hakīm* are working in public and private sectors in the country. There are also approximately 360 *Tib* dispensaries and clinics, which offer free medication and are controlled by the provincial governments. The government has established nearly 95 dispensaries under the provincial Local Bodies and Rural Development departments, and a Directorate of Hakeems that works under the Federal Ministry of Population Welfare Program. The National Population Welfare Program engages around 16,000 *Unānī Hakīm* with diplomas. Around 40,000 homeopathic physicians are also registered with the National Council for Homeopathy (ibid.).

To integrate traditional medicine into the national health system, the government passed the *Unānī*, Ayurvedic, and Homeopathic Systems of Medicine Rules in 1965. The rule covers the registration of practitioners, elections of the boards, and recognition of the teaching institutions. As per this rule, teaching must be competitive; institutions must offer four-year courses in homeopathy and conduct examinations. Furthermore, the government has constituted a Board of Homeopathic Systems of Medicine to maintain these standards and registration of the qualified persons.

According to the same WHO (2007) report, the Ministry of Health controls the Tibbia colleges and Pakistan's *Unānī* teaching institutions through the National Council for *Tib* to maintain education standards, revise the curricula and syllabi, and conduct annual examinations. There are 27 (26 private and 1 public) functioning colleges that offer a four-year diploma in the traditional *Unānī* and Ayurvedic systems. After completion, the National Council for *Tib* registers the graduates and permits them to practice legally. Pakistan is the only country in the Eastern Mediterranean Region (EMR) to formally incorporate *Unānī* teachings.

The Biomedical System

The biomedical system, also known as "Western" medicine or "conventional" medicine, applies biological and physiological principles to clinical practice. It stresses standardized and evidence-based treatment that is validated through biological research. Here treatment is administered via formally trained or licensed practitioners such as doctors and nurses. Some see the development and transformation of biomedicine as primarily occurring during the nineteenth century (Quirke and Gaudillière 2008).

Biomedicine treats each body on universal principles: with similar organs and structures. Joralemon (2017, 19) mentions that biomedicine follows a universal, standardized, or "mechanistic" approach; it separates body and mind, and leaves no room for treating personal imbalances, energy, or spirit. Also, the structure of the body remains viewed as the same, even if the geography or sociocultural settings are different.

As previously mentioned, illness according to *Ayurvedā* and *Unānī-Tib* may be due to a disturbance in the humors or elements; however, in biomedicine, a disease is mainly defined in terms of an organ's failure to appropriately function or the invasion of an external force such as a virus or bacteria. This biomedical thought regarding the body depends on laboratory research, which creates "satisfactory" or "convincing" results. This thought provides a foundation for the comprehensive approach of immunization.

The Government Sector of the Biomedical Healthcare System

Comparable to many other colonized countries, Pakistan inherited its biomedical system from the British colonizers, who aimed to prevent the large-scale epidemics that could halt ecopolitical interests. The British selected the individuals from the elites to be administrators, bureaucrats, and doctors to support the colonizers, and during their departure, they transferred the authority to these "Brown Englishmen" (Zaidi 1988, 2). By this transfer, they "retained considerable influence on the entire health service system of the country by ensuring that the top of the medical profession in India remained heavily dependent on them" (Banerji 1974, 1334).

After the end of British colonization in 1947, both India and Pakistan started building institutions, including healthcare systems. Pakistan's initial phase (from 1947 to 1955) of establishing its medical system faced significant challenges with replacing existing staff. This phase witnessed the beginning of the UNICEF-supported Bacillus Calmette–Guérin (BCG) vaccination campaign and the opening of two biomedical schools in West Pakistan (now Bangladesh).

Afterward, the country made five-year economic plans to set objectives, plan actions, and implement them. The healthcare system became part of such five-year plans. Studying the plans provides a precise indication about the structuring of the biomedical system to fulfill health-related needs and signify political and economic priorities to replace the "old" healthcare system with a web of biomedical institutions. The newly installed system was constantly reformulated by opening academic institutions, producing "qualified" doctors, nurses, paramedical staff, making vaccines, and becoming a signatory of the United Nations (UN).

As a signatory of the UN, the country was bound to follow the protocols and recommendations to translate the Sustainable Development Goals (SDGs) framework into National Development Planning. For this translation, the federal government and four provincial governments have already committed to set up SDG Support Units to coordinate with each other. These Support Units have been established in the Federal Planning Commission and *Punjāb* province; however, other provinces and local governments are also making efforts to do so. The units are responsible for delivering five main outputs: "(i) mainstreaming the SDGs in national policies and plans; (ii) data and reporting; (iii) inclusive budgeting process and tracking expenditures; (iv) monitoring and evaluation of progress against indicators; and (v) innovation" (Government of Pakistan 2017b, 186).

In what follows, I describe the Pakistani Government's economic plans to trace the development of the biomedical system in Pakistan and economic and political investment into it. This description will explain the inequalities in the system, such as a dearth of enough budget, facilities, and staff.

Five-year Plans of Development

After the partition of old India by the British colonizers, Pakistan made efforts to introduce Soviet-style centralized economic plans and targets for attaining the social and economic objectives of the government's policy. The first-ever five-year plan (1955–1960) focused on opening more academic institutions to produce qualified doctors, nurses, and paramedical staff. During this plan (1956), six new medical colleges were established with a nursing school attached to each. One college was exclusively for women. A postgraduate institution and a bureau to produce vaccines and serums were also built.

The second plan (1960), from 1960 to 1965, continued reforming the biomedical system. A Medical Reform Commission was introduced, which recommended forming Rural Health Centers (RHCs) to cover a population of 50,000 for each unit. The commission also recommended developing two Health Technician Training Institutes, introducing family planning, and malaria eradication programs.

Under the third plan (1967), from 1965 to 1970, the government supported the WHO-launched initiative called "Health for All by 2000" and commenced a widespread infrastructure and policy-forming initiative. This phase structured the biomedical system with Basic Health Units (BHUs) to increase the reach at a village level; Tehsil (subdistrict) Headquarters (THQs) hospitals for secondary healthcare; district headquarter (DHQ) hospitals, and teaching and referral units for tertiary care. This phase, therefore, witnessed the birth of the BHU, THQ, and DHQ. The public health campaign under the guidelines of the WHO was also launched to translate and accomplish the given targets. The country introduced several programs: an Expanded Program on Immunization (EPI); Malaria Control Programs; Tuberculosis Control Programs; Smallpox Eradication Programs; Family Planning Programs; and Diarrhea and Pneumonia Control Programs. Afterward, the government established the National Institute of Health (NIH) to implement the policy, monitor the programs as mentioned earlier, and propose further improvements.

The fourth plan, from 1970 to 1975, stressed on the expansion of the biomedical quota for leading hospitals and pioneered a generic name drug system to decrease prices in the country. To avoid inflation, the government founded eight state-owned fair-price drug shops. The focus was also on the production of "human capital." The result was new educational institutions: the creation of six medical colleges, three nursing schools, and one public health school (Government of Pakistan 1970).

The fifth plan (1978), despite its scheduled beginning from 1975 to 1980, started three years later from 1978 to 1983, owing to deficiencies and a more authentic and practical plan being devised. The plan witnessed the formulation of the Country Health Program (CHP) for improving the planning and management of health services. This program recommended increasing the rural health coverage to at least 50%, controlling communicable diseases, combating malnutrition, handling food adulteration (adding another substance to a food item to increase its quantity), and highlighting industrial hygiene.

The sixth plan (1983), from 1983 to 1988, launched an extensive rural development program to provide a stable base to the WHO-led initiative called "Health for All by [the] Year 2000." The fifth plan's objectives remained unachieved due to the inflation rate (Government of Pakistan 1983). The sixth plan, therefore, emphasized a comprehensive, integrated healthcare system by enhancing physical infrastructure that was enriched with required paraphernalia and trained staff and integrating traditional medicine (*Unānī-Tib*, homeopathy, and *Ayurvedā*) in the National Plan (ibid.).

The Alma Ata declaration of 1978 significantly influenced the seventh plan (1988), from 1988 to 1993. Zaidi (1988) critically argues that this declaration brought new directions and protocols for the UN signatories, including Pakistan. During this plan, a female medical technician school, laboratories, and further BHUs and RHCs were established. Community health workers such as semiskilled and trained paramedics for health facilities were also added. The Family Health Project started to improve MCHC services by focusing on female health. The other initiatives included creating national school health services, minimizing drug abuse, and controlling goiter (Government of Pakistan 1988).

The eighth plan (1993), from 1993 to 1998, launched the Health Management Information System (HMIS), Social Action Program (SAP), and Prime Minister Program for Family Planning and Primary Health Care.

There were eight economic plans. Afterward, there was also an attempt at a ninth plan (1998–2003), which concentrated on decentralizing planning, levying the user charges for financing, creating public–private partnerships, and privatizing the healthcare facilities. It also introduced specific changes in the health system to address grey areas in the management and to establish balanced promotional, preventive, and curative measures. These changes were intended to improve the quality of services.

Afterward, the government shifted its focus to reforming programmatic, organizational, and management aspects. In 2010, the government passed the 18th Constitutional Amendment, and transferred power from the federal to the provincial governments: it made health a provincial task. At present, a district health system is the principal target of policy analysis, while the federal level involves a reform unit, which is responsible for making any structural changes.

Currently, the Federal Ministry of Planning and Development, which is also called the Planning Commission, is responsible for making long-term or strategic (5–15 year) plans. According to it, the Ministry of Health and Provincial Health Departments develop appropriate plans to implement them in relation to other social development indicators such as education and gender. Finance comes from the government through the Annual Development Plans (ADPs). The financing also includes external funding derived from foreign aid—given by bilateral and multilateral organizations.

Moreover, Pakistan's population is rapidly increasing. Globally, the country is the sixth most populated with an estimated population of around 200 million (Government of Pakistan 2017c, xvii). Among several other factors, population size plays a considerable role in health planning. It affects expenditures on development sectors, such as health and education, which have always been minimal and unsatisfactory. For the health sector, the country has spent less than 1% of its GDP, except for the last two years. This allocation is significantly low, as per the WHO's 6% benchmark (see Figure 4.1). Per capita expenditure on health is around $36, which is $56 less than the aforementioned benchmark set for the low-income countries (Government of Pakistan 2017b) (Table 4.1).

Structure of the Biomedical System

The country's constitution makes human welfare and development "a basic right of every individual," which is also in the UN's charter (Government of Pakistan 2017c, 182); hence, health provision is a government's responsibility. To carry out this responsibility, the country has a top-down structure in terms of administration and service delivery (Figure 4.1). The top-level, that is, federal, has substantial power and significant facilities. At the local level, especially in rural areas, almost every person working in a BHU, RHC, or THQ is usually called a "*Ddākdār*" (a Sindh version of *Sindhī*, a doctor, though people also use *Sindhī* "doctor"). The local people do not differentiate

Administrative levels		Health Facilities	Referral
Federal and Provincial Teaching/ (Ministry/Dept of Health	⇐⇒	**Tertiary Care Hospitals**	
Districts EDO (H)	⇐⇒	**District Headquarter Hospital**	
Tehsils (DDHO/MS)	⇐⇒	**Tehsil Headquarter Hospital**	
Union Councils (MO i/c)	⇐⇒	**Basic Health Units**	
Community	⇐⇒	**(Outreach Workers: CDC, EPI, etc.) (Health Houses: Lady Health Workers)**	Feedback ???

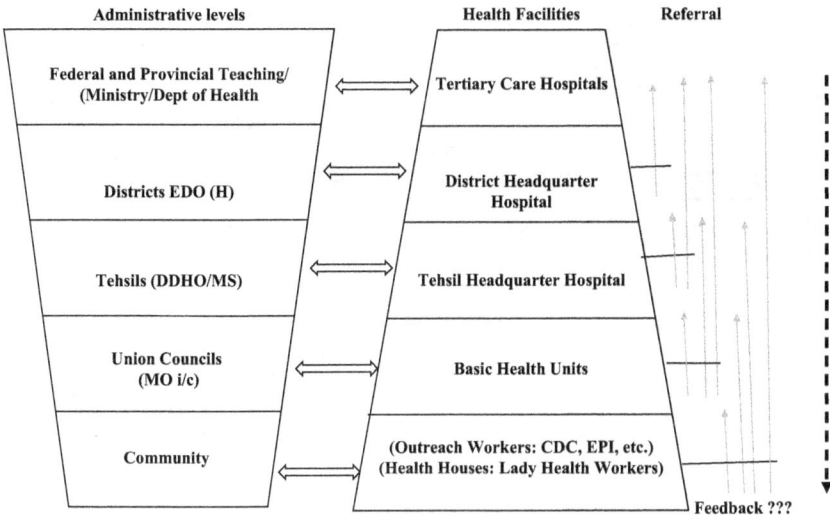

Figure 4.1 Structure of the biomedical system in Pakistan.
Source: World Health Organization 2007a, 32

between the hospital staff. For them, the entire staff are *"Sāhib"* (boss, sir, superior) and *Ddākdār*. Local people often discuss who is an excellent doctor, bad doctor, or doctor with healing power. Word of mouth rapidly circulates such information about a doctor.

To provide healthcare, according to the *Pakistan Economic Survey 2017–2018*, by the year 2017, the country had 1,211 public sector hospitals, 5,508 BHUs, 676 RHCs, and 5,697 dispensaries. The next two economic surveys do not sketch the total number of these facilities, but rather provide the number of healthcare providers and doctor–people ratio. Over time, a slight change has occurred in the quantity of these facilities. Furthermore, a report published by the Pakistan Initiative for Mothers and Newborns (PAIMAN 2005) on the functions reveals scarcities of such facilities in Sindh province (Table 4.2).

The country has horizontal and vertical structures of healthcare. Horizontally, it goes from a provincial level to a district and a community level. However, the categorical or disease-specific programs that the federal government runs are vertical, as I describe below.

The Horizontal Structure of Healthcare

Each province provides healthcare in a three-tiered system, which is then administratively managed at a district level. The first tier of healthcare includes RHCs, BHUs, MCHCs, and dispensaries. This tier is the core of the

Table 4.1 Showing the 2000–2019 budget (in Billion PKR)[a]

Fiscal years	Public sector expenditure (Federal and Provincial)			Per centage change	Health expenditure as % of GDP
	Total health expenditures	Development expenditure	Current expenditure		
2000–01	24.28	5.94	18.34	9.98	0.58
2001–02	25.41	6.69	18.72	4.63	0.57
2002–03	28.81	6.61	22.21	13.42	0.59
2003–04	32.81	8.50	24.31	13.85	0.58
2004–05	38.00	11.00	27.00	15.84	0.58
2005–06	40.00	16.00	24.00	5.26	0.49
2006–07	50.00	20.00	30.00	25.00	0.54
2007–08	59.90	27.23	32.67	19.80	0.56
2008–09	73.80	32.70	41.10	32.21	0.56
2009–10	78.86	37.86	41.00	6.86	0.53
2010–11	42.09	18.71	23.38	−46.63	0.23
2011–12	55.12	26.25	28.87	30.96	0.27
2012–13	125.96	33.47	92.49	128.51	0.56
2013–14	173.42	58.74	114.68	37.68	0.69
2014–15	199.32	69.13	130.19	14.94	0.72
2015–16	225.33	78.07	147.26	13.05	0.76
2016–17	291.90	101.73	190.17	29.54	0.91
2017–18	416.46	87.43	329.03	42.9	1.2
2018–19	421.77	58.62	363.154	0.1	1.1
2019–20	505.411	77.496	427.915	00	1.1
2020–21	657.185	122.867	534.318	00	1.1
2021–22	712.289	207.129	919.418	0.3	1.4

Source: (Government of Pakistan 2017b, 187–188; 2019b, 172, 2020, 2022)[7]
[a] The government has announced the budget for 2019–2020; however, it has not published its document called *Pakistan Economic Survey 2019–2020* that contains the exact figures about the expenditure. Although this table does not contain expenditures for the ongoing year (2020), the current budget has been significantly criticized for decreasing the resources for development and increasing the defence budget.

primary healthcare structure. Such facilities are a focal point for people living in rural settings. The BHUs, RHCs, and MCHCs provide primary obstetric care with community outreach programs offered via Lady Health Workers (LHWs).

An RHC serves 25,000–100,000 people and provides educational, preventive, therapeutic, diagnostic, referral, and inpatient services. One RHC has approximately 10–20 inpatient beds. Providing medical, logistical, and managerial support to BHUs, LHWs, MCHCs, and dispensaries, an RHC performs legal, surgical, dental, and ambulance services. Each RHC contains around 5–10 BHUs.

Furthermore, a BHU with a catchment population of 10,000–25,000 works at a Union Council (UC) level and provides promotional, preventive, remedial

Table 4.2 Healthcare facilities, providers, and ratio 2021–2022[a]

Governmental healthcare facilities				
Hospitals	BHUs	RHCs	Dispensaries	Grand Total
1,276	5,558	736	5,802	13,092
Healthcare providers				
Registered Doctors		Registered Dentists		Registered Nurses
266,430		30,501		121,245
Healthcare services, providers, and population ratio				
One Doctor		One Dentist		One hospital bed
963		9,413		1,608

[a] Drawing on Pakistan's *Economic Survey of 2017–2018 and 2021–2022*, I have created this table (Government of Pakistan 2018, 168). Although the government has updated figures about the total number of doctors, dentists, and nurses in its *Economic Survey of 2019–2020* (Government of Pakistan 2020), it did not mention their ratio per population. Hence, I have provided the (almost old) data in this table.

and referral services, in addition to outreach or community-based services and programs. In other words, a BHU offers primary healthcare and essential services such as basic medical, surgical care, Control of Diarrheal Diseases (CDD), Centers for Disease Control (CDC), Acute Respiratory Infections (ARI), and malaria and tuberculosis control. This unit also controls MCHCs and provides managerial and logistical support to LHWs. LHWs refer a patient to a BHU, which further refers a patient to higher-level facilities, if necessary.

The second tier contains first- and second-level referral facilities (THQs and DHQs) to ensure acute, ambulatory, and inpatient care. A THQ serves a population of 100,000–300,000, and a DHQ a population of 1–2 million. The THQ and DHQ hospitals have specialists to provide comprehensive obstetric care.

The third tier is the tertiary care that teaching hospitals provide. These facilities are present in big cities such as *Karāchī*, *Lāhore*, and *Islāmābād*. This tier also supports the second tier. In addition, some departments, such as the army, railways, and autonomous organizations, provide healthcare to their employees.

According to the WHO (2007a), less than 30% of the country's population consults public healthcare, or on average, one person visits a facility even less than once a year. The underlying reasons include a dearth of health professionals, especially female staff (doctors, gynecologists, nurses), frequent staff absenteeism, unsatisfactory services, and inaccessible and distant locations of Public Health Center (PHC) units (ibid.).

Vertical Programs of Healthcare

To manage functions related to health and interprovincial coordination, the government founded the Ministry of National Health Services, Regulations and Coordination (NHSRC) in June 2011. The ministry's vision, according to its website, is to ensure: (a) a capable healthcare system that provides equitable, efficient, accessible, and affordable healthcare services intending to support people for improving their health status; (b) coordination between national and international stakeholders in the field of public health; (c) oversight for regulatory bodies in the health sector; (d) population welfare coordination; (e) enforcement of drug laws and regulations; and (f) coordination of all preventive programs, funded by the Global Alliance for Vaccines and Immunizations (GAVI) and the Global Fund to Fight AIDS, Tuberculosis, and Malaria (GFATM) or simply "the Global Fund." This ministry also has the Drug Regulatory Authority of Pakistan (DRAP) to ensure the safety, quality, and affordability of medicines across the country. There are several programs that are run under this program, such as the Prime Minister's National Health Program; Family Planning and Primary Healthcare (FP&PHC); the Expanded Program on Immunization (EPI); the Malaria Control Program; the Tuberculosis (TB) Control Program; the HIV/AIDS Control Program; the Maternal-Child Health Program; the Prime Minister's Program for Prevention and Control of Hepatitis; and the Cancer Treatment Program.

The Private Sector of the Biomedical Healthcare System

There are two types of private care: formal and informal. The formal, according to the WHO (2007a) is a modern, for-profit, or a fee-for-service system, which includes biomedical doctors, nurses, pharmacists, drug vendors, laboratory technicians, Indigenious healers, shopkeepers, and unqualified practitioners. The services it provides include hospitals; nursing homes; maternity clinics; clinics run by biomedical doctors, nurses, midwives, paramedical workers; diagnostic facilities such as laboratories; medical stores selling drugs; journal stores selling medicines; and *Hakīm* selling medicines on public transport such as buses and trains.

Some private facilities lack the required staff, skills, technology, and supplies; they also lack a defined structure and regulation (ibid.). Some, however, are hi-tech hospitals and do have skilled staff, supplies, equipment, and transportation. Such hospitals are comparable to any governmental teaching hospital. Businesspersons run them. These hospitals charge visiting fees to patients, in addition to further charges.

Moreover, small structured nursing homes or centers also exist in the country (WHO 2007a). Two or more people run these facilities. Not all nursing homes have skilled staff and equipment. Also, there are clinics run by one person or in a partnership. These clinics provide part-time or 24-hour services. Government doctors mainly run such clinics after office time. Some doctors refer patients to visit them at their private clinics. The staff may be qualified, but not all are legally allowed to practice. The second category is of semi-qualified practitioners, such as dispensers, Lady Health Visitors (LHVs),

LHWs, or technicians, who run clinics after obtaining a diploma or training, although illegal, nonqualified practitioners also practice and provide shoddy services. They may be "ward boys" (those who work in the hospital wards to support the medical personnel), unskilled laborers, or pharmacists, who obtain some skills through an apprenticeship. Also, many homeopaths and *Hakīm* who are practicing do not all have proper qualifications.

Informal private care, according to the WHO (2007a), includes grocery or general stores that sell medicines such as tablets—Aspirin, Paracetamol, painkillers, and antibiotics—in small towns and villages. Legally, this practice is not allowed but is a frequent exercise.

Moreover, other facilities that provide modern, not-for-profit care are (I)NGOs. For instance, Médecins Sans Frontières (MSF) provides medication against Hepatitis C. During the measles outbreak, organizations such as World Vision and Red Crescent were also quite active. The latter organization even provided rooms in hospital wards to keep and treat children who had contracted measles. According to the WHO (2007a), Pakistan has a network of approximately 80,000 NGOs registered under various Acts. The government and international donor organizations in coordination with each other are helping them to become self-dependent, autonomous, and financially sustainable.

In the above sections, I have briefly sketched a picture of the Pakistani healthcare system without going into much detail about the relationships among the state and donor organizations. Sania Nishtar (2006, 9)—a public health practitioner and special assistant to Pakistan's Prime Minister—depicts this relationship as follows: "the role of the State as steward and regulator has become critical as we move to new models of financing health and delivering services as these involve the roles of many stakeholders including the private sector." That means the domain of health has become more complex while involving several stakeholders that can not only be divided as governmental and nongovernmental but also in terms of scale such as national and international (see Hadolt and Hardon 2017).

The Current State of the Biomedical System

Documents and reports of the government and (I)NGOs reveal a good picture of Pakistan's current healthcare system. Yet these documents demonstrate an optimism bias that stretches a crafted impression in which everything seems to be on the desired track. Almost three decades ago, Syed Akbar Zaidi (1988) highlighted the weak areas in the health sectors of Pakistan, yet his identified issues still prevail: a dearth of healthcare facilities; unemployment of doctors; a "brain-drain" of graduates; lack of motivation in medical staff, particularly among those who are working in rural settings; the monopoly of pharmaceutical companies and their profit-centered approaches; and lack of clean tap water and proper sanitation. He has identified "class-bias" as a determinant of Pakistan's health sector, which reflects the overall patterns of the economy. People holding less economic and political power are more prone, in the words of Farmer (1996b), to "structural violence" and remain muted.

This silence is appreciable and is part of enculturation, particularly in Pakistan's rural settings. Active and argumentative children meet harsh punishments—physically, emotionally, and psychologically. Similarly, if an adult complains about anything, then they receive a familial or communal suggestion to stay calm and thankful. However, at the state level, complaints bring various forms of "punishment," for example, a concerned officer would not help anymore; a politician could get someone in trouble; physical punishment could be applied. Consequently, an individual does not report wrongdoings, not even corruption.[8]

Moreover, in Pakistan, for some doctors, seasonal diseases bring patients as well as packages from pharmaceutical companies, whose incentives can be a percentage per sale or trips. For incentives, doctors only need to recommend medicine prepared by such pharmaceutical companies. This bargaining is highly relevant to what Farmer (1996b) calls the "benefits of emerging infectious diseases."

Additionally, a columnist for the English-language newspaper *Dawn*, named Sara Malkani (2016), published an Editorial on Pakistan's healthcare system indicating that it is in an "abysmal state" owing to the government's indifference, which reflects in the allocated budget that a few years ago was a mere 0.9% of the country's GDP. For this figure, only two countries— the Democratic Republic of Congo and Bangladesh—stand below Pakistan. Neither civilian nor military governments have made health a priority in Pakistan.

Although the healthcare system of Pakistan is struggling with challenges and issues, the country is on the list of those countries that do not spend the required resources (WHO 2007a). As mentioned earlier, from 2000–2001 to 2014–2015, the average percentage of its GDP that Pakistan spent on healthcare was 0.53%, and in 2016, it was 0.45% (Government of Pakistan 2016b). In two budgets of 2017–2018 and 2018–2019, that percentage only increased to 1%. Thereafter, it has remained stagnant.

Yet despite paying ample attention to this allocation, the government identifies some underlying hindrances: "the high population growth, uneven distribution of health professionals, deficient workforce, insufficient funding and limited access to quality health care services" (ibid., 187). On Pakistan's healthcare system, another editorial of *Dawn* (2017b, 8) states that Pakistan is "a country beset with issues of poor vaccination practices, hygiene challenges, illiteracy and unawareness, and an extremely patchy healthcare system, the costs may well be staggering. Far from the politics that take up the attention of our legislators and policymakers, these are issues that merit immediate action."

On the one hand, most Pakistanis seek care at these government facilities (WHO 2007a). On the other hand, the situation at DHQs, THQs, BHUs, and dispensaries is further worrying and worsening. Owing to a lack of funding, national healthcare fails to meet the primary needs of people. Thus, people go to private facilities. Malkani (2016) claims that the result of the government's indifference is an inadequate quality of services, which diverts those who can afford it to the private healthcare system.

In sum, several significant issues hinder the health service delivery process. These include the lack of good governance and transparency, a dearth of needed healthcare facilities, poor quality services, a lack of supportive monitoring and required resources, and inefficient use of existing facilities. These problems also include administrative delays, poor management, absenteeism, the unprofessional attitude of staff, extra emphasis on private practice, vacant sanctioned positions, inadequate capacity of staff, lack of incentives for staff, unresponsiveness to community needs, and lack of public intervention and participation. Hence, people consult traditional medical systems. Yet these traditional systems themselves lack adequate facilities, medicines, and staff.

Comparing *Unānī-Tib*, *Ayurvedā*, and Biomedicine

Every medical system has unique ideas, practices, and approaches in dealing with the human body. *Unānī-Tib* and *Ayurvedā* have much in common, such as belief in the "power of the body" itself: a human body is more potent than microorganisms, viruses, and bacteria. Both treat each body as distinctive and as a product of universal humors. Hence, when the humors are in balance, no other organisms can successfully attack it, because a body has a defensive power, called *Quwaat-e-Mudabbira* ("vital force"), to avert any attack and sometimes just needs some support to do so successfully. These medical systems deal with a body according to individual factors such as sociocultural, economic, political, geographical, historical, and interpersonal ones; additionally, they take the whole person into consideration, and not just their symptoms.

Biomedicine, however, believes differently. It views microorganisms as more powerful, which can successfully attack if the body has no external support in terms of medicine. The focus of Western medicine is on the pathogens and how to control them, whereas the other two medical systems concentrate on the body, insisting that it can acquire strength by maintaining the balance among its constituents (Frawley 2001; Ranade 2001). Biomedicine acknowledges the state of the immune system. Yet it pays less attention to the interplays of sociocultural, historical, environmental, economic, and politico-economic factors, which play a significant role in shaping the body and perceptions toward it (see Lock and Kaufert 2001; Lock and Nguyen 2010). It significantly focuses on an "outside-in" approach while emphasizing that the body needs external interventions to be strong.

In contrast, *Unānī-Tib* and *Ayurvedā* practice an "inside-out" approach that focuses on the potential of the body itself. They have specific suggestive patterns such as (1) the air of one's environment; (2) food and beverages; (3)

movement and rest; (4) sleep and wakefulness; (5) eating and evacuation; and (6) dealing with emotions in ways that keep them in a balance; all of these lead toward a "strong body." Biomedicine, however, deems medicine, for example, vaccination, necessary to create power inside the body and improve the immune system to beat any outer attack.

Healthcare Systems Compete: A "Most Wanted" Medical System

Biomedicine, *Ayurvedā*, and *Unānī Tib* can be regarded as either complementary to or as competitive with each other. Yet rather than regarding these time-tested traditional healing systems as complementary, biomedicine considers them to be unscientific, improper, irrational, outdated, ineffective, hazardous, and harmful. Cunningham and Andrews (1997, 12) argue that unsurprisingly, the local systems of former colonies' imperialist states "were judged inferior, stupid or merely superstitious in comparison with this scientific medicine." Likewise, "the natives were in general regarded as dirty, lazy, and as reservoirs of disease, needing the imperialist to bring them health and civilization" (ibid.).

Yet these "natives" tend to greatly prefer their traditional medicinal systems, which they have been using and consulting for many generations. They understand them as identity markers and very much want to use them; the following stories illustrate this wanted-ness. This negotiation of healing patterns and revival of "the Indigenous" relates to a wider movement across the world, as many Indigenous peoples are now strongly speaking out in favor of their traditional healing systems, for example, as Gabriele Alex (2009) finds in the context of a South Indian Narikuravar community, which negotiates and defends its folk medical practices within India. And Langford (2002) links the revival of *Ayurvedā* to the revival of "the Indian" in a global context.

Imagining Indigenous Practices

What do people believe, and how do they differentiate Indigenous practices from biomedicine? There are local stories that prevail in Pakistani society, which reveal how resentment occurs against the Western biomedical system. To make this point, I would like to mention a few narratives. A 50-year-old man, who is quite famous in *Rahīmpur* village due to his folk wisdom, shared two stories regarding the *Hakīm* to explain his knowledge and skills for the diagnosis and treatment of an illness. As the day is incredibly hot (around 40°C), we are sitting under a green tree, locally called *Tāri* (*Dalbergia Sissoo*). Under the tree, two black buffalo are chained, with their eyes closed, chewing grass. The tree made the heat a bit easier on all of us. The older man begins the tale:

> Once upon a time, there were two popular *Hakīm*. Kings used to battle each other to demonstrate their strengths, wisdom, and skills. Warriors

once fought each other to testify their skills, strength, power, and bravery. So do the *Hakīm*, but with different tricks and ways to evaluate the *JJānn* [knowledge], *Hunur* [skills], and *Ddāhap* [wisdom].

So, one day, one *Hakīm Jibrāīl* (pseudonym) wrote a letter to another *Hakīm*, named *Luqmān* (a pseudonym): "I am sending you a sick person, please treat him accordingly and send me back a healthier one." He gave the letter and address to a healthy person who was under his apprenticeship. Besides, he recommended to the person, "When you feel hungry, tired and sleepy, then you must use the wood of the *Aku* plant (*Calotropis procera*) to make fire, cook food, rest and sleep beside it. These are the recommendations that you must follow." The person started his journey on a horse with a cloth bag carrying some food, water, and clothes. The journey lasted around one week. He was following the given directions accordingly, as promised. As time passed, he began to get sick. On the seventh day, he was very ill, unable to move, cook, and eat. Thankfully, he had the horse and just managed to reach his destination.

As soon as he reached the village of *Hakīm Luqmān*, he asked someone to bring him there. Since he was a guest as well as sick, the person obliged him and brought him to the *Hakīm*. They knocked at the door. *Hakīm Luqmān* came outside. The person—who now was very sick—managed to speak while providing him with the letter from *Hakīm Jibrāīl*.

The *Hakīm Luqmān* read the letter and then looked at the face of the person, who was still sitting on the horse. The *Hakīm Luqmān* said, "Well! The *Hakīm Jibrāīl* is extraordinarily intelligent. I have heard good stories of his *Ddáhap*. I have great respect for him. Also, you are very ill, and fortunately, I have diagnosed the illness. Please do not worry, as you will recover soon. I would have asked you to get down from the horse and have a meal, but I must also follow some strict rules. I am not allowed to show you my hospitality this time, but next time for sure. Your *Hakīm* has challenged my *Ddāhap*. The challenge is akin to questioning or doubting someone's prestige. Therefore, please do not get down from the horse, and let me write down the answer to this letter."

The *Hakīm Luqmān* replied, "Thank you for writing to me and sending a sick person. You are a very well-known *Hakīm*, and I am like a student and still learning. I respect your commitment to serving humanity with your *Jjānn*, *Hunur*, and *Ddāhap*. However, with a limited *Jjānn*, I have diagnosed the causes of ill health. I believe that the right diagnosis is half the treatment. Please accept my regards and this recovered, healthy person." The *Hakīm Luqmān* gave the person some food to eat and recommended: "You have to use the Bair the same way that you were using the *Aku* plant (*Ziziphus mauritiana*). Also, please make a promise to be consistent."

The person began the journey back to *Hakīm Jibrāīl*. He followed the recommendations of *Hakīm Luqmān*: resting and sleeping under a Bair tree and using its wood for cooking food. Slowly and gradually, he was recovering. He was sick on the seventh day. On the final day of the return journey, he recovered fully and was healthy again. He arrived home and met the *Hakīm Jibrāīl*. Without any further delay, he handed him the letter of the *Hakīm Luqmān*. After reading the letter, the *Hakīm Jibrāīl* inquired about the whole journey, requesting every detail from the beginning. The person told him everything—how he became sick and healthy again. After listening to the details of the travel account, *Hakīm Jibrāīl* then praised the *Ddāhap* of *Hakīm Luqmān*. In this way, the *Hakīm* used to test each other.

Moreover, my interlocutor asked me if he could share another story. What else would a researcher dream of, if not a interlocutor who was willing to oblige and share knowledge without hesitancy? I replied with a big, "Yes, please! Do tell."

Once upon a time, two *Hakīm*, let us call them *Sārang* and *Sodhal*, were going somewhere. It was sweltering summer weather. The sun was coming down to meet the earth. To protect themselves from the heat, both cover their heads with *Rumāl* (handkerchiefs). On their way, they see a farmer wearing a *Goadd* (a type of sarong that is wrapped around the waist and worn in place of trousers, especially by men from South Asia) only, with no *Qamīs* (shirt). He is cultivating the paddy in the fields, which are full of water. A woman comes to him with a small basket on her head, which [they assume] contains lunch for him. When they see the farmer and the woman, both start an argument with each other about whether the farmer will die or survive. They stop under a nearby tree and continue observing the whole scenario. *Sārang* argues that "These are the last breaths of the farmer" and *Sodhal* refutes it: "he (the farmer) can survive, if ..."

Meanwhile, the female reaches and calls to the farmer, who comes from the middle of paddy fields to the *Bbano* (small pathways intersecting in the fields between small parts so that the fields can be adequately watered and to walk between the fields). He sits down on the *Bbano*, opens the basket, and promptly starts eating the meal. He is eating and simultaneously sipping something. After the meal, the farmer does not die but survives. His survival raises further questions and discussion for both the *Hakīm*. Both start thinking; they want to know the reasons responsible for the farmer's survival. They brainstorm and come to conclusions on his survival. *Hakīm Sodhal* excitingly shouts as if he has solved a big-impossible puzzle. He said: "Yes, the farmer can survive under certain conditions, such as consuming a specific food, i.e., raw onion, that he certainly has eaten, and secondly if his feet remain in the paddy fields when he is eating. Otherwise, there is no other way possible that he could survive." The other *Hakīm* agreed with him and praised his knowledge.

Afterward, they said, "OK, let us go to meet him and inquire if he followed what we have concluded." Both went there and called to the farmer, who was again working in the field. The farmer came and asked them what he could do for them. They asked, "Could you please share with us what food you eat and how you have eaten it since we have a puzzle?" The question surprised the farmer, but he responded to it politely, considering them as guests. He said, "Because we are farmers. We do not have many options to eat, as we cannot afford it. We eat something simple to survive. We eat for survival rather than surviving for eating."

"Similarly, today, my wife brought two chapatis (homemade bread), one onion, and a jug of Lassi. While she called, I came quickly due to hunger, so sat down on the Bbano without going to sit under that tree and started eating with half-washed hands. I could not take my feet out from the wet paddy fields. That is what I ate and how I have eaten." Both the *Hakīm* then looked at each other. Soon after, *Hakīm Sārang* asked the reasons from *Hakīm Sodhal*, who shared that the food, and feet dipped into the water maintained the hot and cold nature in the body of the farmer. The onion and Lassi have a cold nature, and so does the water. After listening to this brief answer, *Hakīm Sārang* appreciated the understanding, knowledge, and wisdom of the *Hakīm Sodhal*. Later on, they also told the whole story to the farmer, who was still looking at them with surprise.

After having told the stories, the older man had a victorious smile on his face and said:

My son, this is called the real *Hikmat* (wisdom). Nowadays, doctors do not even respect humans. If you visit them, then they behave very arrogantly. They cannot even diagnose the illness until you tell them the feelings and problems you are having. However, *Hakīm* used to diagnose people while looking at their faces or just listening to the pulse on the wrist [and not on instinct]. A *Hakīm* was fully aware of the beats and sounds of the pulse.

These vignettes reveal how these local people perceive a healer: how a healer should be. Biomedical doctors do not check them or treat them in this way. According to them, a practitioner should have a thorough understanding of the body and know the causes of illness before asking questions of the sick person. They indirectly resist the biomedical system. This resistance is part of societal memory. They consider the biomedical system as a system of "others." Refusing vaccination, while considering it a "Western plot" to "sterilize" the Muslim females, also relates to this "our" and "their" dichotomy. An overwhelming number of people are still served by these Indigenous medical systems, where practitioners of these systems feel their pulse, inspect a patient, and offer them both a diagnosis and a cure, just as their ancestors have done for centuries. This is not only due to the lack of biomedical facilities but also to the alienation or foreignness of biomedical knowledge and practices.

The existence of such stories reflects the mechanisms of sharing and transferring local knowledges and viewpoints from one generation to another. Stories, folklore, and myths in each culture play a significant function in enculturing its members and preserving knowledge (Miller 1994; Miller and Moore 1989). As Leslie claims, "Human affairs take narrative form through our own stories and those of other individuals, and through stories that account for our customs and place in the world. The inherited forms of these stories guide our selective observation of the world" (1989, 26).

Moreover, some authors have traced the revival of the "Indigenous" medical systems, particularly *Unānī* and *Ayurvedā* (e.g., Alex 2009; Weiss 2008; Langford 2002; Leslie 1963). As Leslie (1963, 72) sketches the revitalization, especially during the struggle for independence, "by 1947 there were 57 colleges, 51 hospitals, and 3,898 dispensaries of Ayurvedic and *Unānī* medicine" in Pakistan. He further mentions that the followers of *Ayurvedā* consider the "golden age" of this system to be before the arrival of *Unānī-Tib*; however, they view the British-imposed allopathic medicine as being to the "detriment of the native systems" (ibid., 73). Advocates of *Ayurvedā* know that the Mughal invaders introduced *Unānī-Tib*, but the Arabic-translated version of Greek medicine has roots in *Ayurvedā* (Leslie 1989). This understanding may be a reason that *Unānī-Tib* and *Ayurvedā* are less threatened by each other than they are by biomedicine.

This coexistence and coordination of *Ayurvedā* and *Unānī-Tib* against the biomedical system during the time of colonization and post-colonization makes a different type of contestation visible, or what is called "the politics of identity" (see Weiss 2008). Despite the differences in their respective ideologies, both traditional systems are united against the "external force" in the form of biomedicine. Both systems want to defeat the latter. This contestation reflects a famous local saying: "[*Sindhī*] *Tray Dost Ain Tray Dushman*" (three friends and three enemies). For instance, a person's friend, their friend's friend, and their enemy's enemy are considered three friends, and thus a person's enemy, a person's friend's enemy, and a person's enemy's friend make the three enemies. The context of *Ayurvedā* and *Unānī-Tib* against the allopathic system is an example of this proverb. Perhaps, if the biomedical system had not challenged both, they might have confronted each other. The fundamental point in both is the body itself, which has the commanding position. This means that external forces or factors are secondary whenever it comes to ill-health. Nevertheless, as I have shown, they have many similarities in terms of geographical practice and theoretical under-standings, and on occasion have competed with each other. No medical sys-tem can cure all illnesses and diseases; therefore I argue that *these systems should act in tandem instead of in competition with each other.*

Concluding Remarks

Pakistan has a wide array of knowledge and practices related to health. This multiplicity illustrates a medical pluralism—encompassing *Ayurvedā, Unānī Tib,* homeopathy, and biomedicine. The country has made efforts to legalize this pluralistic medical system, as it legally incorporated all three of these non-biomedical healing modalities. Illustrating these systems from a historical perspective as well as supplying the data on their current state, I have shown what the government has done thus far to meet people's needs related to health, and what structure of the biomedical facilities exist in the country. After being transferred from the British colonizers to the "Brown Englishman," the biomedical healthcare system has evolved and received considerably more attention from the government than *Ayurvedā* or *Unānī Tib.* Nevertheless, the resources allocated to this system are insufficient when compared to other governmental sectors, most especially Defense. From 2000 to 2022, the country's average budget allocated to healthcare has never crossed 1% of the total GDP. The country's last few budgets for healthcare have remained stagnant at 1% of its GDP.

Consequently, the healthcare sector remains unestablished and over-whelmed: in 2018, according to *Pakistan's Economic Survey,* the doctor–patient ratio was around one doctor for 970 people, one dentist for around 9,540 persons, and one hospital bed for around 1,610 people. These differ-ences in terms of healthcare services and providers further intensify when compared to the rural and urban divide. The former category has fewer opportunities as compared to the latter one. This unfortunate situation dem-onstrates the prevailing inequalities and their substantial implications for the rural people of the country.

Moreover, providing a basic understanding of the local perceptions of these healthcare systems, this chapter has highlighted an ongoing and highly visible contestation. Although the biomedical system is strong in terms of its network, supplied resources, and governmental attention, the Indigenous systems are perhaps even more widely used, especially in rural areas like Sindh province. Despite its hegemonic status, the biomedical system is unable to meet the growing needs of a rapidly increasing population. Moreover, this chapter discussed the competition between healthcare systems: biomedicine on the one side and *Ayurvedā* and *Unānī Tib* on the other. I situate this ten-sion within the broader revival of Indigenous medicine and identity politics, and reiterate that these modalities should work in complementary, not com-petitive, ways.

Notes

1 In Hindu mythology, the *Ashvins* or Ashwini Kumaras are two Vedic gods. In the *Rigveda*, they are described as divine twin horsemen. Their mother is *Saranyu*—a goddess of the clouds—and their father's name is *Surya*. They are symbols of the shining of sunrise and sunset and appear in the sky prior to dawn in a golden chariot. They are believed to bring treasures to human beings and avert misfortune as well as sickness.

2 A milky fluid containing emulsified fat and other products of digestion, formed from the chyme in the small intestine and conveyed by the lacteals and the thoracic duct to the veins, and chyme: the semifluid mass into which food is converted by gastric secretion and which passes from the stomach into the small intestine.

3 A single individual cannot be considered as a founder (Sheehan and Hussain 2002), since the theories of Galen seem influential, as well as the contribution of Persians e.g., Abu-Ali-Abdullah-Hussain-Ibn-Sina (known as Avicenna) (980–1037 CE), and Muhammad-ibn-Zakariya-ar-Razi (called Rhazes) (860–932 CE), who are thought of as central in the establishment and development of Tib (Sheehan and Hussain 2002; Bürgel 1976; Subbarayappa 2001). The contribution of Hippocrates is also undeniable. Additionally, Ibn-Sina developed the system of therapeutics, and his book *Qanoon* (*Canon of Medicine*) is still considered the central text in *Unānī-Tib* (M.H. Shah 1966).

4 It comprises Or (*Ilaj Bitadir*): venesection (*Fasad*), cupping (*Mohajim*), diaphoresis (*Tareeq*), diuresis (*Idrar Baol*), Turkish bath (*Hammam*), massage (*Dalak*), cauterization (*Kai*), counterirritation (*Imala*), vomiting (*Qai*), purging (*Ishaal*), leeching (*Taaleeq*), exercise (*Riyazat*). Other treatment options include diet therapy (*Ilaaj Bil Ghiza*), pharmaceutical or drug therapy (*Ilaaj Bidawa*), and surgery (*Ilaaj Bilyad*) (Sheehan and Hussain 2002, 126), or practices such as 'cupping therapy' against arthritis, asthma, and migraine (Akhtar and Siddiqui 2008).

5 This statement provides a probable ground to the refusals and resentment against vaccination considering it as harmful for the body. Chapters 11 and 12 have further details on this matter.

6 I avoid using "complementary and alternative" medicine because I see them as problematic concepts. Both terms indicate something that is not primary; however, either may complement a primary phenomenon or create an alternative to a primary thing—e.g., biomedicine in the current sense. I see all Indigenous medical systems, including *Ayurvedā* and *Unānī-Tib*, as primary, not as "alternative" systems. They each have their own knowledge, ideas, and practices. If we look from the *Ayurvedā* and *Unānī-Tib* perspective, then, despite its near-global hegemony, biomedicine may be rightly called a "complementary and alternative" medicine.

7 The last calculations for "percentage change" are not mentioned in the governmental document, thus, I have calculated them myself.

8 Nonetheless, there are certain (I)NGOs working to create an awareness of the complaint redressal mechanism at various levels and giving confidence to the people to lodge their complaints.

5 Health and Illness
Sociocultural Understandings

Conceptualizing and Maintaining Health

Local people conceptualize health as being the greatest blessing from a supernatural being. The Muslim population considers it a blessing of *Allāh*, and the Hindus perceive it as a blessing of their gods and goddesses. Thus, they both relate it to supernatural beings. Being healthy in that perspective means that the supernatural being(s) is happy with that individual. The healthy one is richer than the others. This is because the blessing permits the predefined roles and responsibilities to be performed, and essential elements of existence, such as food and sleep, to be accomplished smoothly (Ali 2011). Performances of roles and accomplishment of elements of existence are signs of healthiness and relate to the second perspective. People judge an individual's health by his or her physical appearance. Here, a slim person is believed to be ill and a chubby healthy. Slimness is considered as a sign of malnourishment, and it also reveals someone's economic state. There are numerous ideas and practices to stay healthy—that may be about specific prescriptions and regimens related to food patterns; routine activities; sleeping patterns; hygienic patterns; dress patterns; visiting sacred spaces; time–space relationships; symbolic protection; propitiation; and worship—which one should perform in daily life. Local people believe that failing in any of such practices can cause illness. In order to explain the causes and to decide about treatment type, family members examine an individual in the light of the abovementioned cultural perspective of healthiness.

Local people in Sindh province deal with health in a triadic relationship: human to human; human to the natural environment; and human to the supernatural beings. To maintain their health, they practice the abovementioned sociocultural stock of knowledge and practices. More importantly, one can find connections of the local sociocultural ideas and practices of health and illness to their religion as well as to *Ayurvedā* and *Unānī-Tib*. People think about health and illness in terms of elements and humors and then adopt the related measures to recover lost health (see Chapter 4) (Rafatullah and Alqasoumi 2008; Sheehan and Hussain 2002) (Figure 5.1).

DOI: 10.4324/9781003253716-6

Food Patterns and Health

The food-related guidelines include the type of food, how to cook and eat it, the timing of eating, and the combinations of food. The food prepared at home is regarded as healthy as compared to food available at the market. People who often eat by choice at restaurants or hotels are seen as not "good" for mainly two reasons: (a) the food is unhealthy due to improper usage of spices and because it is not fresh, which disturbs their health; and (b) it is a waste of money. Eating food in a proper routine is necessary. The best timing of food includes a breakfast early in the morning by 9.00 am, *Mānjhāndo* (lunch) around 1.00 to 3.00 pm, and dinner around 5.00 to 6.00 pm.

Similarly, a combination of a particular food is avoided; for example, fish, beef, other meat, and chiefly chicken are not eaten after drinking milk. Foods such as butter, milk, fish, meat—and specifically beef—are considered as healthy in *Rahīmpur* village. In contrast, in *Rāmpur* village with a higher Hindu population, everything remains the same, except that the meat is replaced by vegetables.

Following these food patterns plays a pivotal role in staying healthy. In contrast, those who breach the stated guidelines may get sick. Yet eating healthy food is not the only way to remain healthy; other practices are equally important.

Conducting Life Affects Health

It is widely known that health is related to the way one conducts life, and so it is believed in Sindh province. Emotions, intentions, and concrete actions can influence health. There are many abstract actions, such as *Sārr, Hasad, Baimānī,* and *Munāfiqat* (literally: jealousy, envy, dishonesty, and hypocrisy) that are not only perceived as bad for one's overall life, but also as harmful due to their significant effects on one's health. It is impossible not to have these negative states of emotion. Other practices include performing physical activities regularly, such as walking and doing physical work. Local people use an expression *Hadd-Harām* (one who is lazy and does not perform physical tasks such as cutting grass, carrying some weight, and cultivating crops in order to support his family in survival), which also has sociocultural and health-related implications. Believing that a working (physically) body is a healthy body, one should actively participate in the stated activities and not lie in bed during the day as that brings misfortune and ill-health.

Sleeping Patterns and Health

Sleeping patterns relate to timing and space. Sleeping late or not sleeping during the night are considered to be unhealthy. Deliberately sleeping late is highly discouraged, as people in the villages follow the routine of sleeping and rising early. The majority fall asleep by 9.00 pm and wake up before sunrise, that is, around 5.00 am. Someone who sleeps until sunrise, unless they are ill, is highly criticized and considered as a source of attracting misfortune and trouble. Some local expressions and proverbs exist related to sleeping patterns (metaphorically). The expressions are not limited to the villages, but one may observe these across the province and the country. These include [*Sindhi*] *Sawair Sumho Ain Sawair Utho* ("sleep early and rise early") or [*Sindhi*] *Suta Uthi Jagg Nind Na Kajy Aitri, Sultani Suhagg Nindon Kandy Na Mili* ("avoid excessive sleepiness, if you want to achieve the crown"). A change in sleeping behavior indicates that either the person is ill or will fall ill. Hence, if someone sleeps longer than a culturally prescribed routine, family members inquire about the person's health. Besides, space for sleeping alters seasonally in order to protect against seasonal changes such as heat and cold. During summer and winter, the villagers sleep under an open sky within the premises of the house and inside the house, respectively.

Hygiene Patterns and Health

Locally, hygiene patterns are related to cleanliness, purity, and pollution. Semen, excretion, dogs and pigs, dead animals, and menstrual blood are among the impure entities. After releasing semen, a person is considered *Mathy-Mero* (a person who has not taken the necessary ritualistic bath after intercourse). It is because the said person can be harmful to the person him/herself and also others and bring misfortune until ritualistic ablution is observed. Likewise, the menstruation period makes a woman impure. In both the mentioned states, an individual must not visit a child who has contracted measles. Furthermore, to maintain cleanliness, people use water after excretion. Water, sunlight, air, and fire are the sources for obtaining purity.

Moreover, human–animal relations draw a different picture. Touching specific animals such as dogs or cats is strictly avoided; if so, then washing hands is strictly necessary. On the contrary, it is reasonable to touch, live with, and share spaces—and even sleep—with buffalo, cows, camels, goats, and sheep (as discussed in the previous chapter). The dung of cows and buffalo is used, after drying under the sun, to fire the oven for cooking food, and as fertilizer on agricultural fields.

Flies that fly inside the house, or sit on food and children, which emerge in the thousands during the summer season are another hygiene-related issue. People who are weak in terms of economic resources do not even consider that flies might spread viruses (as the etic perspective says). Pictures of children, circulated in the media during the measles outbreaks of 2012 and 2013, show flies sitting on their bodies, and exhibit the circumstances under which people are living. On the contrary, flies perhaps are nonexistent in the houses of rich people—those who can afford bungalows, air-conditioning, and vehicles. These economically rich people are also well aware of the harm that such flies can bring.

Dress Patterns and Health

People also directly link health to the dress patterns that are followed. There are recommendations for dress patterns in terms of colors, designs, and wearing patterns. These recommendations vary further according to age and gender. For little children, bright colors, such as green and red, are avoided. This is because of the belief that children can easily catch *Nazar* (literally: "sight," however, it reflects a belief that every human contains a power which is often transmitted through the eyes; thus, a person can be affected by anyone else and become ill by the evil eye). The colors make children more attractive, as they are already innocent and beautiful. However, for women, such bright colors are acceptable. But they should be highly careful, mainly when they go to dark and unpopulated places such as the graveyard, as such places are abodes of supernatural beings, including *Jinn-Bhut*, which can be enchanted by women and ultimately be possessed by them. For men, light colors are recommended. In the village of *Rahīmpur*, wearing green and black dresses is subject to specific conditions. People prefer not to wear them, but if they do, they take strict purity measures. It is because green is associated with the color of the Prophet Muhammad's tomb and black with the color of *Qabā*, the sacred building for Muslims in Mecca. Yet during the Islamic month, Muharram, they usually wear black clothes to show pain and sadness in relation to the event of Karbala, in which the Prophet Muhammad's sister's son Hazrat Hussain was martyred, along with his family and friends. The strictness of green and black is further uncompromising for a woman who must not wear these colors during the menstrual cycle.

Additionally, gender and age significantly shape the recommendations about covering certain body parts. A woman must wear a headscarf, cover her chest, avoid exposing the body, and wear trousers down to her ankles. A man must wear a vest and sarong. He must not visit a graveyard, especially in the evenings, without wearing a full-sleeve shirt and trousers or a sarong.

The prescribed patterns of dressing are considerably related to religious teachings and practices. For instance, if a woman ignores such recommendations, *Allāh* will be angry and may punish her. The punishment may be ill-health. Although punishment is not limited to ill-health, it can have other adverse consequences such as poverty, illness to her children, and family members.

Supernatural Beings and Health

Moreover, people believe in supernatural beings, for example, *Jinn*, who they believe live in dark and unpopulated places such as thick forests, ancient trees, and graveyards. These beings return to their abodes at sunset. They do not deliberately intervene in human affairs until disrupted. They especially get disturbed after sunset, which makes them malicious. Therefore, going with specific dresses, colors, and, in particular, at a specific time—after sunset—is strictly avoided. Women and, specifically, children must not go to such places because they can enchant a *Jinn* on his way back to the abode. *Jinn* most commonly possess women, though they can also possess men and children. It is always a *Jinn* (masculine) that possesses a woman and a *Jinrrī* (feminine) that possesses a man. When the volume of a voice increases, such as during music or crying at death, a possessed woman faints, dances, and enters a trance, and then she speaks with a different voice. For people, it is not the woman, but the supernatural being that speaks: *Jinn* called *Faqīr* (a term used to address the male *Jinn*), or *Jinrrī* called *Faqīryannī* (a term used to address the female *Jinn*). During that trance, the people (who are present there) ask *Faqīr* via the possessed person for prayers or inquire about their problems and misfortunes. After the trance, the woman falls to the ground, and a family member accompanies her until she comes to herself. Usually, these are women who are possessed rather than men. Also, whenever a possessed woman visits a shrine, she goes into a trance.[1]

Sacred Spaces: Shrines as Centers of Hope and Health

Sacred spaces, such as shrines of saints, are sources for attracting fortune, good health, and solutions to all sorts of problems. Shrines function as centers of hope and health across the country. People visit shrines to receive blessings and to avoid misfortunes and solve problems. These problems may be sociocultural (such as issues in getting married), economic (poverty), political (unresolved disputes), and biological (having a baby and especially a male baby) problems, or the aim may be to treat illnesses. The shrines prove to be the last hopeful resorts to seek miraculous help when everything else has failed. The devotees visit and observe *Manat* (literally: imploration or beseeching), make a vow, perform specific rituals, and give votive offerings.

As noted in Chapter 4, the inhabitants of *Rahīmpur* village do not merely visit the shrines in the province. However, each year, some—not always the same ones—travel to Iran, Iraq, and Syria to pay visits to the shrines of *Ahal-Bait* (the family of the Holy Prophet Muhammad), such as the shrines of Imam Ali (the Prophet's cousin), Imam Hussain (the son of the Prophet's daughter, Fatima), and Hazrat Zainab (the daughter of the Prophet's daughter, Fatima). The visitors are considered the luckiest. People share stories of miracles of the *Ahal-Bait*. There is, for instance, a famous narration that Hazrat Ali gave eyes to a blind person, or he gave seven sons to a formerly barren woman. A common perception is that the seeker's intention and way of making vows matter most; otherwise, the *Ahal-Bait* are kind. On the other hand, in *Rāmpur* village, people visit shrines of saints—irrespective of religion—in the province and go to Mandar.

People of various religions visit shrines. The shrines are synchronized centers where Islam, Hinduism, Sikhism, and Christianity intersect. The province is home to famous saints—such as *Qalandar Lāl Shahbāz, Shāh Abdul Latīf*

Bhittaī, Sachal Sarmast, and *Shāh Ināyat Shahīd*—where people come from across the country. Similarly, there are also *Mandar* in the province such as the *Kālkā Devī Mandar* near to the village of *Rahīmpur;* and the Shiva *Mandar* in the mountains of *Kārunjhar*. Moreover, the Thar Desert also has several shrines, temples, "memorial stones," and *Marrhī* and *Māth,* where people make vows about their good health and fortune (see Kalhoro 2015; Chapter 3 of this book).

Zayārāt, meaning pilgrimage, is a local concept of paying a visit to a shrine. During *Zayārāt,* people pay respect by kneeling, touching, and kissing the shrine, especially the saint's grave. According to them, saints are closer to *Allāh* than ordinary people. Saints become God's friends through unceasing worship. In return, God bestows on them *Karamat* (miraculous power). People specifically visit shrines when they remain ill despite treatment at a healthcare facility.[2] A single visit to a shrine is sufficient in some cases; otherwise, staying for three, five, or seven (or more) nights is a prerequisite.

Although not a single person from the selected villages stayed at a shrine during my fieldwork, while living in the province (since my childhood), I have been observing shrine-related rituals and practices. By visiting a few shrines during fieldwork, I also observed numerous people staying there. After interacting with the people, I knew that people who had hepatitis, cancer, and ulcers were staying for healing through *Karamat*. The stay continues until these people receive *Niā* (we can call it a piece of news). The Nia reaches them through dreams during sleep, irrespective of timing, that is, the day or night. The dreams often include a saint, mostly with a white beard, who comes to the person carrying something in his hands. The saint operates on or touches the problematic part of the body and permits the person to go afterward, as everything will now be all right.

During the stay, people do not take any preventive measures pertaining to eating. They eat whatever food—called *Langar*—is distributed there. This applies even if the food is otherwise prohibited. People avoid eating rice during some internal or external injuries, but at a shrine, rice in the form of *Langar* is regarded as sacred and potent for healing. They drink *Sabīl* (it can be explained as water served at the sacred places and associated with the saints),[3] and eat *Khāk* (clay) available at the shrine. The association with the saint makes this food, water, and clay sacred and a remedial measure. Moreover, they clean the premises of the shrine, offer prayers, make vows, and sleep waiting for a remedy. They also receive verbal healing from the *Mujāwar* or *Faqīr* (a religious ascetic with some mystical powers) of such shrines.

Besides *Zayārt, Faqīr* at shrines do verbal healing. They chant some verses and blow over the body of the person. They also give people threads, on which they blow some verses. In return, people pay them some money. Consider the following vignette from my fieldwork:

> I am with one interlocutor, *Dil Murad* (pseudonym) from *Rahīmpur* village, at his *Katchā* (literally: unbricked) house. He is in his late thirties,

works as daily wage laborer, and cultivates his land. The temperature is above 40°C. Although it is a sweltering summer's evening, children are playing hide and seek: the silence and yelling occur at intervals. The hen with her fledglings, which nowadays is called an organic chicken in the West, especially in Europe, is moving here and there. Countless flies are sitting, flying. One brown-colored dog is half-sleep under a small neem tree. Her mother, who is around 50 years of age, was wearing floral printed lawn clothes with the dominant blue.

While having a cup of tea and having *Kachaharī* generally about the usual daily activities and measles, the discussion came to fever. We start talking concerning fever because *Dil's* wife, Ms. *Sārān* (v) has a fever—locally called *Purānno Bukhār* (literally: an old fever). On the one hand, she is not recovering, and on the other hand, she performs her routine work. Through word of mouth, they learned about a *Faqīryānnī* (a female religious ascetic with some mystical powers), who performs verbal healing at a nearby shrine. She recites some chants to heal the *Purānno Bukhār*. These days they are visiting her. I ask regarding the reasons behind the preference, as they could afford biomedicine.

Her mother, Ms. *Gulān* (pseudonym)—who is a gentle lady, in her fifties—the skin of her face and hands was losing its grip, but she still seemed a healthy person as she brings the grass and fodder for the animals (two buffalos, one cow, and seven goats). She does this work, especially for the goats. She today is wearing cotton, floral-printed lawn clothes that are predominantly blue. She joins the *Kachaharī* and shares the underlying reasons to visit the *Faqīryānnī*. "I tell you, my son, that we have been consulting government hospitals and private doctors, but they are of no benefit, including the expensive doctors, who charge 200 PKR just for the receipt to allocate a waiting number. We have done all *Hīlā-Wasīlā* (made all possible efforts), but nothing has worked. The fever is complicated now and has turned into a *Purānno Bukhār* or *Waddo Bukhār*, that is when fever remains hidden in the bones and makes a person weaker. There are two other types of fever: *Mudy Jo Bukhār* when fever occurs with an interval; and *Halko Bukhār* is a slight fever, which lasts for one or two days, and the person recovers without any medication." (This specific type of fever is explained below.)

Ms. *Gulān* continues, "Since last month, my *Nuhn* (daughter-in-law) is suffering from a *Purānno Bukhār*. We have consulted a doctor, first at a government-run-dispensary, and then a private MBBS doctor, but her fever continues. She is not eating due to sour saliva in her mouth as in this fever saliva becomes sour. Due to not eating, she has lost weight.

Eventually, some of our relatives informed us of a girl who recites some verses and blows over the person. She belongs to a *Faqīr* family of a Dargah (shrine) named *Ubhan Shāh*. His father was a healer, too. He died around a year ago, and now she has that *Hudo* (power, skill, authority). She is in her thirties. After holding the right hand of the person, she recites verses and blows over him/her. The minimum requirement is three visits: morning, evening, and the next morning. We (she, her son, and her *Nuhn*) went yesterday in the morning and evening but missed the visit the next morning due to the marriage of our relatives. We will, therefore, go this evening. After two visits, my daughter-in-law is much better. During our visits, we paid the girl some money. Yesterday we paid 100 PKR in the morning and 50 in the evening. Since we pay in the hospitals, why not pay her? She neither asks for nor checks the given amount. This girl is popular. Many people visit her. Yesterday, two women brought their little children.

The described case illustrates people's belief in shrine behavior and verbal healing. The local people visit shrines when they have illnesses, mostly when biomedical doctors dismiss a patient after declaring them as incurable, or what local people call *Ley-Dāwā* (literally: unclaimed). Thereafter, family members bring that person (sometimes due to a person's desire) to a shrine for *Karāmat* to heal illness. Some people spend a maximum number of *Ākhrī Dīnh* (which could be translated as "last days to live") at a shrine with the belief that the saint will cure illness, or otherwise, he will be a source of *Nijāt* or *Chutkāro* (literally: forgiveness) in the grave and on the day of judgment. There are some famous shrines across Sindh province, where people go to seek health. The most famous shrines include *Qalandar Lāl Shahbāz*, *Shāh Abdul Latīf*, and *Saeedī Mussānī*. During my fieldwork, I met two persons. One of them was from *Rahīmpur* village, who was suffering from stomach cancer, and the other person was from another nearby village who was suffering from hepatitis. Both were in a critical condition. The biomedical doctors declared them *Ley-Dāwā*. As a result, both the persons visited shrines. The former spent a couple of weeks of his life at *Ubhan Shah* (he also died), and the latter person stayed at a shrine until the night he died. These anecdotes illustrate how local people consider the shrines as a last resort to seek health. They believe that saints can heal them.

Symbolic Objects, Chanting, Worship, and Health

Symbolic objects such as *Tavīz* (amulets) or certain verbal spells are used primarily to avoid a *Jinn* attack, misfortune, and to ward off a *Nazar*. They also attract luck. A *Tavīz* is created by a religious person or a person who has some *Hudo* (required skills, knowledge, and permission). The *Tavīz* contains the holy verses, names of *Allāh*, the holy prophet, and *Ahal-Bait*. Packed in a small box of steel or enveloped in a leather piece, it is tied around an arm, waist, or neck. *Tavīz* is commonly used for children.

Although verbal chanting also has the same purpose, this is done more for health than protection. Prayers and supplications—a form of verbal chanting— serve both prevention and healing. Mostly, the old people recite *Tasbih* (a set or string of 33 or, mostly, 99 beads to recite) specific phrases such as "*Allāh-u-Akbar; Shukur Al-Hamd-u-Lillāh; Subhān Allāh* (God is great; all thanks to *Allāh*; and glory to *Allāh*). Furthermore, with a similar purpose, houses contain objects such as horseshoes, posters of the holy verses and pictures of shrines and saints. The charts in *Rahīmpur* contain the Quranic verses, and names of *Allāh*, the prophet, and his family; while in *Rāmpur*, the posters carry pictures and motifs from Hinduism, such as gods and goddesses.

The propitiation and worship, such as *Namāz*, function as a protection against evil, troubles, and as a source to attract blessings, luck, and good health. In *Rahīmpur* village, there is a mosque where people observe daily *Namāz*. However, in *Rāmpur* village, people worship gods and goddesses at home and at the nearby Mandar (see Chapter 3).

Furthermore, alms, giving charity, and sacrifices protect against or ward off troubles, tensions, and misfortunes. In *Rahīmpur* village, a 30-year-old male interlocutor shared the following story on the importance of these practices:

The prophet Moses used to communicate to God daily on the Mountain Sinai. One day, a wood collector asked him about his death. Moses replied, "Yes, today, I will inquire from God and will tell you tomorrow." On the very next day, the Prophet Moses informed the person that tomorrow morning he would die. The person was shocked but accepted the revelation. As usual, on the next morning, he went to collect wood for his home. On his way back, he was engulfed in deep thoughts about his approaching death.

Meanwhile, a beggar shouted, "Please give me something in the name of Allāh." The person offered him something valuable as a charity. The whole day passed, but he was still alive with a bundle of wood, carrying it on his head. He met the Prophet, Moses, by chance. He asked the prophet why he was still alive, while the prophet informed him about his death. Moses was surprised to see him alive. Promptly, the Prophet Moses ordered him to bring the bundle of wood down and open it. After opening it, both saw a big snake with a stone in its mouth. Moses told him that your death has been traveling with you, and you could have been dead by now. However, you have done something extraordinary that has consequently protected you and prolonged your life. Now please tell me what you have done after meeting me since yesterday. The person shared each detail, including giving *Sadqā* to the beggar. Moses replied: "This is the leading cause that you are alive."

Dealing with Illness

As stated earlier, illness is the opposite state of health, which shows that something wrong has happened in maintaining the triad relationship: human to the supernatural, human to the natural environment, and human to human. Thus, people raise questions to determine the reasons for illness. The leading question can be, why did a specific illness occur to that specific person at that specific time? The preliminary conclusions may be that the illness is due to an *Imtehān* (literally: test); a *Sazā* (literally: punishment, curse); *Qismat* or *Taqdīr* (literally: fatalism); *Sāyā* (literally: invasion, possession); *Nazar*; *Jādu* or *Ddooh* (literally: magic); or due to consuming improper food, wearing an inappropriate dress, or seasonal variations.

Imtehān, Sazā, *Qismat, and Illness*

Imtehān is a belief in *Allāh*. He conducts an *Imtehān* to test someone's tolerance, strength, or relationship with Him. *Allāh* thus makes a person ill. A true believer shows strong faith in *Allāh*. S/he remains calm, thankful, never complains, and considers an illness an act of charity through the body. Nonetheless, *Allāh* also punishes evil deeds—individual and communal— dishonesty, deception, lying, oppression, and murder.

Qismat (literally: fatalism) is also a prominent discourse related to life events, including illness. It is written in the *Qismat* that illness is unavoidable. There are several expressions on this, but I merely mention two of them, which are directly related here. First, "[*Sindhī*] *Jaiko Qismat Jo/Me Likhio/ Likhyal Huyo*" (God already wrote it in fate), and second "[*Sindhī*] *Qismat Jo Likhyo Kair Tāry*" (no one can avert a decided fate). Muslims commonly believe that fate is decided on the evening of *Chatthī*. The *Chatthī* is a ritual. It is performed for a newborn on the evening of its sixth day to give it a name. The celebration depends much upon the baby's gender, sibling order, and the socioeconomic position of the family. If the newborn is a son, particularly the first son, first child, or a long-awaited one, then the celebration engages many participants. Likewise, the socioeconomic standing of the family determines the scale of *Chatthī*. Except for the extent, the content of *Chatthī* remains the same. The following is a description of the *Chatthī* of a baby boy that I attended. My choice is not gender-based but selected to exhibit both the content and scale of a *Chatthī*.

The first step is to invite relatives and break the news. The *Dai* (traditional midwife) invites the guests by visiting each house while simultaneously distributing locally made sweets such as sugar candies or jaggery. The receiver of the sweet pays some money (PKR 10–50). On the sixth day, close relatives such as siblings of the baby's mother and father arrive, either a day before *Chatthī* or at least in the morning of a *Chatthī*.[4] The remaining relatives arrive in the evening to eat or collect the food.

For the food, a male member slaughters a rooster, buck or bull (from his animals). Otherwise, he buys beef, other meat, or fish from the market in addition to rice, oil, spices, and sugar. Fabric is provided to be sewn for dresses. This is white for the baby, and there is also fabric for the mother and Dai to wear on that day. When the baby wears new clothes, the women sing folk songs. In the evening, food is prepared to be ready around 6.00 pm. There are two options for meals. The meal either comprises sweet rice called *Chāshnī* (cooked with rice, sugar, oil, and cardamom) and spicy rice called Biryani (cooked with rice, meat, beef, spices). Alternatively, there is *Chāshnī*, curry with beef, goat, buffalo, or fish, and *Chapāti* and Biryani.[5] *Chāshnī* is an essential part, in any case. The food is then distributed among the participants. Those villagers who are not close relatives send a child to bring money and a pot of sweet rice. The Dai distributes the sweets, which is mandatory, or at least stays there to collect the money. After that, the discussion revolves around choosing the name. Different proposals for a suitable name are offered. The parents and grandparents have the right to select the name. Around 9.00 pm, the naming ceremony begins. A small pot carrying the *Chāshnī* and milk is kept beside the head of the baby.

Every relative comes; gives pocket money (not obligatory) to the baby; dips five fingers of the right hand into the pot and places the fingers on the forehead of the baby; chants the chosen name and supplicates. The common supplication is "*Chatthī Māī, Tun* ... [Given Name] Jo *Sutho Likhyo Kajāns. Sehat, Izat, Shuhrat, Ilam Dijāns. Bhāgg Bakhat Wāro Kajāns. Kehn Jo Muhtāj Na Kajāns.*" (Oh! Mother *Chatthī*, may you decide the best for the (name of baby). Please bestow upon him health, prestige, popularity, and knowledge. Please make him the luckiest person. May you please make him an independent person). Once the naming is over, the ceremony ends, and the baby has a name.

There is a tragic story pertaining to *Qismat* that people share in the village of *Rahīmpur*, about how fate is decided during a *Chatthī*.

One day, a king met a contented and beautiful old lady and asked her who she was. The lady replied that she is called *Chatthī*. The king asked what she did. "I decide the fate of a person on the evening of *Chatthī*. What's more, I am now coming back from doing the same task," *Chatthī* replied. The king inquired, "What have you decided, then?" "On his marriage day, the person will die from a lion's attack," she answered. "Oh! However, I will not allow it to happen. I will keep the person safe," the king replied. After that, the king always looked after the family by providing resources, food, and security. Finally, the child becomes an adult, and his marriage day comes. Without sharing the reasons with this family, the king comes to them, brings his whole army along with weapons to surround the house. There was a belief that when a lion attacks, the attacked person quickly dies if he sees a mouse. To avoid this danger, the king also ordered four cats to be tethered at each pillar of the groom's *Khat* (Charpoy). Everything is under surveillance. So far, so good. The king is proactive and worried. It is midnight now. The escorting security is vigilant, ready to hunt the lion when it arrives.

All the rituals have been performed. The groom has brought his bride to his room. The bride and groom converse. During this, the bride asks the groom if he can create a model lion. The groom happily replies with yes. Both ask someone to bring wet wheat flour. Receiving the flour, he makes a lion. Once he finishes putting the tail to the lion, it becomes a real lion and severely attacks him. Although the cats are present, a mouse quickly jumps over the groom, and he dies. The bride loudly laments. Everyone arrives, including the king. The bride tells the whole story. The king is shocked and now shares the whole story with the bereaved family. The king salutes *Chatthī*, repents and confesses in front of *Allāh* to seek forgiveness for intervening in the act of God.

This story depicts a systematic appropriation of certain beliefs to relate every good or bad thing in life to fate. Similarly, as previously mentioned, the new-born's health is also believed to be decided on the evening of the naming ritual. However, this is not merely limited to health or illness but extends to other desired or undesired happenings in life. Considering an unwanted event as fate and accepting its occurrence reduces the pain or suffering and helps divert attention toward the solutions. This belief in fatalism is structured by influential stakeholders so that an ordinary person can justify all suffering without holding those who cause the suffering accountable. The aforementioned ritual of *Chatthī* clearly shows how such structures have been created, which nonetheless can be seen in the light of critical theories of anthropology—the theories which question these structures in order to explore the root causes of any suffering.

Sāyā, *Nazar, and Illness*

Sāyā is when someone is possessed by supernatural beings; these can cause illness. Mull (1991) found that *Sāyā* is a cause of malnutrition in *Katchī Ābādī* (a ghetto) of *Karāchī*. *Nazar* means a gaze, with the belief that everyone carries invisible energy that can exert an effect on other people. The energy is released through the eyes in a state of jealousy or happiness. That may not only be an evil eye, but also an eye that is pleased. In specific situations, someone catches the attention of someone else and becomes vulnerable to *Nazar*. These situations include wearing attractive clothes (especially for children) or performing an activity in a very precise way makes someone vulnerable. A child who is wearing new, attractive, and washed clothes and performs a *Nakhrā*—in which a child copies someone or is playful—catches the *Nazar* of others. A person's own family, neighbors, relatives, or even an unknown person can cast *Nazar*. In the villages, there are a few individuals best known for *Nazar*-casting.

To avoid a *Nazar*, a *Tavīz* works as a great protector. However, there are different ways to heal or what is locally called *Nazar Khan'an* (literally: absorbing *Nazar* to undo it)—to ask the *Nazar*-casting person to put saliva on the body of the *Nazar* receiver or to chant something and blow on the water for the latter to drink, or to visit a faith healer for chanting and *Tavīz*.

Gender and age make a significant difference in etiology and treatment choices. The etiology regulates decisions of whether and what treatment is required. It determines the suitable medical system(s) to be consulted for the treatment. People may consult one or several types of healthcare.

Concluding Remarks

This chapter has described some of the guidelines and orientations that culture provides on how to live, which are learned, shared, and passed on from one generation to another. These specific ways can be a source of health since the guidelines can encourage adopting or avoiding specific practices, which are related to daily life activities: for example, food, dress, character, sleep, hygiene, and supernatural beings. The people in the two villages I studied, along with others in Sindh province, believe that not following them may result in ill-health. I described: (a) conceptualizing and maintaining health; and (b) dealing with illness to recover the lost state of health. Needless to say, these ideas and practices related to health and illness are substantially shaped by sociocultural and economic and political factors, which again are a result of current as well as past circumstances. One can also find the roots of such guidelines and orientations in *Ayurvedā* and *Unānī-Tib*. People dealing with ill-health can sometimes involve only one or more medical systems: *Ayurvedā*, *Unānī-Tib*, biomedicine, homeopathy, home-based remedies, and shrine behaviors.

Notes

1 Pirani (2009) has studied several therapeutic measures related to this possession that are taken at shrines in Pakistan.
2 See Pirani (2009). Pfleiderer (2006) has described the procedures and occurrences at a Muslim shrine called *Mira Datar Dargah* in northern India. Another significant work on shrine behavior is from Frembgen (2011), who elaborates on one of the famous saints of the country situated in Sindh province, called Qalandar Lal Shahbaz.
3 During *Muhram* (the first Islamic month), the practitioners of Shia-Islam distribute water, syrup made of milk, sugar, and juices in the memory of the event of *Karbala*, in which the *Ahal-Bait* (family) of the Prophet Mohammad was martyred. They also distribute *Langar-Niaz*. They use terms *Sabīl* and *Langar* during this entire month for all drinks and food.
4 As in most cases, baby's grandparents from the father's side live together in a joint family.
5 It purely depends upon the socioeconomic position of a family.

6 Local Rituals of Containment
Emic Perceptions and Practices around Measles

Measles in Local Cultures

Measles is not a new phenomenon. It has been overwhelming the world and attracting discussions for many centuries. I operate under the assumption that most people are rational. Few operate without exercising judgments that derive from a set of values. Yet explanations and perceptions are distinctive, demonstrating the orientations and experiences of engaged stakeholders. Throughout history, measles has been subject to debate, especially on its prime causes, and received different rationales and responses as it has significantly affected populations worldwide (Morley 1969; Furuse, Suzuki, and Oshitani 2010; Rāzī 1848; Koplik 1962; Cunha 2004).

Five decades ago, David Morley (1969, 297) provided background information about the local perception of measles across the world. He writes that in Europe measles was perceived as "the failure of the mother to menstruate during pregnancy," and that "bad blood" enters the fetus and emerges after birth as rashes of measles (ibid., 297). He further describes that in Africa, people believed measles occurred because of sorcery. Nonetheless, some people linked it with heat and eating certain foods, for example, snails or beniseed (also known as sesame seed). Owing to fears that the rash may not come "out," people avoid both traditional and scientific medicines. Morley further mentions two "dangerous" customs: restricting fluids during measles in many African areas, and an astringent fluid made from roots or herbs for the eyes in the Zambesi valley.

On the perception of measles in Asia, Morley describes a few proverbs collected from West Asia: (a) "A child that gets out of measles is a child that is reborn" (Arabic); (b) "Count your children after the measles has passed" (Arabic); and (c) "Smallpox will make your child blind. Measles will send him [her] to his [her] grave" (Parsee) (ibid., 297).

Moreover, in Asia, people usually consider measles in relation to a "malignant goddess," thus, parents may hide their children from neighbors. Considering it useless and dangerous, they do not bring the measles-infected child to a hospital. Moreover, if a child who is brought to a hospital due to some other health conditions develops measles there, the parents promptly

DOI: 10.4324/9781003253716-7

bring the child home. Based on ancient medical systems, they prefer to treat the child with special foods having "cold" properties (ibid.).

Morley's description demonstrates that measles has been received and perceived differently in local cultures. These perceptions vary, yet resemble each other. As mentioned earlier, Morley's words, such as "malignant goddess," are loaded with specific meaning. Second, he has not touched upon factors that lie beneath these ideas and practices.

Besides, there are a few more examples of measles in local cultures. For example, the following Aztec painting (Figure 6.1) shows a person who is sitting on a wooden stool with the marks of the measles rash. On the right side, a woman is checking the measles rash. The painting reflects a ritual for healing measles.

Moreover, in Uganda, people believe that measles occurs twice in a lifetime. A colleague from Uganda shared this information when he was working on his doctoral research in medical anthropology, during our discussion at the Medical University of Vienna (Ronard Mukuye 2013, personal communication). To deal with measles, they perform certain rituals. During the measles outbreak in 2013 in Uganda, local people preferred to heal measles by using local herbs than opt for a hospital cure (Mafigiri, Nsubuga, and Ario 2017). These people were "blamed" that their ideas and practices were the cause of outbreaks. In contrast, people in Sindh believe that measles occurs once in a lifetime, and then the person who had measles is *Pakā* (immunized). For them, measles is a necessary and sacred illness, which I discuss below.

Measles in the Grave: A Manifestation of *Mātā* in Sindh

From the village of *Rāmpur*, a 40-year-old interlocutor stated: "Measles certainly will occur to a person. Mostly during one's childhood. However, if it

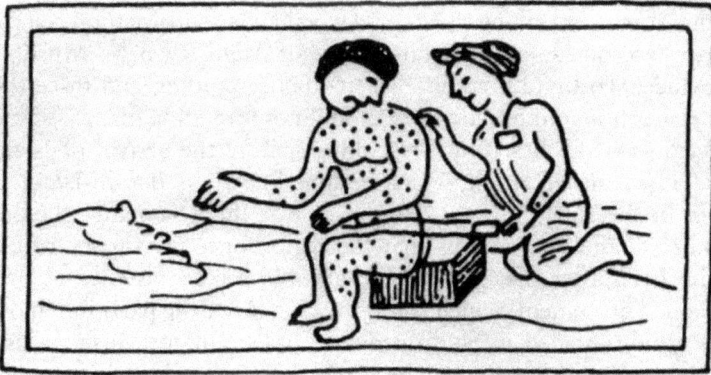

Figure 6.1 Oldstone, Michael B. A. (2009) *Viruses, Plagues, and History: Past, Present and Future*, Oxford University Press, USA, p. 144.

does not occur during life, then one will even contract it in the grave. There is no way that it will miss someone."

This statement illustrates an underlying belief in the necessity of the occurrence of measles. The grave is a metaphor indicating the cultural belief in this inevitability. People perceive that measles will unquestionably occur in everyone. If it does not occur during life, one may not escape it during the grave after death. They draw its etiology from Hindu mythology, irrespective of religion, and give a supernatural explanation of the occurrence of measles. Hindus and Muslims both believe that measles is a manifestation of the goddess *Mātā*, and she visits everyone. Despite a similar perception, there are a few differences. Hindus have a name for this goddess's manifestation in the form of measles— *Sitālā Mātā*—while Muslims use the more generic term *Mātā*.

Two questions arise: Why do people consider that measles will necessarily occur, and why do they consider it a sacred illness?

One reason may be that before the work of *Rāzī* or Rhazes, there was no proper differentiation available across the world between smallpox and measles until the tenth century (Kaadan 2000; Rāzī 1848). If the scholars of that time were unable to distinguish between the two diseases, then, how could a layperson do so? This lumping together of these two diseases compelled people to contemplate measles as sacred, link it with *Mātā*, and give it a supernatural explanation akin to the one they had for smallpox, due to the similarities in the symptoms and vague differentiation between the two, and to the power attributed to both diseases, which still prevails. The memories and stories related to smallpox outbreaks and the extraordinary infection and implications they caused have not vanished. I suggest that their fear of the overwhelming implications of both measles and smallpox pushed people to categorize them in the same domain of sacredness. Humans tend to place all phenomena—that overwhelm and frighten them or cause death—into the extraordinary category: the supernatural (see, e.g., Foster 1978). When people believe that a disease's primary cause is supernatural, they also believe that control over it can only be possible through making vows, performing rituals, and worshipping supernatural beings.

Why is measles considered a manifestation of *Mātā*, even by Muslims in Sindh province? To build a comprehensive understanding and trace the roots of this perception and practice, we should not forget the history of the region in which Pakistan lies. Briefly speaking, before the arrival of Islam in South Asia, especially in Sindh, which became known as *Bab-ul-Islam* (a door to Islam in the subcontinent), Hinduism was the dominant religion. The oral history of the area reveals that the region once used to be called "Sindh-Hind." Even after the Indo-Pak separation, the coexistence of two religions remained prominent, which still is the case. After the partition, most of Pakistan's Hindus stayed in Sindh province, where many Muslims also reside; some were ancestrally Hindu. The etiology of measles provides a vivid example of cultural assimilation and religious syncretism.

There are at least a few more cultural traits related to Hinduism that people are practicing in the province despite being Muslims. The case of measles is one among them. Measles seemingly helps to refute the principal grounds for the separation of India. People, irrespective of the fact that their primary religion is Islam, still retain Hindu traits that are contrary to the critical event of Indo-Pak separation, which happened in part because their leaders at the time considered the "two nations different." Consequently, the old geographical "Sindh-Hind" region split into two countries in 1947, and the third one Bangladesh separated in 1971 (Wynbrandt 2009).

This brief description helps to holistically comprehend the local ideas and practices of measles and provides a base for contextualizing measles as a phenomenon. The purpose behind mentioning this history is neither political nor economic but to highlight cultural connections still existing between the two countries. Otherwise, it would be difficult to answer the research question regarding the etiology of measles drawn in Hindu mythology, especially by the people of Sindh province who live primarily in rural areas, irrespective of their religion.

In *Rāmpur* village, people link measles with *Sitālā Mātā*, while inhabitants of *Rahīmpur* village use a generic word *"Mātā."* The name *"Sitālā"*—taken from Sanskrit—means "one who cools," as mythologically, she was born from the cold ashes of the sacrificial fire (Stewart 1995, 389). She is also known as *Roga Raja* (the king of diseases), *Basanta Raya* (mother of poxes), or *Vyadhi Pati* (lord of pestilence) (Ghatak 2013, 120). According to Fabrizio Ferrari (2015), it is not only Hindus who worship her but Muslims, Sikhs, Buddhists, Christians, and Adivasis in the villages across Pakistan, North India, Bangladesh, and Nepal.

Why *Mātā*? According to Flood (1996), a glance at Hinduism shows that the concept of a goddess is not less important and visible than the conception of Shiva: various goddesses exist, who are benevolent or malevolent. The *Kālī* (the "black" one) is among them. She is garlanded with severed heads, girdled with severed arms, with rolling, intoxicated eyes, and a lolling tongue. That means *Mātā* worship has remained in the region.

Cultural Knowledge and Healing of Measles

According to the local people, the preliminary bodily signs of measles include reddish eyes, a bad-smelling mouth, fever, and eruption of small red spots on the body. The last two signs are significant precursors. Mostly, the first identifier usually is a child's mother who reads these signs.[1] For surety, she needs an older woman's affirmation, as an older woman has witnessed and dealt with numerous cases. After confirmation, they observe a series of rituals, which constitute what Van Gennep (2013 [1960]) terms *"rites de passage"* in which an individual leaves one group and joins the other.

Measles implies a transition. After contracting measles, a child is no longer believed to be the same, but to be in a transition to join a *Pakā* (mature, strong, and stable) group. For a successful transition, people perform certain "dos" and "don'ts" without hierarchizing them. All are essential actions to offer a pleasing welcome and grand farewell to *Mātā* for a child's successful transition to become *Pakā*. Commonly, the total duration of this passage is seven days. The rites have various parts, which I describe in the following sections.

Chillo *as Preliminal Rites*

After contracting measles, the next step is what Van Gennep (2013 [1960]) calls a "rite of separation." For quarantining, the child is separated and put into *Chillo* (quarantine) in a specific place in the house. The place depends upon the economic situation of the family. For instance, if the family owns a big house, the child is kept in a separate room. In contrast, if people are not wealthy enough to have a separate room, they keep the child in the same room where they live. In *Rāmpur* village, they have *Chanworā* or *Jhuggi* (huts); thus, they keep the child in one of them.

A red thread is tied at the room's entrance to signal to the people that a person with measles is living inside. The red simultaneously symbolizes life, as it is the color of blood, and indicates danger or a "no-go" area. If entering the room is necessary, then one must perform a specific measure, especially related to purity. For example, *Mathy-Mero* (a person who has not taken the necessary ritualistic bath after sexual intercourse) or *Uhto-Kuhto* (a person with a bad intention, e.g., evil eye, jealousy, dishonesty, or of bad character— e.g., a magician) cannot enter the house, specifically into the child's room (I deal with this in the next few paragraphs).

The child wears clean, soft, and thin clothes to observe purity and avoid irritation—caused by the heat of rashes—to the body. The child receives money, jewelry, and toys from his/her family members, especially from the mother. Dealings with the child are conscious, careful, and reverent. Family members, including any visitor, try their best to entertain the child, as entertaining the child is thought to be pleasing to *Mātā*. The child's living space is cleaned continuously to ensure cleanliness and purity. During the phase of measles, vocabulary in the whole house substantially changes. Everyone uses reverent language to address the child: respectful phrases are used such as [in *Sindhī*] "*Bhāgg Wāri Āi Āhy*" (one that brings blessings or luck has arrived). In actuality, these words address an invisible supernatural being: *Mātā*. Abusive words and loud voices are strictly avoided.

Cooking and eating patterns also change. The family practices a strict regimen. Muslims stop consuming meat, beef, fish, and chicken and even bringing meat to the home. Moreover, some Hindu groups such as *Bāggrrī* and *Bhīl*, who consume meat, also observe this regimen. There is a direct link between the regimen and *Mātā*, as in Hinduism, meat consumption is forbidden (generally speaking). Meat makes *Mātā* malevolent. As a 40-year-old Muslim female respondent from *Rahīmpur* village said:

A ten-year-old child was not yet diagnosed with measles. He was usually behaving, such as playing, eating, moving, and walking. One day, he ate meat with neighboring relatives. As he returned home, he got a high fever. His whole body became reddish. The next day, measles appeared on his body with severe intensity. Eating meat displeased *Mātā*.

Furthermore, regardless of religion, people refrain from cooking food with onions, garlic, and spices, called *Dāgg*. It creates a robust smell that spreads through the house and reaches to a child. These ingredients make the smoke spicy too, which then hurts and irritates the rashes on the child's body. This also irritates *Mātā*, and then she increases the intensity of pain for that child. People avoid intercourse because it pollutes an individual and requires ablution. Prompt ablution is not possible after intercourse as one needs to walk toward a bathing place or hand-pump. This walk brings impurity, and the impurity makes *Mātā* vindictive.

Similarly, three types of people are never permitted to enter the house. First, an outsider, irrespective of blood relationship, denotes a person who is not living in the same house or sharing the same space. For example, if there is more than one house and people share the same space to fetch water, and often go to see each other, they are not considered outsiders. Or, to make it more comprehensive, an outsider is a person whom a family member needs to greet or shake the hand with—which they do not need to do with insiders.

Second, *Mathy-Mero* (a person who has not taken the necessary ritualistic bath after sexual intercourse), and third, *Uhto-Kuhto* are forbidden to enter the house, specifically into the child's room. In cases of extreme necessity, a person can observe a ritualistic ablution to enter. If the person engaged in sexual intercourse, then the requirement is a ritualistic bath while chanting holy verses from the sacred texts, for example, *Qurān* and *Geeta*. However, if the person is just a regular outsider, then s/he needs ablution, which includes washing the feet, hands, rinsing the mouth and nose, and washing the face. Usually, such people never intentionally enter the house because they share the same culture and know the expected consequences.

After the onset of the rash, Muslims bring the child to visit a Hindu person in order to please *Mātā*. Then the child is brought to a Hindu healer for a check-up and remedies. The underlying reason is that *Mātā* is a goddess of the Hindus. Therefore, a Hindu healer knows the revered ways to deal with her. This treatment subsequently pleases *Mātā*, contrary to biomedicine, which displeases her. The child is not left alone, especially by the mother, who accompanies the child and sings a *Lorī* (lullaby) for him/her. The *Bhajjan* (Hindu religious songs) are played (Kawrani 2013; Sachanandbaghzai 2011) to please *Mātā*. An audio cassette with *Bhajjan* is bought from a market or borrowed from a Hindu family. Although smartphones have replaced stereo players, many people do not have such phones in this locale. Also, there are a few people who have stereo players.

Furthermore, the child is given a bath with clay obtained from the mountains and goat milk.[2] Almost equal quantities of water and milk are mixed for the bath. Both ingredients have cold properties and effects, so the bath provides comfort to the child by reducing the body's heat. During this transition, people observe a ritual of the *Chando*, which has two parts: *Katcho* and *Pako*.

Katcho Chando as *Liminal Rites*

On the third day of measles, people observe *Katcho Chando*—a rite of transition. Etymologically, *Katcho* denotes unripe, weak, pre-, initial, the beginning of another phenomenon that will follow it, and *Chando* means to sprinkle. The term *Katcho Chando* connotes that the child is weak and must go through a transitionary process to be strong again. Usually, an older woman leads the ritual. She can be from the same family, village, or a neighboring village, as long as she is known for her ability to perform such rituals. In some cases, the child's mother, mother's sister, or mother's or father's mother observes the ritual. The criteria are that she must know the *Lorī* (*Bhajjan*) and the necessary steps. To participate in these rites, the child comes outside his or her room for the first time after the rites of separation[3] but remains inside the house. Constituents of the rites include cow's milk and sweet flat *Chapāti* made from a mixture of wheat flour, jaggery, and water prepared during the night on a flat pan, and chickpeas that are left to soak in a pot full of water during the night. Importantly, water is sprinkled on the stove where the sweet bread is prepared. Sprinkling symbolizes coldness and soothing, which indirectly brings comfort to the child. The rites commence after the mother holds the child in her lap (if the child is young in age or weak), or the child sits while holding sweet bread in her/his lap. The older woman leads the ritual and chants the following *Lorī*:

Sindhī (in Latin Letters) English Translation by Author

Sindhī (in Latin Letters)	English Translation by Author
Thār Tharī	Soothe [*Mātā*] Soother
Amarr Mehr Kandīn	Mother bestow your kindness
Jagg Thār Amarr Tharī	Soothe the whole world mother soother
Mokhy Dhari Dhurāi Day	
Jag Khān Agy	We beseech to heal the child before the world
Jagg Thār Amarr Tharī	Soothe the whole world, mother soother
Thār Tharrī	Soothe [*Mātā*] Soother
Khāshā Gulrrā Kandīn	Beseeching to make good flowers [rashes]
Pahnjy Gulrran Ji Parwarsh	
Pān Kandīn	Please grow them by yourself
Jagg Thār Jījal Tharī	Soothe [*Mātā*] Kind Soother
Shikarpur Jun Chokron	Girls from *Shikarpur*[4]

Amarr Māī Māī Kan	Mother calling thee repeatedly
Hath Me Lotā	While holding pots in their hands
Mathy Tay Chapotā	While wearing headscarves
Dar Dar Chandrro Dīan	They observe the ritual at every house
Jagg Thār Amarr Tharī	Soothe the entire world, thee soother
Thār Tharī	Soothe [*Mātā*] Soother
Asān Jo Paitrro Thārīn	Soothe our inside (belly)
Asān Jā Bachrrā Thārīn	Soothe and heal our children
Jagg Thār Jijal Tharī	Soothe the universe, thee soother
Tuhnjo Sij Chand Bhāī	Sun and moon are your brothers
Tuhnjo Kokal Bhāī	*Kokal* is your brother[5]
Pahnjan Bhāirn Jay Sadqy[6]	In the name of your brothers be kind
Mukhy Dān Diār	Give me the news of health [of my child]
Thār Thārī	Soothe [*Mātā*] Soother
Khāshā Gulrrā Kandīn	May thou grow beautiful flowers (rashes)
Panhjy Gulrran Jī Parwarash	
Pān Kandīn	May thou ripen your flowers
Thār Tharī Asān Jā Bachrrā	
Thārīn	Soother [*Mātā*] Soothe our children
Tuhnjo Sij Chand Bhāī	Sun and Moon are your brothers
Tuhnjo Seharr Bhāī	Rabbit is your brother
Tuhnjo Jāhāl Bhāī	*Jāhāl* is your brother
Tuhnjo Kokal Bhāī	*Kokal* is your brother
Satan Bhāiran Jay Sadqy	In the name of your seven brothers
Moky Daan Diār	Give the news of health [of the child]
Jagg Thār Jejal Tharī	Sooth the entire world, Kind Soother
Sāggion Ghitrrīon Sāggrrā Sair	Same pictures, same tours
Bachrrā Dai Ghumandum Pair	May the children walk again
Thār Tharī	Soothe [*Mātā*] Soother
Asān Jā Bachrrā Thārīn	Soothe our children, please
Thār Tharī	Soothe [*Mātā*] Soother
Amarr Mehar Kandīn	Be a benevolent mother to us (please)
Mehar Kandīn	Bestow mercy upon us
Asān Jā Paittrrā Thāraīn	Please soothe our belly (inside)
Jagg Tharī	Mother! The healer of the world
Oh! Rānni Jo Āi Muhnjy Taddy	Oh! The queen has visited me
Amarr Bachrrā Widhā	
Mun Tuhnjy Taddy	Mother I submitted my children thee
Mokhy Dhārāi Dhurrāi Dday	Please heal them
Jagg Khān Aggy	Before the rest of the world
Jag Thār Amarr Tharrī	Soothe the entire world Mother Soother
Jeejal Aayam Muhnhy Taddy	Mother visited my (poor) house
Amān Bachrrā Widham Tuhnjy	
Taddy	Mother (I) presented my children thee
Sāgīon Ghītyon Sāggrrā Sair	Same streets, same trips

Bachrrā Dai Ghumdam Pair	Make them able to walk again
Thār Thāri	Heal (you) the healer
Muhnjā Bachrrā Thārīn	Heal (soothe) my children, please
Jagg Thār Amarr Tharrī	Soothe the whole world, Mother soother
Thār Tharī Amarr Mehar Kandīn	Soothe soother, mother, be benevolent
Mehar Kandīn	Have mercy (upon us)
Khāsha Gulgrrā Kandīn	May you grow beautiful flowers (rashes)
Pahnji Gulrran Ji Parwarash	May you look after them (rashes)
Pān Kandīn	
Thār Tharī	Heal (you) the healer
Muhnjā Bachrrā Thārīn	Heal (soothe) my children, please
Jagg Thār Amarr Tharrī	Soothe the universe, Mother soother
Oh! Rannī Jo Āi Muhnjy Taddy	Oh! The queen came to my (poor) house
Amarr Khanī Diān Mehmānī	A warm welcome and homage to host you
Channān Pusāyān	(I) put chickpeas in water (for her)
Mithrrā Lolrrā	(I) prepare sweet bread
Āun Thadhrro Kayān	(I) make it cold (during the whole night)
Māi Rājā Khay Tharyān	To make Mother King blithe and kind[7]
Māi Rājā Thāry	May mother king be soothing
Asān Jā Bachrrā Thāry	May then she soothe, heal our children
Thār Tharrī Asān Jā Bachrrā Thāry	My Soother heal our children
Adī Mubarak Hujy	Sisters congratulations to all of you
Māi Rājā Tun Wanj	Mother King, you may go, please
Bāggan, Amban, Tutan	To gardens of mangoes, mulberries
Mokal Athāi	We permit you: say goodbye
Asān Jā Bachrrā Thārion Wanj	Please go while soothing our children
Pān Bhī Wanj Daryāin Main Thar	You may go to the rivers to soothe them
Māi Rājā Asān Jā Bachrrā Thārion Wanj	We request, leave after soothing our children

During the incantation of the *Lorī*, the chanter regularly sprinkles cow's milk on the child's whole body, especially on his/her face through a filter that is usually used to filter wheat flour. Using cow's milk is more respectful, as a cow is a sacred animal in Hinduism. In the absence of cow's milk, milk of a buffalo, goat, or camel might be used. Milk is a ritual prerequisite. After completion, sweet bread is distributed among participants and, in some cases, also in the neighborhood. Although paying money after receiving the bread is not mandatory, most of the receivers give money to the child according to their financial capacity. The family members, such as father, mother, or grandmothers, often give money. Some of them put the remaining milk, chickpeas, and some bread into running water, preferably in a nearby river or a small watercourse; the running water symbolizes life, and the water cools down the heat caused by measles. After that, they bring the child back to the room s/he stayed before. Thereafter, following the dos and don'ts continues. This rite is followed by the *Pako Chando*.

Pako Chando *as a Postliminal Phase*

The *Pako Chando*—which can be understood as "rite of incorporation" in Van Gennep's terms—is usually observed on the seventh day. *"Pako"* in my translation means *ripen, strong,* or *stable*—the ending of a thing that started earlier and *Chando*. In some cases, it may be performed on the fifth day, determined by the situation of the child. For example, this is the case if the rash is not severe, and the child is active and able to eat. As a 50-year-old mother shared, "When we see that *Mātā* has started returning [to her abode], then we observe the ritual earlier. If treated worshipfully and reverently, she returns quickly. Otherwise, on day seven, her *Mudo* (tenure, duration) is completed."

The procedures of these rites are analogs to those described above. However, *Katcho Chando* contains a few additions to the required elements. Before these rites, the child receives a bath with clay (obtained from mountains) mixed with goat milk and water. The inherent belief is that this clay has a cooling quality, which soothes the body by reducing the pain of the rash. After this bath, the child wears new clothes, which in most cases, are newly bought or sewed.

Akin to the *Katcho Chando*, a woman leads the ritual while invoking the *Lorī* mentioned earlier. However, the child, either in the mother's lap or elsewhere, receives one piece of bread on the forehead, two on the eyes, two on the feet, and two in the hands. Cow's milk is continuously poured on his/her body during the invocation. After accomplishing this ritual, every participant congratulates each other, especially the child's mother and his/her family members, for the successful completion of the transitionary phase. Again, the child receives some money, especially after this final ritual. This completion is no less than a celebration showing an appropriate farewell to *Mātā*, who was pleased and has therefore now gone. The child now receives the title of *Pakā*. Considering the meanings of the term *Pako* that denotes mature, strong, or accomplished, the child has successfully gone through the passage and completed the transition.

Until the performance of *Pako Chando*, during the whole course of measles, the child is addressed with reverent words and actions. Every effort is made to please and keep him/her calm. There is generally no negligence in observing the aforementioned 13 steps. The child is never left alone. Notably, the mother accompanies him/her and sings the *Lorī*.[8] The cassette of *Bhajjan* is played. When I conducted the current research, people still had a small number of mobile phones. Yet, nowadays, there are good chances that many of them may have mobile phones to play *Bhajjan*. During my fieldwork, they were still playing cassettes in the stereo players.

Although performing the regimen becomes a bit lenient thereafter, it does not stop after the *Pako Chando*. The child still receives intensive care to prevent the disease from recurring. Also, an old Muslim woman, when talking about the elements of rites, claimed that in the past, pouring of cow urine, instead of milk or as an addition to it, on the body of the affected child was also common. Nonetheless, over time, it was realized that this was impure. They therefore now either use cow milk or goat milk for this purpose.

The dos and don'ts of treating a child with measles index certain aspects of underlying cultural knowledge. Quarantining a child demonstrates cultural awareness of the infectiousness of measles, especially for people who are *Katchā* (plural form of *Katcho* in *Sindhī*). Treating the child with "cold" substances shows the cultural belief in the hot/cold system of beliefs. Covering the child with clay can have the medico-therapeutic benefit of relieving the itching and drying up the rash. Maintaining cleanliness could further indicate the cultural acceptance of germ theory even as it also honors the culturally perceived sacredness of measles as a gift from *Mātā* to make the child strong.

Lorī *or* Bhajjan: *Musical Healing*

During the course of measles, the importance of music is undeniable.[9] People play cassettes of *Bhajjan* and women, especially the mother, sing the *Lorī*. People perceive measles as one of the toughest and most testing phases of life. They are afraid of it as measles leaves only a few parts of the body unwounded. The passage of measles is believed to inflict wounds inside the body more than the outside. Measles is considered to be one of the toughest times for a child, especially when its intensity increases. The child falling unconscious is the peak of measles—a woman, often the child's mother chants the *Lorī* that is a *Bhajjan*.

Interestingly, Muslims call it a *Lorī*, not a *Bhajjan*, for religious reasons. That means Muslims do not have a problem with the inherent properties of a *Bhajjan*, such as the use of the word *Mātā*, but they do not like the term *Bhajjan* because of its strong association with Hinduism. Therefore, uttering the term *Bhajjan* may make someone a *Kafir* (a nonbeliever, usually connoting a Hindu). During the ritual of *Chando*, women sing the *Lorī* without any instrument, but as melodiously as possible. The *Lorī* soothes.[10]

Visiting Kālkā Devī Mandar

Although shrine behavior, including *Mandar*[11] (a Hindu temple), was mentioned earlier in Chapters 6 and 7, my focus in this section is on the *Kālkā Devī Mandar* itself. The *Mandar* is an historical place where Hindus have been coming to worship for several centuries. The *Mandar* is associated with *Kālkā Devī* (the black goddess or mother), who is an incarnation of *Durga*, who is a Hindu goddess of war, and whose mythology centers around combating evils and demonic forces that threaten peace and prosperity.

The *Kālkā Devī Mandar* is one of the oldest and most venerated *Mandar*s of the province. It is located in a mountain cave where the goddess is believed to have made an appearance during her *Hinglāj Yatra*. *Hinglāj*, about 250 km from *Karāchī*, is another famous sacred place of pilgrimage for Hindus that is situated in *Taluko* (subdistrict) *Lyāri* of Pakistan's *Baluchistān* province. The *Kālkā Devī Mandar* is believed to have two tunnels that connect it to the *Hinglāj* temple in *Baluchistān*.

The *Kālkā Devī Mandar* is at a distance of around 60 km from the village of *Rahīmpur* in *Sakhar* district and is located about one mile south from the capital city of *Arorr* (old name of the present-day *Rohrrī* city in *Sakhar* district). According to legend, a devoutly religious woman, named *Kālkā*, used to live in these caves and the hills were called *Kālkā* hills during Roe Dynasty (that ruled modern-day *Sindh* and northwest India from 450 BCE). The entrance to the cave is hardly five to six feet high. The smell and the smoke of *Agarbatī* (incense) creates a mystic aura around the area. The priest sits on a stone platform next to the statue of *Kālkā Devī* with a dagger in one hand and a chopped head in the other. One can sit and chat with the priest.

Most Hindu devotees pay homage to *Kālkā Devī* on the night of the first Monday of every month. According to the caretaker of the temple, 60% of people who visit this temple are Muslims or belong to other religions. During my fieldwork, many families paid a visit to this sacred place. They made vows, cooked food, ate it, and distributed it among the people present there.

When the 2012 and 2013 outbreaks of measles occurred, many people, irrespective of their religion, despite the usual quarantine, brought their children with measles to this *Mandar* or fetched water from the *Mandar* to be brought home for the children to drink and also to spray over their bodies. This sacred place has long been central for attaining healing. Bringing children to the *Mandar* shrine simultaneously serves two purposes: for the child to meet a Hindu person, and to heal the measles. Generally, the underlying purpose was to make *Mātā* benevolent. The child, first, was brought to a *Pujjārī* (leader of Hindu rituals) of the temple for various verbal chanting, and then to the statue of *Mātā* inside the cave.

At the *Mandar*, people also applied lamp oil and water on the child's forehead and got the child to drink some of the water. Carrying water back to home in a bottle in order to mix it with other water to increase the quantity to spray across the house—particularly in the child's room—and getting the child to drink it is also done to please *Mātā*, and consequently to decrease the intensity of the measles, helping it to become "cold," or bearable.

Consulting a Hindu Healer

For apprehensions about measles, people preferably bring the child to a *Hakīm*. The older women, especially, work as the primary healers to diagnose measles by reading the child's face and other symptoms. The reddishness of the face is one of the first signs and symptoms of measles. Therefore, whether measles is recognized or suspected, the child may be brought to any Hindu healer.

When parents suspect that the face of the child is red and has a fever, but there are no rashes on the exterior of the body, then they think that the *Mātā* has hidden herself. In some cases then, the child thought to have measles is brought to any Hindu person. Considering this person believes in *Mātā*, this act ultimately pleases *Mātā*, who will afterward manifest and make the measles visible. The invisibility of measles inside the body is highly dangerous. In local expressions, this inconspicuousness demonstrates that *Mātā* has hidden herself. Bringing the child to a Hindu *Hakīm* also serves at least three essential purposes. The first is that causing *Mātā* to choose to make herself visible will also make the measles visible. Second, the *Hakīm* knows the esteemed ways to deal with *Mātā*, since he is Hindu by religion, and thus is unlikely to do anything that might displease *Mātā*. The third purpose includes the treatment of measles. He gives the child some syrup and recommends necessary preventive measures such as avoiding intake of meat and prohibiting a *Uhto-Kuhto* person from visiting the child.

As mentioned before, people avoid biomedical medication as it makes *Mātā* uncongenial. Given this, whenever fever occurs due to measles, parents bring their child to a local Hindu healer. To reiterate, a Hindu *Hakīm* practices Hinduism, he thus knows the required ways of dealing with *Mātā*, who appears in the form of measles. In contrast, biomedical doctors lack this knowledge and orientation. Generally, these doctors treat measles with injections. Consequently, Mātā becomes malevolent and augments the severity of effects since the injection is believed to be not targeted at the child but at *Mātā*.

Hence, in *Rahīmpur* village, during the outbreak of measles, the local people consult the local healers first. These Hindu healers had been practicing *Hikmat* for several generations. There are two Hindu *Hakīm*, as mentioned in the previous chapters, who are quite famous in the area, not merely for dealing with measles but for treating other illnesses as well. These *Hakīm* were reluctant to share their views with me, as the outbreak attracted the government's attention, and the Expanded Programme on Immunization (EPI) personnel directed them to refer the affected individuals to biomedical hospitals. They saw me as a person from the EPI or the media or belonging to an inspection team who could get them into trouble by inquiring about their views.

A *Hakīm* was initially extraordinarily reticent in sharing his views about measles. After building a rapport, he claimed that measles is an infectious disease that spreads rapidly from one person to another and that it gets more intense after three days. People of the area bring those suffering from measles to him because of their beliefs. During the outbreak, around 40–50 cases were brought to him, which, so he told me, he refused to treat and referred them to the Tehsil Headquarters (THQ). Much against his claim, local people told me that this *Hakīm* never referred any child to a biomedical hospital but treated them himself.

Nevertheless, after ensuring privacy and confidentiality and stressing that this was not an inquiry for an institution but instead that this was research in which his (*Hakīm*'s) name would be kept highly confidential, he comfortably shared his opinion in the following way:

> Measles is the arrival of *Mātā*, and we also call it *Devī Mātā*. We Hindus observe an associated Sao Mangal (Green Tuesday) in her name. That means this is the day of *Mātā*, in which we perform certain rituals on that day. We sprinkle milk on every person's face, mainly unaffected children/people in advance to respect and please *Mātā* so that if she comes, she should be benevolent.
>
> We have been practicing *Hikmat* since our forefathers.[12] We treat a person as per our orientation and belief system. Our religious teachings teach us how to deal with *Mātā* respectfully. People believe, too, that measles is a manifestation of Mātā. This belief drives them to bring their children to us and to the *Kālkā-Devī-Mandar*, where they offer water of that *Mandar* to the affected children. People also play the cassettes of *Bhajjan* in their homes, which are a *Lorī—Thār* Mātā *Thār*. Since they believe that it will heal the person, it heals in actuality. It is all about one's *Waisah* (beliefs). (...) If someone believes in a *Choddo* (bark) of a Bair tree (*Ziziphus Mauritiana*) to cure some illness, it does indeed cure this. In Sindh province, people, for example, believe in several Sufis (puritans) such as *Qalandar*, *Bhittaī* or *Sachal*, and make vows there. Resultantly, their wishes come true, but the wishes of non-believers never come true.

This fascinating quote clearly shows this *Hakīm*'s belief in the power of belief itself, along with his high degree of reflexivity. It is quite reminiscent of the *Kwakwaka'wakw* shaman Quesalid, who entered shamanic training to prove its falsehood, yet ended up understanding that shamanic healing techniques worked because people believed in them and so continued to practice it for many years (Whitehead 2000). Quesalid, originally named George Hunt, was the long time key informant of Franz Boas and remained a key figure to develop a theory on shamanism, magic, symbolic healing, and healing and religion (Whitehead 2000, 166). He eventually received significant attention in anthropology (Lévi-Strauss 1963; Brumble 2008; Briggs and Bauman 1999).

Another *Hakīm* has been practicing for approximately 20 years at a 50-year-old clinic, where his father used to practice.[13] He is, therefore, the second-generation practicing *Hikmat*. During the outbreak, people brought around 70–80 children to him for treatment. Simultaneously, he was reporting the cases to the THQ, as the government had issued a recommendation letter that measles should be referred. Talking about the outbreak, he remembers:

> It was a massive outbreak in which five children died. People were frightened. They believe that *Mātā* causes measles. We Hindus call her *Parwati*. *Kālkā Devī Mandar* in *Arorr* is associated with her. People brought their children to this *Mandar*. The children that were brought to the *Mandar* and given a bath (there) survived. Interestingly, most of them

were Muslims. People prepared sweet bread to be offered to *Mātā* to please her. When people visited *Mandar*, the intensity of illness reduced, and no other deaths occurred after that. It means that bringing children and showing respect to her pleased *Mātā*, and she became benevolent afterward. In their houses, people play cassettes of *Mātā*, based on some religious chants for worshipping and pleasing *Mātā*. Some women, in particular, chant those words over affected children for the same purpose. Whenever measles occurs in a household, people chant *Bhajjan*, perform *Chando* on the seventh day, prepare sweet bread, and pour goat or cow milk, cook vegetables to eat, avoid sex, and worship more.

These two quotations from the *Hakīm* specify similarities in the belief system. Both *Hakīm* and people believe in the sacredness of measles and deal with it with equal respect. Avoiding an injection for a child with measles, *Hakīm* give syrup and *Kakh* (a ground form of specific plants) and prescribe pharmaceutical products, such as paracetamol and antibiotics. The medical representatives of various pharmaceutical companies regularly visit to mobilize them to recommend the medicines these companies produce.

Not only this, but these *Hakīm* also deal with other diseases and suggest the medicine of these pharmaceutical firms. They also have a stethoscope, thermometers, an oxygen machine for asthma patients, syringes, and medicine. The clinics—one and two rooms—of these *Hakīm* are notable examples of the coexistence and syncretism of various medical systems such as *Ayurvedā*, *Unānī*, and biomedicine. The walls of these clinics include several pamphlets encompassing the Quranic verses and pictures of Hindu gods and goddesses right beside advertisements for biomedical products.

Briefly Comparing Both the Villages

As I have shown, both Hindus and Muslims of the selected villages believe in measles as something necessary and sacred that is a manifestation of *Mātā*. In Hinduism, it is believed to be one *Mātā* or *Devī*, *Durggā*, and she is called "Mahadevi" (great goddess), and then she manifests in different forms (Dowson 2000, 90). However, a slight variation exists in the names of measles in these villages. In *Rahīmpur* village, the term for measles is "*Ur'rrī*," while in *Rāmpur* village, it is "*Ourhī*." In *Rahīmpur*, no specific name of *Mātā* prevails among Muslims to show which specific manifestation of *Mātā* it is.[14] However, in *Rāmpur*, a particular name exists—*Sitālā Mātā*.[15]

Although rituals are performed during measles, Muslims do not conduct any worship, unlike Hindus. In *Rāmpur*, as a preventive measure, people often invoke *Mātā* to keep her pleased. As a 40-year-old Hindu lady from *Rāmpur* village shares:

In our native language, we call it "*Ourhī*" and believe that it is a *Sitālā Mātā*; therefore, worshipping her is a regular practice to receive her blessings. We observe a ritual called *Thadrrī* (my translation: soother) fortnightly. For this, we prepare *Thadrrī* from a combination of wheat flour, sugar, and water on a flat pot, which is identical to *Chapāti*. Sometimes we prepare sweet rice instead. After that, water is sprinkled over the stove to cool it. Once the *Thadrrī* is ready, we bring the deity mentioned above under a tree to worship and implore it to prevent or cure an illness, including measles and problems—whether social, psychological, or economic. However, whenever, measles appears, the ritual is delayed, and a person is kept on a waiting list to see if any other family members get the symptoms to observe the *Thadrrī* then together. Once the measles appears, the very second day, no food considered to have a hot or cold effect is cooked at home or eaten by the affected person. The person eats ground wheat grains prepared in milk and with dates.

In both the villages, whenever measles occurs to one person in a home, the family members wait to see whether the symptoms are appearing in any other family member before performing the rituals of *Chandā* mentioned earlier. Observing the ritual may have severe consequences for the next child(ren) contracting measles, such as *Mātā* hiding herself inside the body of the next child. Her hiddenness causes problems, including death. Because, as an old lady from *Rahīmpur* claims, when "*Mātā* hides herself, we neither behave with that child reverently nor take required care of him/her. This unawareness also causes failure to follow the regimen, which makes *Mātā* malevolent. She becomes angry."

As I have shown, in both villages, during measles, the child receives complete attention and devotion. The child is given no food of hot or cold nature during that phase, except ground wheat grains cooked in milk containing dates. In *Rahīmpur*, they also give fruit such as apples to the child. Also, inhabitants of both the villages accentuate that seeking biomedical healthcare is strictly forbidden. It displeases *Mātā* and makes her malevolent. They, therefore, do not bring the child to a biomedical hospital but perform the rites at home because *Mātā* becomes malevolent due to biomedicine, particularly the injections and an impolite attitude of doctors. The injection is perceived as not directed toward the child, but indirectly toward *Mātā*. During those days, the child is "possessed" by *Mātā*, and she lives inside the child's body. Biomedical treatment provokes her to be unkind and aggressive. As a result, she chooses hostile reactions. Consequently, the child suffers due to the vindictiveness of *Mātā*.

During the outbreak, the resistance against bringing the children to modern hospitals, in general, came from the women and the older women in particular. They were appealing to their male counterparts: "Since you do not obey and listen to us while carrying these children to the hospitals, please, in the name of the Holy *Qurān* and *Allāh* at least, do not allow the doctors to inject our children."

Despite these strong beliefs, the change did occur. When parents did take children to a hospital, they could see that the children returned to their homes healthy. Women of *Rahīmpur* village strongly said:

> If measles occurs again in any other children (in our home or village), we will bring them to the hospitals for the treatment and observe the *Chillo* and *Chando*. Whatever [the conditions], we will never hesitate and compromise on the [bio] medical treatment. The outbreak and the (biomedical) treatment have opened our eyes that there is no harm in bringing the affected persons to the modern hospital.

Nonetheless, despite the said determination, in the village of *Rahīmpur*, measles occurred in an infant during my fieldwork who was not brought to a hospital. Her family treated her with traditional healing in the form of observing dos and don'ts and performing the ritual. The child was also brought to the *Kālkā Devī Mandar*, and the water of the *Mandar* was used as a remedy. Simultaneously, they consulted a Hindu healer. After performing these practices, the infant got well.

I enquired about the fact that after the outbreak, people were determined to bring every child who contracted measles to a biomedical facility, while still taking traditional measures. One woman I spoke to explained that this was because the government provided ambulances during the outbreak of measles to transport their children to the hospital for treatment. This mattered because the hospital is quite far away, so bringing a child there always consumes time and resources. The provision of ambulances made it much easier to bring an infected child to a hospital.

Measles as Mātā in Media: Print Media Reports

The people of other districts also believe that measles is a sacred illness associated with *Mātā*. The central purpose of their response is to please *Mātā* by performing rituals. The newspaper *Dawn* (2014) wrote about the measles outbreaks in 2012 and 2013 with the caption "Sindh's measles nightmare."[16] This English daily published the views of a medical doctor working at the *Sijāwal* district government hospital. The doctor claimed:

> When it comes to treatment, many in the rural sector turn to superstitions for the management of measles. For them, measles is a "Hindu" disease, and thus, only a Hindu faith healer can handle it easily. Per cultural practices, children are not to be taken outside the house when symptoms of measles—spots on [the] body, inflammatory eyes, or reddening—first appear. Villagers usually bring a child to us [at a hospital] after they start suffering post-measles complications, such as high-grade fever, diarrhoea, or acute respiratory infections.
> However, the child arrives late on, and complications become the ultimate cause of death. A child is brought to a hospital covered in

rallies (bedsheets) so that he or she is not exposed to the external environment. This handling is part of many people's belief[s]. Many villagers strongly believe that an injection cannot and must not be administered to a suffering child on the pretext of it aggravating the illness. Measles is a highly contagious disease (…) if a child in a village suffers from it, the disease is bound to affect other children of the same village.

This doctor argues that poor health literacy and lack of education are substantial causes of this "ignorance" in the rural sector. The same newspaper also published the views of a Sindh EPI Project Director named Dr. Mazhar Khamisani:

> During our visit to upper Sindh in 2012–13, we were in *Saleh Pat* [a *Talukā*, where *Rahīmpur* village is also located], which had been adversely affected by the measles crisis. We c[a]me across a family that told us that they followed the advice of a Hindu faith-healer, who wanted them to listen to *Bhajjan* to treat measles. However, it is not a rural community alone that has a different set of belief systems. In the urban sector too, residents deal with measles much the same way as their rural counterparts, before eventually going to doctors. Many urban families hold the belief that measles completes its influence before disappearing, so it's better not to touch the rash lest the disease gets "annoyed" and causes more complications for the patient.
>
> (M.H. Khan 2014)

The newspaper *Dawn* in the same report also presented the ideas of Ms. Sofia Iqbal—a resident of *Karāchī*: "Measles usually disappear in two-and-a-half days or seven days at the most. People keep a piece of the neem tree's bark underneath the pillow of a child and dangle it on the main entrance of their homes. A small piece of gold wrapped in white cloth is often also used, sometimes kept in a patient's pocket."

This newspaper then mentions the problem of infrastructure in Sindh that "not all districts have a fully functioning hospital. The accessibility and affordability go together: everyone cannot bear the hefty expenses of transportation to travel from the far-flung villages." One villager shares his thoughts with the newspaper. Bābu Kand[h]rā—a social activist from the Rāwal Kand[h]rā village—claims, "It becomes challenging for us to hire transport first from the main road and then shift our patient, adult or child, to a hospital. Also, there is the cost of medication."

The newspaper *Express Tribune* (2012b) also printed the views of Dr. Jay Ram Das—EDO Health district *Sakhar*: "In rural areas, people mostly live in single-room houses and are not able to quarantine their ailing children" because measles spread through sneezing and coughing. Dr. Das further says, "That's not all. People irrespective of their religion don't want to offend

Mātā Rani, who, according to Hindu mythology, takes over the body of a child [during measles] for five to seven days. We are trying to convince the people to bring their children for proper treatment."

The same newspaper (2012c) also reported a similar understanding of measles in a different district of Sindh, called *Khairpur*. During the outbreak, there were also parental refusals to receive medical help for measles while believing that the "disease" is a test of faith in the *Khairpur* district. These Muslim families believe strongly in Hindu mythology and link the high fever and the red spots signs to the goddess *Mātā* Rani [in Sindh it is pronounced as *Rānnī*], who controls the child's body. Several families, many of them Muslim, therefore, do not allow doctors to vaccinate their children.

According to a *Talukā* headquarters (THQ) hospital's superintendent, Dr. Qurban Sahito, people in rural areas still adhere to old customs and beliefs of Hindu mythology although the majority are Muslims, who then chant songs for five to seven days to appease the goddess who helps to restore the child's health.

About the ritual, the *Express Tribune* (2012c) mentions the view of a resident of *Thul* named Mukhi Baksho Mal, who is a Hindu. He claims:

> When Mātā Rani takes over a child, he/she should be treated very politely. During the stay of the goddess, the child should not be given any kind of meat or fish and only served vegetables and boiled rice. The families also sing hym[n]s to appease Mātā Rani. [Mal further explained that] Hindus avoid giving medicines to children suffering from measles and prefer using their faith during the healing processes.

The same English daily produced another story from *Kandhkot* district about measles as a manifestation of *Mātā*. The newspaper (2012c) mentions,

> The villagers adhere to Hindu beliefs which state that a goddess enters the child during this period and using medicine may offend her. They believe that she would leave the child's body on her own, and the child only needs to abstain from wearing red or eating red meat. Specific bhajans are also sung to the affected child.

The paper then quotes Dr. Jay Ram Das, who

> criticised the prevalence of old customs and methods of treatment in villages. He said that some people didn't even know the difference between a qualified doctor and a quack. He also advised that parents should not hide their children during visits from the vaccination teams or take them to Hakims.

The above-cited news reports illustrate local conceptualizations of measles. The reports also reveal the occurrence and associated perceptions toward measles across Sindh province (without generalizing). The newspaper describes the etiology of measles in terms of "superstitions" and Hindu mythology. Interestingly, the focus of these reports is on other districts of Sindh province, such as the *Sijāwal, Sakhar, Khairpur*, and *Kandhkot*. The reports hint at the persistence of perception of measles as a sacred illness. However, there are some variations compared to the selected villages of my project. For instance, in *Sijāwal* district, people dangle the bark of a Neem tree, a small piece of wrapped gold, at the entrance to their homes or the entrance to the infected child's room, but not the red cloth. The gold falls into the category of jewelry. Hanging the bark or gold at the entrance is similar to practices in the selected villages, which signify that someone with measles is in the home, that room in particular.

Concluding Remarks

Among the central bodies of the thesis, this chapter explained the local rituals of containment in Sindh province: that it is a necessary sacred illness, which requires extraordinary measures to deal with it. I elucidated rituals to deal with measles that reveal a transition from an unimmunized state to an immunized state. Observing the symptoms of measles, the local people put the child into *Chillo*. Thereafter, different rites and regimens start. The major among them are *Katcho Chando* (preliminal rites) and *Pako Chando* (postliminal rites).

An older woman leads them and chants a *Lorī (Bhajjan)*. Although both rites are performed at different phases of measles, constituents of these rites remain the same to a greater extent. They include cow's milk and sweet flat *Chapāti* made from a mixture of wheat flour, jaggery, and water prepared during the night on a flat pan, and chickpeas that are left to soak in a pot full of water during the night. Importantly, water is sprinkled on the stove where the sweet bread is prepared. Sprinkling symbolizes coldness and soothing, which indirectly brings comfort to the child. The rites commence after the mother holds the child in her lap (if the child is young in age or weak), or the child sits while holding sweet bread in her/his lap.

After focusing on how local people deal with measles and what measures relevant stakeholders take to deal with it, the chapter illustrated measles as a process of transition, a disease, and an issue that requires intervention. Through the content of print media, I have elaborated on how the government officials and doctors "blame" the meanings the local people give to measles for these outbreaks. In the forthcoming chapter, I will deal with the two outbreaks while emphasizing the perspectives of local people, the government, and the global stakeholders.

Notes

1 Throughout the thesis, the term "child" is used for an individual who contracts measles, because measles usually occurs during childhood.

2 In *Rahīmpur* village people use water, not milk. This is mainly due to the lack of milk, in contrast to *Rāmpur* village where people have herds of goats, sheep, and cows.

3 As during the course of measles, the child is kept in a room, except when the child needs to excrete. That sometimes is done in the room and the excrements disposed of. It completely depends upon the child's individual situation.

4 Shikarpur is the name of a city, which was one of the popular settlement centres of the Hindu population prior to the partition of 1947. At the moment, there are a couple of places named with Hindu owners. The names of government hospitals are Hindu names. This may be a reason for using the name of this city in the *Lorrī*.

5 It is unclear who *Kokal* is. However, mostly he is known as a supernatural being.

6 *Sadaqāh* is an Arabic term—a kind of voluntary offering or charity according to the position of the giver.

7 This is quite interesting that here *Mātā* is addressed with a masculine term *Rājā*, perhaps to show the "power."

8 One of my editors from the USA made a comment that is highly relevant to my project, so I would like to mention here: "Wow, if we treated kids with measles in these ways, I think everybody would want to have measles! I remember that when I had measles, my mom put my favourite coral sheets on my bed and served me beef broth in a gorgeous antique cup and saucer. She made me feel very special and loved—but that was nothing compared to all this!"

9 Appreciable work has been done on musical healing across cultures (Gouk 2017), specifically in the subfield of medical ethnomusicology, which has cast full attention on the powers of music impacting social, cultural, psychological, emotional, spiritual, and biological aspects of human life (Lloyd, Barz, and Brummel-Smith 2008; Koen 2006; Boyce-Tillman 2014). Anthropology has also invested its efforts and energies in this domain (Laderman and Roseman 2016; Friedson 1996; Feld and Fox 1994; Roseman 1991).

10 In classical Hindu music, as there are seven *Chakras*, there are also seven *Swarā* (notes). Each note stimulates a specific Chakra inside the body. According to Koen (2006), music generates different vibrations by affecting the tympanum, body, and thoughts simultaneously. Hence, this dimension of singing *Lorī* or *Bhajjan* makes this connection of sounds and body occur. Music is often used to cure various illnesses—for instance, the usage of *Falak* and *Maddāh* musical forms in a hospital in Tajikistan as complementary healing to anesthesia (Koen 2006), or using music in various spiritual healing rituals in Baluchistan for diagnosing, curing, and preventing ill-health mainly caused by supernatural beings (Sultana 2013).

11 In Urdu/Hindi and sometimes in *Sindhi*, *Mandar* is pronounced as *Mandar* ['mændɪr] not *Mandar* ['mændər].

12 I have used "forefathers," as according to them, in their family, only male members practised *Hikmat*. Nonetheless, I understand that their women might have (even to a lesser extent) helped them during preparation of herbal medicine.

13 Presently, one of his nephews has completed a biomedical technician course, and now works with him at his clinic.

14 It is interesting that in Karachi, Mull (1997) found that the Muslims associate measles with *Mātā and* know the name of *Sitālā Mātā*.

15 *Sitālā* is a deified *Mātā*, who is worshiped by Hindus, Muslims, Sikhs, Christians, Buddhists, and "Adivasi" across Pakistan, India, Bangladesh, and Nepal. Ferrari (2015) mentions that worshiping her is not determined by any fear, but rather because of her gentleness, compassion, and lovingness. Her name itself denotes "Cold"; he claims. She is invoked to protect against poverty, illness, injustice, and misfortune. See Chapter 5 for more details concerning invocation.

16 All these names are the original names, which were published by the newspapers.

7 Social Dramas

Two Measles Outbreaks and Multiple Narratives in Pakistan

The Local Perspective

Sakhar was the second most affected district. As repeatedly mentioned in the book, it witnessed a higher incidence of children contracting measles and experiencing deaths during the severe measles outbreaks of 2012 and 2013. These outbreaks also significantly affected *Rahīmpur* village within the stated district, with regard to infections, including some deaths. However, measles had been occurring in the village earlier too, which was always dealt with local measures, for example, the ritual of *Chando* (see Chapter 6). The outbreak was overwhelming. Although the local people performed the ritual, the number of children contracting measles rapidly escalated. The rising spread and the severity of outbreaks, particularly deaths, created chaos, fear, and anxiety in the village. In response, they started making sense of the phenomena and sorting out possible options. The male members of the village decided to opt for modern medicine; however, there was no hospital in the nearby surroundings, except a dispensary at a distance of around 10 km.

Perceiving the outbreak as extraordinary, they delibrated on doing something unusual. They staged a protest on a nearby small road with the dead body of a child who died from measles. The aim was to seek local media coverage—print and television—and thereby to garner the attention of the relevant health officials. The most influential person of the village *Sāhil* [a pseudonym], who was in his late thirties, had a secondary school education, and was working with a local *Sindhī* newspaper. The *Sāhil* used that platform to approach the local press. The protest's aim was fulfilled when coverage sought the attention of the healthcare officials and politicians, who then visited the village. The responsible vaccinator also accompanied those officials. The *Sāhil* recalls the "outbreak event" in the following way:

> When cases rapidly increased, and there was no response from the health officials and politicians, then we staged a protest with a dead body of a child suffering from measles to seek the attention of stakeholders concerned. I invited the media to record our protest, later on, the politicians, including a provincial president of one of the political parties of the country, government health officials such as District

DOI: 10.4324/9781003253716-8

Coordinator (DC), Executive District Officer (EDO) health reached us along with police protocol. Meanwhile, the vaccinator responsible for our village also came, who was not visiting us according to his schedule, and even he was not aware that our village was part of his assigned field. When we inquired, he was lying. Therefore, we physically beat him in front of all the politicians and health officials, since we were highly concerned about our children, who were suffering and dying. This way, our village secured full attention, and we received an ambulance to carry our children to hospitals in *Sakhar* city, e.g., the government civil hospital, Red Cross hospital, where wards were reserved for the measles-infected children.

Two more interlocutors, *Ibrāhīm* and *Ismāīl*, both in their forties, recalled the outbreak in the following way:

Before a swift escalation in cases and especially in deaths, we perceived the outbreak ordinary and following the cultural measures taken by the older women. However, the rapid spread of measles overwhelmed us with fear and anxiety. In the face of a significant outbreak, we started searching for effective measures to deal with it. There seemed no other option, but biomedical care. These overwhelming circumstances led us to hold a demonstration of the required care of our children. The protest was successful in seeking the attention of responsible officials. The politicians and doctors visited us and provided an ambulance. At the time of taking our children to the hospital, the women, particularly the elderly females, were showing a high resistance and did not want us to bring the children to modern hospitals. The elderly women were repeatedly saying, "Please, we give you the oath of the Holy *Qurān* and the *Allāh Pak* (God), do not allow the doctors to inject our children; otherwise, *Mātā* will be vindictive." The doctors, however, made the treatment according to their knowledge and understanding.

During the outbreak, when our children were dying, and the number of affected children was increasing. We decided to bring our children to the doctors because we wanted no more deaths—the deaths of children, which had already occurred, scared us. However, our old women were saying that we breached the required dos and don'ts, especially we became careless about cleanliness—that is why measles spread quickly from one child to another. Owing to negligence, measles happens and spreads rapidly. Moreover, during that time, a local politician started paying around 10,000 PKR (around US$90) to parents whose children died due to measles and 5,000 PKR to every affected child in the civil hospital of *Sakhar*. He paid the amount from his pocket. His offer played a significant role in mobilizing the parents, who started to bring their children to the hospital because of money. The politician encouraged us to change our attitude towards the measles.

Zamīr, a 40-year-old male interlocutor from *Rahīmpur* village, shares his view about the outbreak in the following way:

> As soon as we knew about the vaccinator—that he was the person responsible for vaccinating our children—we without any delay started beating him severely due to not visiting our village to vaccinate our children. We did not know it was him earlier. He was continually making excuses that our village was not his field while uttering that he was unclear as to whether (or not) this was his responsibility. We were frantic after observing the overwhelming situation of our children. He enraged us. Nevertheless, we spared him because health officials and politicians protected him and requested us to let him go.
>
> After the arrival of politicians and health officials, we were given an ambulance to bring our children to *Sakhar* Hospital. One ward in Red Crescent Hospital and one in the Civil Hospital in the *Sakhar* city were reserved for us. We formed two teams of volunteers from our village. One team was responsible for bringing the children to the hospital, and the second team's duty was to stay at the hospital to look after the children. We commenced bringing our children to the hospital, which was almost 40 km away. The doctors were waiting for us. Upon our arrival, they started the medication of our children. Steadily children were recovering. Moreover, a politician from our area started giving a stipend to the parents who were bringing their children or allowed their children to be brought to the hospital. He also gave the double amount to the parents of deceased children.

Moreover, after transporting all the children of *Rahīmpur* village to the biomedical hospitals, these volunteers approached nearby villages to carry the children infected with measles to the said hospitals. The measles outbreak was not merely limited to that village, as stated earlier, but the outbreak occurred in the whole *Taluko*. While visiting those villages, volunteers encountered hesitancy and resistance from the parents to bring the children to hospitals because they were considered "outsiders." People were uncertain as to whether these volunteers were *Uhta-Kuhta* (plural of *Uhto-Kuhto* in *Sindhī*: that means, persons with a bad intention, e.g., evil eye, jealousy, dishonesty, or of bad character—e.g., a magician) or *Mathy-Mero* (plural of *Mathy-merā* in *Sindhī*, which means an individual who has not taken the necessary ritualistic bath after intercourse). About the hesitancy of parents, *Sāhil* and *Jamāl*—in their thirties with higher secondary school certificate (intermediate) education who volunteered for health officials during the outbreak to locate the measles-infected children and mobilize parents to bring the children to the hospital—shared their views in the following way. *Sāhil* said:

> After taking our children to the hospitals, we surveyed nearby villages to find the affected children and take them to the hospital. However,

people were not allowing us to see their children as they were scared that our visit would cause the deaths of their children, as *Mātā* becomes angry when someone impure and an outsider meets or visits the child. Even our simple looks were considered as harmful. It was the same perception and belief as inhabitants of our village used to have. However, EDO briefed us that measles is like a viral disease that starts with fever, rashes, and can rapidly spread to other unaffected persons, especially children. We were using our dead and cured children as a source to mobilize inhabitants of nearby villages. Owing to our constant mobilization, they permitted us but requested us to be pure before visiting their children. They gave us water for ablution.

[*Jamāl* continued:] The parents were not allowing us to see their measles-infected children. They were afraid that perhaps some of us might be a *Uhto-Kuhto* and *Mathy-Mero* person, which can lead to the *Mātā*'s malevolence. We experienced that resistance throughout the area we visited. We introduced ourselves and started mobilizing people by giving them a reference to our village. After receiving awareness of measles from the health officials, we stated to people that measles was a viral "disease," not a manifestation of *Mātā*. Despite massive mobilization, parents were still hesitant to let us meet their children. Some of them did not even allow us, who steadfastly refused and believed that their children would recover through observing rituals.

In terms of how this purity and impurity works, and how people practice these concepts, particularly during measles, *Sāhil* and *Jamāl*—the two volunteers—shared one story about a teenage girl who was severely affected by measles.

We reached a village where villagers informed us about a teenage girl who had contracted measles and was in critical condition. We quickly reached that house and called[1] for the head of the household; a woman appeared. In response to her inquiry about our visit, we informed her that we were volunteers carrying measles-infected children to the hospital. After our briefing her concerning the visit, we learned that she was the mother of that girl. First, she completely denied the presence of a person having measles and then accepted, but she showed a great reluctance to let us visit her daughter. Her refusal was straightforward, "I cannot permit you to see my daughter, because this will lead towards the anger of *Mātā*, and as a consequence, my daughter could die."

We assured her that we were neither *Uhtā-Kuhtā* nor *Mathy-Merā* [plural form of both in the *Sindhī* language]. Instead, we had observed prayers five times a day and that we know what purity was. After a discussion and mobilization of half-an-hour, she agreed, however, with the condition that we must perform ablution before entering her house and seeing her daughter. She brought water for us to perform ablution to maintain the purification before entering the house. We followed her instructions accordingly. She afterward brought us inside her house, where her daughter was lying in bed in a critical condition. The girl was in a critical situation: weaker and wrapped in clothes. She was unable to speak. The family was economically poor.

After looking at the critical situation of her daughter, we asked the lady to permit us to bring her daughter to the hospital promptly. She should also accompany us to stay with her daughter. Concerning her permission, she would receive some money as well as free medication for her daughter. Otherwise, the consequences might be quite severe, including death, as some of our children had already died due to measles. We told her success and critical stories from our village to allow us to bring her daughter to the hospital.

Although she resisted bringing her daughter to a doctor, something worked, and she agreed for the treatment. We took both the mother and the daughter in an ambulance to the mentioned civil hospital. The doctors, after inspecting the girl, informed us that the situation of the girl was substantially critical, and thanks to God that we brought her at the right time. Otherwise, there were high chances that due to extreme severity, she could have succumbed to death. These words made the girl's mother cry.

Doctors allotted a bed to her and started medication. Gradually, the girl recovered enough to speak. After some days, she became entirely healthy and was discharged from the hospital. Then her mother was praying for us.

The views of these interlocutors illustrate the intensity of the measles outbreak and how these local people made sense of a challenging situation. The uncertainty and fear caused the local people to seek the attention of politicians and health officials. Undoubtedly, whenever an overwhelming situation occurs, we cannot merely sit and view how that situation impacts us. Instead, we humans make some best efforts to deal with it. Responding to a challenging situation is part of our enculturation. It has continuously evolved and is preserved in "societal memory." Analogously, when the outbreak's scale considerably increased, people had to make a suitable choice to contain the disease. They understood that local measures were proving to be ineffective to deal with measles. Hence, despite their elder—socially respectable— women, they protested against receiving the necessary attention of officials and bringing children to hospitals. This response may better be understood as concerning our sociocultural and biological history, in which we have learned how to make sense of a challenging situation and deal appropriately with it.

Moreover, the anecdote demonstrates the way politicians and officials dealt with the outbreak and how it changed the perception people had of measles. On the one hand, local people's children were overwhelmed by the infection, and on the other hand, they got a chance to earn some money. Hence, in the face of an overwhelming situation that made them helpless and in the absence of relevant resources (money, hospital care, and the ambulance), the provided money and the ambulance played a pivotal role in changing local perceptions and practices of measles to bring children to modern hospitals. The money as a "token" from the politician reflects how economic and political factors structure the inequalities and then shape the views of people. One can easily see how an unequal distribution of resources, facilities, and awareness have created a sense of "aid," and "greed" in the village of *Rahīmpur*.

Furthermore, the punishment inflicted on the vaccinator by the local people demonstrates how the poor (in terms of economic) manipulate their equivalents without understanding who is the main responsible person or institution for such a testing situation. The vaccinator was also not wealthy, and he lacked enough funds and facilities to reach a far-flung village.

Views of Medical Doctors and Local Health Officials

Riaz (2013, 189) cites an interview with Zulfiqar Bhutta[2] in the *Lancet*: "This was a tragedy that was waiting to happen. We have been predicting for a while now that without adequate cover with routine immunization in many parts of Pakistan, notably in rural populations, that there was bound to be a situation where you would have an outbreak like this." He further shared that they saw an outbreak of a preventable "disorder" that was happening in the country's south. Likewise, the BBC (2013) broadcasted the views of a *Punjāb*-based medical doctor from *Lāhore*, named Dr. Raza Hasan, who argued that he had been working for over two decades and had not seen a measles epidemic of this severity. Parents refuse modern medication, and when they come, it is late, so doctors cannot do anything.

A district-level government health official, Mr. *Rānno*, boldly claimed during my *Kachaharī* (see Chapter 3) with him that people of this *Taluko* [referring to the subdistrict, in which the village of *Rahīmpur* is located] are economically poor. They practice "cultural taboos," yet not all of them refuse vaccination. Some people openly welcome it, as they do not want to see their children suffer and die. Nonetheless, children still go unvaccinated not only due to parents' refusals but because of some other factors, too, such as lack of access to people due to unestablished road infrastructure, inaccessible vaccination, officials' deficiency of sincerity, and commitment and ownership at service delivery level.

Mr. *Rānno* further shares that lack of sincerity, commitment, and ownership—of the health officials—at the service delivery level are among the primary reasons for the outbreak. For example, there are five tiers: vaccinator, supervisor *Talukā* Superintendent Vaccination (TSV), District Superintendent Vaccination (SV), focal person of EPI, and the Project Director at the provincial level. Routine vaccination is facing problems in this chain of responsible people. There is a lack of commitment and proper supervision and monitoring. If staff conducted work candidly, then it is possible to control the vaccine preventive diseases (PVDs) and outbreaks would not occur. Even if a microorganism causes disease, then its intensity will be not as severe.

For example, if a doctor or staff member of the EPI learns about a case of measles anywhere in a respective field, then s/he must reach there as soon as possible; otherwise, that one case of measles will affect another 22 children/ persons. The official must keep an affected child in an isolated room and give him/her a vitamin A capsule promptly, which will help to reduce the chances of death. Afterward, the official has to give the same capsule after one month, which will help to further decrease the chances of mortality. This way, we can avoid an outbreak, and if we do not do this, outbreaks will occur.

Mr. *Rānno* further continues that the government of Sindh has employed Health Education Officers (HEOs) to change people's attitudes and behaviors that are harmful to their health. In other words, HEOs will change their views toward modern medicine. Strictly speaking, if there were no vaccine refusals, then what would the HEOs do? How can I tell you because [in *Sindhī*] *"Zubān Tay Tālā Āāhin, Pairan Main Bairryion"* (tongue is locked, and legs are chained)? Hence, he told us what he could.

The expression is used metaphorically to convey a sense of constraint or restriction. In this context, he is suggesting that they are unable to freely express themselves or provide detailed information. The metaphor implies a sense of being bound or restricted, as if their ability to speak openly or act freely is limited. The explanation follows that Mr. *Rānno* shared what information he could within the confines of these constraints. The use of the metaphor suggests a fear of punishment or repercussions if they were to disclose more details, perhaps due to the sensitive nature of the information or potential consequences related to their job or position. Despite these limitations, he provided some information by sharing a sheet containing cases of refusals, offering what insights they could while adhering to the perceived restrictions.

Politicians' Debate Outbreaks

The consecutive outbreaks of 2012 and 2013 remained the center of attention not only in the media but also in political circles: it became part of the government's discussions and debates. The rumors had it that the government did not provide the province with a sufficient amount of vaccine, or the government used an expired vaccine. Consequently, a debate was held in a Senate meeting of the Upper House of Pakistan's Parliament.[3] As mentioned earlier, the newspaper *Dawn* (2013) reported that during that meeting the Federal Minister for Inter-Provincial Coordination at the time accepted that the measles outbreak was a result of "poor handling" of measles infections, which resulted in deaths of over 200 children in 11 districts of Sindh province. Contending that the federal government supplied 10.7 million doses of the vaccine, against the province's need of 4.1 million, the minister claimed that shortage of vaccine was not the issue, but "access to people" insofar as 40% of the area was under the vaccination coverage.[4]

To the minister's second inference, one Senator argued that if shortage of vaccine was not the prime reason, then outbreaks were "a case of severe [governmental] mismanagement." An opposition Senator argued that the measles outbreak did not result in 200 deaths, but approximately 1,000 deaths. The ruling minister labeled it as an "exaggerated" claim and stated that the real figure is 232 deaths.

The senator's discussion shows how an outbreak was negotiated via quantification. Fewer numbers reflect here a success story of the government— "the proper management"—of the outbreak. For instance, a thousand deaths demonstrate more "value" than over a hundred. This "valuation" and quantification of loss is highly prominent in political circles as well as with governmental and nongovernmental health officials. Interesting enough was the end of the discussion: since the home district of this minister was also among the eight areas severely affected by measles, he promised that the government would supply further vaccines after administering the ones supplied. Summing up, he asked the elected representatives to play a significant role in increasing the coverage of vaccination against the "deadly disease."

Furthermore, seizing the opportunity presented by the upcoming elections, political parties aside from the ruling political parties used these outbreaks and rumors surrounding the "expired" vaccine as a pretext. It is essential to mention that the measles outbreak occurred when the first-ever democratically elected government in the history of Pakistan was completing its five-year tenure, and the next general elections were approaching.[5] Hence, during election campaigns, other parties were citing the measles outbreak and mentioning in their election campaigns that the present government mismanaged the vaccination in general and the outbreak in particular, which consequently led to the high morbidity and mortality of the children.

The government authorities, especially at the federal level, accepted that measles could have been controlled with proper handling of the cases and ensuring an ordinary person's access to healthcare. This access and "poor handling of the outbreak" signify several existing disparities in the country, which are related to the availability of the healthcare services and providers, and ineffective checks and balances. For instance, competent dealing with an infectious disease requires the following actions: (a) the vaccine, (b) a routine vaccination, (c) an appropriate cold chain to maintain the temperature of the vaccine, (d) well-informed and well-resourced vaccinators to administer the vaccine, and (e) adequate supervision of the vaccination. Once the infection spreads, then it is highly necessary to carefully handle it, which necessitates: (a) a thorough survey of the area to identify the infected people, (b) a careful and effective medication of the infected people, (c) a well-established and resourced medical facility that has the required capacity (beds, services, and providers) to accommodate the infected people, and (d) well-trained medical staff to treat the infected people.

These entire preventive and curative measures considerably depend on those policies, which make a difference to have an (in-)effective healthcare system. These policies are devised and implemented at national and global levels. Yet, they negotiate the outbreaks in a way that most likely makes the local people appear as the "culprits" for epidemics. The following letters, which two politicians and parts of the government wrote to the federal government, highlight how they were negotiating the outbreaks and inferring those underlying causes.

The first letter was written to the President of Pakistan on 10th January 2013 by Dr. Azra Fazal Pechuho, who was a Member of the National Assembly, Chairperson of the National Assembly's Standing Committee on Defense, and sister of the country's then president. Mentioned in the report of *Wafaqi-Mohtasib* (Federal Ombudsman), the details of the letter are as follows:

i) The Federal Government through the Federal EPI Cell was responsible for the uninterrupted supply of vaccine to the provinces till June 20, 2013. Due to inordinate delay in [the] supply of vaccine to the provinces, the target children could not be protected with the measles vaccine which resulted in a nation-wide epidemic and hundreds of deaths which could have been averted.

ii) Monitoring and surveillance system[s] clearly failed to forewarn and inform the authorities at the Provincial and Federal level with the result that no timely intervention could be made. Deaths of hundreds of children from measles were brought to the light by the media. More deaths of children are being reported every day from across the country and the toll is unfortunately likely to rise manifold.

iii) In her view, the Federal EPI Cell, Ministry of IPC had failed in its duty to process the case[s] and arrange for release and disbursal of funds to the UNICEF for purchase of vaccine. This has resulted in [an] interruption in [the] supply of vaccine to the provinces which continues to persist and there is no clear time frame in which vaccine[s] will be made available to the provinces despite the deaths of hundreds of children across Pakistan.

iv) From the above, it is clear that the responsible officials failed to perform their duties in [the] timely purchase of measle[s] vaccine[s], timely release of funds and effective monitoring and surveillance of measles in the country. This criminal negligence has cost the country hundreds of precious lives and brought a bad name to the Government

(Government of Pakistan 2013, 10–11).

Ms. Pechuho, in her letter, holds the federal government responsible, not the provincial government, because she belongs to the Pakistan People's Party (PPP) that has been active in the province for many decades and ruling the province from 2008. She criticizes the federal ministry for an untimely procurement and supply of the required vaccine and views government officials as having failed to perform their due roles effectively. Moreover, in her view, the problem also exists in surveillance to detect the outbreak prior to the media. She does not mention the provincial government. Nonetheless, as stated above, the federal minister argued that the requirement of the vaccine was fulfilled. This also highlights the aspect of contestation between the provincial and federal governments.

Another letter that the Ombudsman's report contains was written by Mr. Haleem Adil Sheikh, who was the Advisor/Minister for Relief Department, Government of Sindh. The following are the details:

a) Parents were not bringing the infected children to nearby hospitals.
b) [The] Medical staff was found misreporting/hiding facts, as people could not afford the treatment.
c) Measles has spread mostly in the areas which were badly affected in three consecutive rain flood disasters.
d) Financial constraint is also the prime factor, as people could not afford the treatment.
e) Malnutrition combined with measles have caused fatalities.
f) Lack of prompt treatment and improper isolation procedures [are] also cause of [the] spread of measles.
g) Children were not vaccinated [in] proper time and immunisation was compromised.
h) Privately administered clinics and hospitals were not having sufficient well[-]trained staff to treat the increasing epidemic.
i) Government hospitals did not take [the] widespread epidemic threat seriously and no plans were made or prepared for [a] micro[-]level immunisation plan.
j) Medicine [was] not available in OPD [Outpatient Department] to fight the measles virus and post measles complications on [an] immediate basis.
k) Improper handling of vaccines compromised their quality and efficacy.
l) More than 50% of cases were not reported mainly because of [the] nondeployment of health teams in the field.
m) As per rural custom[s], symptoms of measles in children and women, [e]specially female child[ren], are not taken seriously.
n) Classical taboos of [S]tone [A]ge treatment are adopted in houses, based on superstition.
o) Measles is not a life[-]threatening disease but due to lack of awareness, improper treatment and increase in post[-]measles complications, it can cause fatalities in children

(Government of Pakistan 2013, 10–11).

Mr. Shaikh starts with the parents, who could not bring their children to modern hospitals. Afterward, he mentions the following reasons behind the outbreak: medical staff's misreporting/hiding of facts, impacts of floods, economic factors, malnutrition, untimely treatment, low-vaccination uptake, lack of staff at the private clinics, government hospital's negligence to understand the outbreak's scale, a dearth of medicine at the hospitals, improper handling of vaccines, "rural customs," "classical taboos of Stone Age," and the local perception of measles that it is not life "threatening." Nonetheless, Shaikh does not mention the government as he was also part of the provincial governing system.

Report of the Federal Ombudsman on the Measles Outbreak

Based on these letters and informed by the media, the *Wafaqi-Mohtasib* (Federal Ombudsman) of Pakistan took notice of the outbreak, and considered "mal-functioning and negligence of the government departments and their functionaries" behind the 20,000 suspected cases of measles and 463 deaths from January 2012 to 2 February 2013 (Government of Pakistan 2013, 4). Considering this outbreak as important and a result of the government's "neglect, inattention, and delay," the notice was taken under "Article 2(2) of the Establishment of the office of *Wafaqi-Mohtasib* (Federal Ombudsman Order, 1983)" and under its motion following Article 9(1). To detail the causes behind the outbreak, the Ombudsman constituted a committee to compile the statements of national and global stakeholders responsible for vaccination in the country, such as the Sindh government, the Ministry of Inter-Provincial Coordination (IPC)/Federal EPI Cell, the NIH, the Pakistan Medical Research Council (PMRC), Aga Khan University, Accountant General of Pakistan Revenues (AGPR), and the WHO, UNICEF, and USAID. The following were terms of references (TORs) to (a) know the underlying causes of the measles outbreak, (b) "fix the responsibility of the government departments, and their functionaries for their failure" to procure measles vaccines in a timely fashion, to immunize children throughout the country and to recommend suitable actions "against the delinquents," and (c) recommend appropriate measures for averting the possibility of such outbreaks in the future (Government of Pakistan 2013, 5).

To obtain perspectives on the outbreak, this committee held several meetings with the above-stated stakeholders. The following perspectives concerning the measles outbreaks of 2012 and 2013 are based on this Ombudsman's *Report on Measles Outbreak in Pakistan*, which reveal contestation between the engaged stakeholders.

When considering the critical role of the provincial functionaries to implement the EPI in the provinces, the Ombudsman asked the Ministry of IPC and National Program Manager of the Federal EPI to hold a meeting with provincial Health Secretaries and EPI heads. On 31 January 2013, the Ombudsman's committee held a meeting with the concerned provincial functionaries and senior representatives of USAID and the WHO. The agenda points included the provincial vaccine requirement for the entire year 2012, the number of vaccines provided by the Federal EPI Cell, underlying reasons of the outbreak, suggestions to improve the vaccine procurement and vaccination, and ideas to halt such "disasters" in future (ibid., 34).

The Sindh Government's Viewpoints

In 2012, Sindh aimed to vaccinate 2.74 million children aged 9–15 months, and the required vaccine was 3.570 million doses. Against this requirement, the federal EPI Cell provided 5.504 million doses (Government of Pakistan 2013). However, Sindh province stated several important reasons for the measles outbreak: the federal EPI failed to (a) supply the required vaccines, syringes, safety boxes, and other logistics in a timely way; (b) develop an efficient surveillance system to monitor the burden of disease; and (c) formulate an effective monitoring and evaluation system to monitor coverage of routine immunization and give appropriate feedback; further, (d) the performance of the concerned districts that were severely affected during the outbreak was inappropriate.

To improve the performance of the EPI and avoid any future outbreaks, Sindh suggested that the procurement and timely provision of the vaccine is the responsibility of the federal government. The federal government should buy vaccines from UNICEF because it provides quality vaccines at affordable prices. Otherwise, there are only three manufacturers, GSK, Sanofi Pasteur, and Novartis, who hold sub-offices in Pakistan, and other manufacturers which have their agents in the country. Owing to this low competition, the manufacturers practice a monopoly in the county that leads to an unbearable economic burden on the EPI. Not merely the federal government, but the provincial governments should also pool their resources for centralized procurement through UNICEF, which is necessary for the smooth functioning of the EPI. It is crucial that the Ministry of IPC, in collaboration with the provincial EPI, should formulate an active surveillance system for detecting an early outbreak. This ministry should also focus on building an appropriate monitoring and evaluation mechanism to check the routine immunization activities often (Government of Pakistan 2013).

The Opinion of IPC and the Federal EPI Cell

At the federal level, the central EPI cell under the Ministry of IPC was primarily responsible for the planning and implementation of the EPI throughout Pakistan. However, after the devolution (the transfer of power or authority from a central government to a local government) of the Ministry of Health in June of 2011, the provinces/areas were supposed to procure vaccines on their own. In February 2012, the Planning Commission decided, in consultation with the provinces, that provinces would do the actual procurement, as the federal entity of EPI had ceased to exist. It was as late as mid-October 2012 when the provincial governments showed their inability to procure vaccines, and the EPI had to be resurrected in October 2012 (through the extension of PC-1) to perform this vital function. The federal EPI floated tenders four times to purchase the measles vaccine through open bidding as per Public Procurement Regulatory Authority (PPRA) rules. However, open bidding did not work. Therefore, the government bought all the vaccines through UNICEF during the year 2012.

Since October 2012, provinces had not sent an official request to the EPI for vaccines or informed them of the unavailability and shortages of the vaccine stocks. Nonetheless, the federal EPI fulfilled their demand quarterly. The federal EPI is mostly concerned with supplying vaccines to continue routine immunization. The World Bank indicated pathetically low routine immunization during that period.

The federal government has regularly developed Standard Operating Procedures (SOPs) for ensuring active routine immunization through combating the decision gaps between the provincial, district levels, and further downward. Despite that, the actual coverage remains lower than 50%, except for *Punjāb*, where it is around 60%. The EPI further took a stance that vaccines for 100% coverage reached provinces as per their demand, but the provinces did not send utilization reports to the federal EPI. That means that it was not a shortage of measles vaccines that led to the deaths but pathetically low routine coverage (less than 50%) and a failure of implementation at district levels and below (Government of Pakistan 2013).

NIH's Views

There is now a WHO-supported Disease Early Warning System (DEWS) in all provinces to report suspected cases. The DEWS recorded a total of 17,338 suspected cases from 1 January 2012 to 19 January 2013, with 413 deaths. The case fatality rate was 2.38%. Most deaths are attributable to post-measles complications. The cases and deaths reported from other provinces make it a generalized issue. However, Sindh province was the worst affected. The NIH had already alerted all stakeholders, including provincial and district health authorities, for measles preparedness through Seasonal Awareness and Alert Letters (SAAL). The present measles episode highlights the critical inability of the healthcare delivery system: a failure to find and vaccinate the vulnerable populations; and the inability of the EPI monitoring and surveillance system to identify, investigate, and respond to the issues related to the measles outbreaks from district to district (Government of Pakistan 2013).

Position of PMRC

The present outbreak is a result of overall low vaccination coverage, which did not exceed 60% for many years. The WHO's coverage data imply better coverage in the urban areas than the rural. The stock shows that there was no shortage of vaccine stocks in any province. Also, there is no doubt in the efficacy of the vaccine as no other country has reported such an event. All the neighboring countries have excellent coverage of EPI vaccines that made them successful in the eradication or control of these diseases such as polio, besides measles, much earlier on. Now, the government should procure a future supply of vaccines through UNICEF, because it gives a standard rate, and supplies on time with a guarantee of quantity and quality (Government of Pakistan 2013).

The Standpoint of Aga Khan University

A pediatrician's team from Aga Khan University visited the profoundly affected areas of Sindh during the outbreak. During their week-long visits to health facilities, areas, and observations in the field, the team discovered pressing issues in cold chain maintenance; capacity of the health staff, coordination among the vertical programs and the engaged health officials, such as between the medical officers and vaccinators; attendance of the vaccinators; and great emphasis and incentive for polio vaccination. Aga Khan University proposed short- and long-term plans such as vaccinating all the children (six months to 15 years) during March and April 2013; ensure vaccines; staff training; fixing the cold chain and filling the vacant positions at the health-care facilities (Government of Pakistan 2013).

Views of the Accountant General of Pakistan Revenues (AGPR)

According to the Federal Ombudsman's (2013) report, the Ministry of IPC/Federal EPI Cell sent a cheque to UNICEF for an advance payment of Rs. 633 million against UNICEF's cost estimation for the measles vaccines that was valid until the 31 December 2012. However, the funds did not reach UNICEF as per the said date, as the AGPR issued the cheque on 7 January 2013. UNICEF then refused to accept the cheque, because the prices of vaccines had varied by then. Consequently, there was a delay in the advance payment and vaccine delivery. Therefore, the Ombudsman asked the AGPR to clarify its stance.

The AGPR stated that bills of such substantial amounts require a processing time of at least seven working days. While the bill was processed the following day, the System Applications Products (SAPs) server of AGPR encountered delays due to legal issues, specifically related to a Writ Petition filed by the Pakistan Medical Association (PMA) regarding the purchase of vaccines. The AGPR communicated to the Secretary, IPC Division, seeking specific clarifications. The bill, afterward, was resubmitted after almost 15 days. Meanwhile, the National EPI manager visited the AGPR, and the bill was "expeditiously" passed on the same day on 7 January 2013 (Government of Pakistan 2013).

The WHO Perspective

According to the views that the WHO provided to the Federal Ombudsman (2013, 18), the WHO had already alerted all the provinces about the possibility of a future measles outbreak. To avert that outbreak, a vaccination campaign was held to vaccinate 4.5 million children in 23 districts of Sindh. Despite that, the measles outbreak occurred, and the primary reasons behind the outbreak and the deaths are: "(i) low rate of the routine vaccination in the field particularly in Sindh province; (ii) poor health services management; (iii) untrained staff at health facilities and in the field; (iv) inability and incapacity of the health personnel in the hospitals and in the field [required] to treat post-measles complications." Post-measles complications—pneumonia, encephalitis, and diarrhea—were the leading causes of many deaths (Government of Pakistan 2013).

One of the WHO officials during my interview indicated a dearth of political will, as Closser (2010) also found in her work *Chasing Polio in Pakistan: Why the World's Largest Public Health Initiative May Fail*. His views are:

> The Health Department did not perform its job as required. It [the outbreak] occurred due to their negligence. A family member can make the health department accountable for their roles and responsibilities. The government did not take the proper measures, but it was just busy in blame games. Everyone was saving their skin. During an outbreak, politicians were speaking silly stuff, as they were saying that measles has occurred because of malnutrition. At the same time, they even do not know that the virus is the main reason for measles, not malnutrition. Malnutrition can aggravate the situation but cannot cause the measles.

The official strongly contends that the Health Department failed to meet its responsibilities adequately. The use of the term "negligence" suggests a substantial lapse in performing duties, indicating a failure in the department's preparedness or response to the outbreak. Emphasizing transparency and responsibility, the official suggests that family members (of those who suffered or lost their lives) have the right to hold the Health Department accountable for its roles and responsibilities. This highlights the importance of mechanisms ensuring that government bodies, particularly those in public health, remain answerable to the public. The official criticizes the government for insufficient measures in response to the outbreak. Reference to "blame games" implies a lack of coordinated action, with individuals prioritizing the shifting of responsibility over addressing the crisis effectively. Moreover, the phrase "everyone was saving their skin" suggests a prevailing sense of self-preservation among involved individuals, potentially hindering proactive and effective response measures. This sentiment highlights the urgency and severity of the situation in contrast to a perceived lack of commitment to public welfare. Politicians inappropriately linked measles to malnutrition, highlighting the need for accurate information dissemination in public health crises, and emphasizing the virus as the primary cause. The WHO official clarifies malnutrition's potential impact, underscoring the necessity for an informed, science-based approach to communicating outbreak causes.

The UNICEF Viewpoint

According to UNICEF's viewpoint, as expressed to the Federal Ombudsman, the province was not allocated any measles vaccines for 2012 and 2013 because it reported 118% coverage during the measles supplementary immunization activities (SIAs) between October 2010 and March 2011 (Government of Pakistan 2013). However, the current outbreaks tell another story: it is "suggestive of poor quality of the measles SIAs as well as Routine EPI coverage" (ibid., 19). In most of the cases, post-measles complications such as pneumonia, encephalitis, and diarrhea affected children and caused deaths, and approximately 20% of these children were malnourished (ibid.).

In March 2012, according to the views of UNICEF to the Ombudsman, Sindh province witnessed a rising trend of measles cases, mainly in the Southern districts and *Karāchī* city (ibid.). In that year, cases increased again from October onwards, and reached a peak in December 2012. The last rise of cases and deaths were reported from the Northern districts, such as *Qamber Shahdādkot* district, which reported 777 cases (the highest number), and *Sakhar* district with the second-highest number of deaths—33. The same report mentions that several SIAs have been conducted in the province like the National Measles Catch-up Campaign during the nationwide campaign in 2007–2008 and the National Measles Follow-up Campaign in Sindh Province in 2010–2011.

For the measles follow-up SIAs, Sindh received 4.26 million doses of bundled measles vaccines on a loan basis for case response activities from the existing UNICEF vaccines stock. Then, the Provincial Health Department conducted measles campaigns in eight of the most affected districts from 31 December to January 2013 and further requested support from UNICEF and other development partners in reaching the remaining districts.

According to the Federal Ombudsman's report, the UNICEF Communication Network staff for Polio Eradication (COMNet) played a significant role in Measles Outbreak Response during measles outbreaks in 2012 and 2013 (Government of Pakistan 2013). The report (2013, 20) further mentions that UNICEF:

(a) provided technical assistance for Measles outbreak response activities from planning to implementation, including social mobilisation. (b) facilitated the supervision and monitoring of the activities along with social mobilisation sessions in the community; (c) used [the] local FM radio channel in Larkana [in *Sindhī Lārrkānno*] for messages about Measles and presentations on air by District Heath Communication Support Officer (DHCSO) alongside Executive District Officer (Health) focal person covering the entire district. Coverage included parts of *Kamber* [*Qamber*], *Khairpur* and Jacobabad district; (d) distributed UNICEF proposes that a technical forum comprising of the EPI stakeholders including UNICEF, WHO, Federal EPI and Provincial EPI should be established and made fully operational to jointly discuss the situation and response at regular intervals.

The Ombudsman's report further discussed that on 29 January 2013, the Ministry of Inter-Provincial Coordination (IPC) and the federal EPI requested UNICEF to procure vaccines. On 1 February 2013, UNICEF submitted a cost estimate for these vaccines that the said governmental departments approved on 2 February 2013. During this process, UNICEF negotiated with the head office for procurement—UNICEF Supply Division—"trying to ensure that the most cost-effective vaccine source could be assessed given maximizing the utilization of funds bearing in mind that the measles vaccine in the previously expired Cost Estimate for delivery in 2013 was quoted at a unit cost of USD 2.40 per vial" (Government of Pakistan 2013, 21).

Although the UNICEF measles vaccines were out of stock, UNICEF managed to secure 18 million doses that were not included in the UNICEF global forecast. Each unit costs US$ 2.40 per vial as compared to the previous availability of un-forecasted measles vaccines at US$ 4.25 for the same unit. Around 6.1 million doses were delivered to Pakistan as the first urgent delivery during February 2013.

Moreover, UNICEF urged the establishment of a technical forum comprising the EPI stakeholders, UNICEF, the WHO, and the federal and provincial EPI. The forum must be fully operational to collectively discuss the situation and the response at regular intervals to challenge the measles crisis.

USAID Standpoint

High-level political commitment and technical leadership are necessary to strengthen the EPI system at the federal and the provincial levels. The immediate epidemic and long-term collapse of EPI systems require both short- and long-term financing, commitment, and accountability. This is possible through several measures. First, UNICEF should have the authority to procure all the vaccines for the immediate future. Second, the federal and provincial levels must clarify and build consensus on responsibilities under devolution, including procurement, planning, cold chain maintenance, resource mobilization, adequate operations funding at district levels, agreement on the installation of supply chain systems, monitoring, and reporting at subdistrict and district levels. The current situation needs rapid regional assessment.

Third, for the failure of agreed targets, federal and provincial EPI program managers and EDO health should be held accountable. The provincial governments should ensure the provision of adequate resources such as generators with petrol and solar panels in high-risk districts to ensure the cold chain integrity in the face of constant electricity load-shedding. Fourth, there is a need to report and revise the definition of a fully vaccinated child. For instance, currently, the districts report a once-vaccinated child as a fully covered one. The new protocol, however, recommends the second dose of anti-measles vaccine at 15 months of age. Fifth, there are three levels to generate information for the EPI: DEWS, District Health Information System (DHIS), and EPI Cell. There is a need to revise these mechanisms so that the generated information can function for managing and analyzing the outbreaks and program response. Sixth, capacity building is needed for the provincial governments for smooth planning and transparent procurement.

Concluding Remarks

Supplying the comprehensive standpoints of several stakeholders regarding the outbreaks, this chapter highlighted the intricate negotiation processes. The negotiations started when local politicians incentivized parents through monetary support and an ambulance to the local people to bring their children to the biomedical hospitals. The same politicians wrote letters to the federal government, which initiated discussions and debates that took place in the Senate—the Upper House of Pakistan's Parliament. These politicians, who were part of that government, avoided criticism toward their provincial government while directing it toward the federal government, health officials, and the local people.

Considering it a critical problem, the Federal Ombudsman formed a committee to pay thorough attention to the matter and find out the underlying reasons for these outbreaks. The committee consulted numerous national and global stakeholders, such as the Sindh Government, the National Institute of Health (NIH), the Federal Cell of EPI, the WHO, and USAID. Despite differing views, the consensus is that the EPI system's failure was the primary cause of the measles outbreak due to inadequate vaccine coverage, accountability, and surveillance. Pertinent challenges encompass power disruptions, inadequate investment, and a reallocation of resources toward polio, diverting attention from diseases like measles. This report reveals a visible contestation among these engaged stakeholders while highlighting the outbreaks' significant reasons. It not only demonstrates the negotiation among national and global stakeholders but also between provincial and federal governments.

Since there is a dearth of reliable and active surveillance systems, it should be activated at the national, provincial, and district levels; otherwise, the signals cannot systematically reach the health managers. Due to this lack, the outbreak gets reported first in the media. Moreover, the lapses in the cold chain make the quality and efficacy of even the appropriately procured vaccines questionable.

Although this is an immense waste of national resources, nobody was held mainly responsible. The lucid gap between the reported vaccine usage and actual immunization outcomes requires accountability because the health administration, district administration, and provincial governments are responsible for ensuring the coverage. Such stakeholders should be held accountable for this failure in performance. One EPI district official, during a

Kachaharī with me, highlighted that the outbreak's root cause was a lack of sincerity, commitment, and ownership among health officials at the service delivery level.

In the next chapter, I discuss the vaccination in detail—from the historical development of vaccination to the commencement of EPI in Pakistan with the issues that are surrounding the vaccination in the country.

Notes

1 In villages, it is a normal practice to call (shout) the name of the family's head or any other male member. Because sometimes there is a doorway but no door, or because of voices inside the house, or the width of the house, knocking at the door does not work. There are no doorbells.

2 He is founding Chair of the Division of Women and Child Health at the Aga Khan University, Karachi, Pakistan.

3 Pakistan's Parliament is based on two houses: The Upper House (the Senate) and the Lower House (the National Assembly).

4 During the debate, the minister praised the governments of two other provinces, *Punjāb* and KPK, for their effective steps and the better case management that was lacking in Sindh.

5 During the entire political history of the country, this was the first democratic government about to complete five years of governing. Prior to it, although elected governments ruled the country, they could not complete the five-years tenure due to military coups.

8 The Critical Geopolitical Events
Making Sense of Anti-Vaccination Sentiment

British Colonization: A Brief Overview

The rise of extremism in the country is a result of past and present geopolitics. Colonizers subjugated the colonies and dehumanized the colonized regularly and treated them as commodities in the world market. Pakistan (when it was part of the same country as India) long remained under British colonization. Although the colonization ended, the damage it caused has continually persisted in terms of weaker economic and political systems (see sections on Pak–Afghan relations; Indo–Pak relations) (e.g., Zaidi 1988; Imran Ali 2002; Easterly 2006). Zaidi (1988) has explicitly documented the impact of British colonization on the healthcare system of Pakistan, explaining how "Brown-Englishmen" affected the systems once the British left India (see Chapter 5). After the colonization, new forms of imperialism emerged (see the section on Pak–US relations).

Over time, the strategic importance of the territory that is now Pakistan and its resources attracted the British colonizers and other prior invaders such as Greeks and Mongols. For the resources, the British colonizers came to India and ultimately established the East India Company or the English East India Company in 1600. Taking advantage of India's fragile economic and political situation, they invaded India to rule. Briefly, the British enormously impacted the sociocultural, economic, and political situation of South Asia, internally and externally. Internally, the countries were involved in civil wars and separated. The old India separated into three countries—India, Pakistan, and Bangladesh. Indo–Pak partition occurred in 1947, and Pak–Bangladesh separation in 1971. Externally, animosities emerged between neighboring countries such as Pakistan vs. Afghanistan, specifically due to the Durand Line (see the next section), and Hindustan vs. Pakistan (there are several reasons), mainly due to the Kashmir issue. The latter relations are less related to this project on measles. Hence, I focus instead on the former events and relations for tracing the roots of extremism or anti-West, anti-American, and anti-vaccination sentiments.

DOI: 10.4324/9781003253716-9

Pak–Afghan Relations and Vaccination

The British triggered a critical event when they divided the borders of Afghanistan and the old India (present-day Pakistan) in accordance with the Durand Line,[1] which created unfriendly relations between the two countries. The British's 1893 division sketched the 2,640 km border between Afghanistan and British India that separated the region of Pashtun or *Pathān* settlements. Bruce Riedel (2011, 22)—who is an American expert on US security, South Asia, and counterterrorism—views that for Afghanistan, it was an injustice with the country; therefore, since then, neither the people nor any Afghan government has ever recognized the legitimacy of this British-drawn line.

After the departure of the British colonizers from the old India in 1947, Afghanistan was the only country that refused to accept Pakistan's independence in the United Nations (UN). Riedel (2011, 21) mentions that more importantly, Afghanistan demanded the revision of this division and voted against Pakistan receiving a seat in the UN while demanding an independent *Pashtunistān* to be carved out of Pakistan. Such events aroused animosity between these two countries, which worsened during the USSR invasion in 1978 when the Marxist officers in the Afghan army overthrew the Afghanistan government to introduce Communist ideology and politics there (ibid.). As an event, this invasion ignited rebelliousness in Afghanistan's rural parts and mainly in the areas with long-standing contacts with Pakistan's Inter-Service Intelligence (ISI) and religious parties, especially the *Jamāt-i-Islamī*. During this movement, rebels received arms from the ISI while the USSR supported the new Communist government in terms of arms and advisers (ibid., 23).

Nirode Mohanty (2013) traces the roots of this intervention to the "Great Game" that was a political and diplomatic confrontation between the British and Russian Empires over Afghanistan and other neighboring countries.[2] The game commenced in the nineteenth century when the Russians extended their empire in the south to the border of Afghanistan, and British imperialists wanted to halt Russia's continued expansion in the direction of India. Mohanty (2013, xii) further claims that the British aimed to make Afghanistan a buffer state between both these empires. Notwithstanding, the USSR restarted this game in 1979, but after that, America revitalized it during 1989 as soon as the Soviets departed from Afghanistan (ibid.).

Western Imperialists Make Pakistan an Ally

After British colonization, imperialism dominated South Asia. Tariq Ali (1983, 188–89) stated that the area seemed vital due to two main reasons: (a) its geographical location adjacent to the USSR and China; and (b) it being close to the oil-rich Arab Gulf that held a crucial significance for the resources and was vulnerable to any regional political unrest. In the South

Asian region, Pakistan emerged as a suitable country to approach; thus, the new Western imperialists moved to make it an ally in the 1980s (ibid.). We can classify the underlying reasons into four categories: (i) Pakistan's internal situation, (ii) Pakistan's geographical location, (iii) the Iranian Revolution, and (iv) the USSR's invasion of Afghanistan.

The first, after independence in 1947, Pakistan encountered huge socio-economic and political problems, especially after two big wars with India in 1965 and 1971 and a civil war in which Bangladesh separated in 1971. Both events overwhelmed Pakistan's confidence to develop its significantly affected economy. Ali (1983) claimed that the country was on a quest for the resources and support to recover and progress, and to achieve parity with India in particular. As soon as the USA offered its support in the 1980s, Pakistan accepted it.

Second, as already mentioned, Pakistan was believed to hold an essential strategic position in South Asia, as it shares borders with Afghanistan and Iran in particular where new political events were happening, mainly the fall of the Shah of Iran—an American ally—and the gradual spread of communism.

Third, the Iranian Revolution overthrew Nadir Shah despite the West's material aid, the USSR's tacit support, and China's public endorsement (T. Ali 1983, 182). The people throughout this geographical region celebrated the Shah's collapse as a victory because the Shah interfered in the internal political life of Afghanistan and Pakistan (ibid., 181). In contrast, in the collapse of the Shah, the USA lost its old loyal friend, and a great ally in a vital zone for influencing events throughout the region and America also saw the Shia-Islam's government as a significant threat due to an emerging anti-American sentiment in Iran (ibid.). Hence, the USA wanted an ally in that geographical area—the weakest ally was the most desirable to manipulate. As noted earlier, the USA approached Pakistan.

Fourth, during these substantial changes in the regional power structures, the USSR invaded Afghanistan, which was yet another threat: the spread of communism. In December 1979, Leonid Brezhnev—who was the Secretary-General of the Community Party and the de facto leader of the country—issued orders to the Soviet forces to invade Afghanistan. He initially did this to support the Communist regime of Hāfizullah Amin in Afghanistan. Despite its reluctance to engage in an emerging civil war and a possible quagmire, the deteriorating situation compelled the USSR to protect a client state through an intervention (Riedel 2011). Subsequently, on the evening of 25 December 1979, around 85,000 Soviet troops entered Afghanistan by advancing the army to Pakistan's western frontier (ibid., 23) to fight against the tribal resistance groups. In particular, it conducted a rapid surgical operation to secure Kabul—the Afghan capital—and safeguard communication lines linking Afghanistan and the Soviet Union (Mohanty 2013, 68; Wynbrandt 2009, 218). Soon after the invasion, the Soviets wanted to have a more compliant leader. Amin was therefore assassinated on 28 December 1979, and Babrak

Kamal became the new president, who was a Soviet protégé and puppet (ibid.).

Such regional political events cultivated a context in which Pakistan received a massive amount of attention from the strong geopolitical actors, especially the USA and the USSR. Pakistan was already standing at a crossroads to seek external support. Hence, besides the big players, the third and fourth events mentioned above—the Shia-Islam's dominance in Iran and the arrival of communism in Afghanistan—emerged as rising threats to Pakistan. Ali (1983, 164) notes that for Pakistan, (i) the Iranian Revolution that occurred after defeating the Shah in February 1979, (ii) the left-wing coup in Kabul in 1978, and (iii) Mrs. Gandhi's reemergence as the head of a victorious Congress Party in India, posed new challenges that led Pakistan to seek external assistance to deal with them. In this search, "the military-bureaucratic complex," and its favored politicians, "sold their souls" to the USA (ibid., 189).

Contrary to Pakistan, India cultivated the idea of "positive neutralism" from right after the Indo–Pak partition (ibid.). India kept a distance from joining the American-sponsored military alliances, and the orientations of the Soviet leadership, and Jawaharlal Nehru—an Indian leader—made efforts for a "Third-World" nationalism, which was "anti-imperialist."

The internal and external challenges made Pakistan a suitable ally. America approached Pakistan and supported it from 1954 to 1965 in the shape of weapons and vivid infiltration of armed forces to defend against "communist aggression." The USA promised to India that the weapons would not be used against it, but the weapons were used in Indo–Pak wars, e.g., 1965 and 1971. Harrison (1981) states that for breaching this promise and seeking India's sympathy, the USA cut its military aid to Pakistan, which resumed after Kissinger and Nixon softened toward the country. America also supported the Pakistan army during the civil war in Bengal in 1970–1972 while considering it "as a more reliable defender of [the] US interests in the region" (T. Ali 1983, 189). This American backing made Pakistan's army more influential than the civilian governments, who then ruled the country.

Support was given to the dictators to receive their cooperation, which was required for strategic American interests. The Central Intelligence Agency (CIA) intervened, Ali (1983) argues, because of America's dominant regional obsession with maintaining its status quo in the Gulf. The support arrived to defeat an enemy, not to support a friend. Countries encouraging Pakistan to stand against the USSR were following their vested interests and playing their politics. The USA, James Wynbrandt (2009) notes, was engulfed with the Iranian hostage crisis when the USSR was invading Afghanistan; thus, it was challenging for the States to take more decisive steps. Despite that, Carter had signed a secret deal to support the rebels fighting against the Communist government in Afghanistan six months earlier. As soon as the Soviets invaded Afghanistan, the USA mobilized Muslim countries around the world to lead a propaganda campaign and provide covert aid to work against the Soviets. This move was intended to trigger the Muslims' religious fervor in terms of believing that the Soviets are infidels and that fighting against them would be a holy war (ibid., 218). For the USA and its allies, no other country was as suitable as Pakistan to fight that holy war. Soon after the Soviets invaded, the USA approached Pakistan to be its ally to wage war against the USSR through its assistance to produce "*Mujāhidīn*: the holy warriors" (Mohanty 2013, 68; Cordovez, Harrison, and Harrison 1995). According to Wynbrandt (2009, 218–19), Pakistan accepted the generous offer and consequently "money and matériel were routed through Pakistan" to support the *Mujāhidīn*, "who were organized to battle the infidel invaders" and the country "received most-favored-nation [sic] trading status" for supporting the US plans.

Moreover, after the USSR invasion of Afghanistan, it was not only the USA, but Saudi Arabia and its allies were also extremely concerned about Soviet designs in the region. They significantly supported Pakistan in deepening its activities against the Soviet invasion (Jones and Fair 2010, 11; Mohanty 2013, xiv). Riedel (2011, 23) notes that the Saudis were already panicked due to an expected Marxist threat in Afghanistan. Therefore, Prince Turki, Saudi Intelligence Chief, immediately agreed to engage his General Intelligence Directorate (GID) with the ISI and provide funds to support the *Mujāhidīn*. Furthermore, the Saudi government also stimulated citizens to lend private financial support to the *Mujāhidīn* to join an ongoing *Jihād* (ibid., 23). Concerning the aid to Pakistan, Yousaf and Adkhin (1992) indicate that approximately half of this money came from US taxpayers, and the rest came from the Saudi government and its wealthy Arab individuals.

Mohanty (2013) mentions that Pakistan's Directorate for ISI, worked as a liaison between the governments of Pakistan, the USA, and the *Mujāhidīn* to maintain the relationship. He further (2013, xiii) claims that the military dictator General Zia-ul-Haq, Pakistan's President, used *Jihād* to defeat the Soviets—the *Kafir* (infidels)—with an enormous amount of external support in terms of "money, military hardware, and training" to produce *Mujāhidīn* so that radical Islam resurged with thousands of radical Madrassas and mosques.

Riedel (2011) ascertains that with the support of the Saudis and the CIA, the ISI became capable of training *Mujāhidīn* by arranging training camps along the Durand Line to effectively fight against the Soviet invaders. Pakistan engaged its elite Special Services Group (SSG) in the training camps to train around 100,000 Muslims who came from a dozen countries to fight a "holy war" (Wynbrandt 2009; Riedel 2011).

According to Riedel (2011), the Soviet invasion offered Washington an opportunity to renew its cold war "love affair" with the Pakistan army and its intelligence agency. Carter's national security adviser, Zbigniew Brzezinski, visited Pakistan and offered more assistance for the *Mujāhidīn* and Pakistan. General Zia refused the first offer, considering it "peanuts," which was subsequently increased and took the form of trilateral relations—the American

CIA, Saudi's General Intelligence Directorate (GID), and Pakistan's Inter-Services Intelligence (ISI). As a result, Washington and Riyadh provided matching grants of money and arms, and *Islāmābād* dealt with distribution and training (ibid., 27).

Riedel (2011) additionally claims that Charles Nesbitt Wilson was an early enthusiast of the war effort, the Afghans, and especially of General Zia. He was part of the US White House committee for funding covert operations, providing the CIA with more money than they demanded, and equipping the *Mujāhidīn* with the Stinger surface-to-air missile system to ensure the defeat of the USSR by making it difficult for the Russians to control air traffic (ibid., 28).[3] Moreover, American President Ronald Reagan "waived the aid sanctions imposed on Pakistan under the Symington Amendment," that "assistance" "helped Pakistan's economy, removing the financial problems that had beset earlier regimes" and made the Pakistani army "able" to be modernized "with a $3.2 billion military-assistance package and the US provided weapons and training" (Wynbrandt 2009, 219).

A decade's involvement in the Afghan war made the USSR no longer able to continue the war that it was losing due to massive international support provided to the *Mujāhidīn*. Thus, the Union started negotiations to withdraw from the war under Zia's tenure (S.G. Jones and Fair 2010; Wynbrandt 2009). As a result, the Geneva Accords—an agreement to end the war—were signed on 14 April 1988. The USSR faced a defeat in Afghanistan in 1989 and disintegrated in 1990. The Soviets departed while leaving behind an unstable Communist regime, which was hardly in control of Kabul. Wynbrandt (2009, 219) states that the *Mujāhidīn* and the West interpreted this collapse of the Kabul government in April 1992 as a grand victory for Islam and a significant defeat for communism, respectively. With the enormous external support of the USA and its allies, the trained *Mujāhidīn* made Afghanistan into what became known as the USSR's Vietnam, as the war killed over one million Afghans, and created five million refugees (ibid., 219).

Impact of the USSR Invasion on Pakistan

The war ended in 1988. Notwithstanding, its adverse impacts remained in the region. The effects resonated continuously across Pakistan in the form of drug trafficking and gunrunning, which had formerly played a role in the fight against the USSR. Wynbrandt (2009) argues that the *Mujāhidīn* or "freedom fighters" started fighting with each other in Afghanistan and transformed the country into a lawless society. Eventually, the *Tālibān* "Islamic fundamentalists" controlled Afghanistan and created a safe abode for the "militant Islamists" (ibid., 219). Mohanty (2013) argues that the *Tālibān*—a mixture of *Mujāhidīn*—fought in Afghanistan against the Soviets in the 1980s, they emerged as a significant force in Afghan politics amid a civil war between forces in northern and southern Afghanistan in 1994. *Tālibān* initially controlled the southern city of Kandahar, and in

1996 they reached Kabul through a mixture of force, negotiation, and pay-offs to form the national government (ibid., 82). After that, the *Tālibān* took over Afghanistan.

According to Mohanty (2013), in 1976, with the support of the ISI and the CIA, Gulbuddin Hekmatyar—the Prime Minister of Afghanistan in 1993–1994—founded the *Hizb-e-Islamī* (Party of Islam, HeI) in Pakistan. Mohanty also writes that during the Soviet invasion, Hekmatyar received substantial American and Saudi aid to fight against the Soviets. Then he was involved in drug trafficking and advocated for a centralized Islamic State. Once the Soviets departed from Afghanistan, he declared the USA as Afghanistan's greatest enemy (ibid.). The HeI was associated with the deaths and destruction that paved the way for *Tālibān* rule. After that, during the *Tālibān* regime, Hekmatyar took refuge in Iran and declared to fight against the coalition forces until foreign troops left Afghanistan, and an Islamic government ruled Afghans. Meanwhile, Hekmatyar attempted to assassinate Afghan President Karzai, and in December 2002, the CIA revealed he had joined *Al-Qāidā* and helped Osama bin Laden to escape to Pakistan. In 2003, the USA declared him a terrorist (ibid., 84).

The micro-story mentioned above illustrates the production and spread of the *Tālibān* in the region, mainly in Afghanistan and Pakistan. On the one hand it was "the defeat and departure of the Soviet Union," and on the other, the USA abandoning Pakistan with "thousands of weapons, train-ing camps, and hundreds of thousands of well-trained *Mujāhidīn* terrorists," that caused havoc in this region such as suicide bombings (Mohanty 2013, xiv). This war helped Pakistan to expand its armed forces merely through the weapons given by the USA. To pursue the *Jihād*, the country employed religious institutions and parties, for example, the *Jamāt-e-Islamī* (JI) and the *Jamīat-e-Ulemā Islamī* (JUI) to establish Pakistan-based militant groups for operation in Afghanistan (S.G. Jones and Fair 2010, 11).

After the war, yesterday's *Mujāhidīn* have posed extreme challenges for the country. As on 8 June 2014, the TTP and the Islamic Movement of Uzbekistan (IMU)—an *Al-Qāidā* linked military organization—claimed responsibility for an attack on Pakistan's Jinnah International Airport in *Karāchī* (Golovnina 2014). Consequently, on 15 June 2014, the country's army launched Operation *Zarb-i-Azab*—a joint military offensive—against several militant groups in the North Waziristan region of Pakistan along the Afghanistan border. This operation targeted the TTP, the IMU, the East Turkestan Islamic Movement, *Lashkar-e-Jhangvi*, *Al-Qāidā*, *Jundullah*, and the Haqqani network.

Against this operation, six militants carried out an appalling massacre of schoolchildren of the Army Public School of Peshawar that occurred on 16 December 2014. Many media reported that the militants were foreign nationals: one Chechen, three Arabs, and two Afghans. This deadly inhu-mane assault killed around 150 people, including 132 schoolchildren. The *Guardian*—a UK newspaper—called this attack "Pakistan's 9/11" (Fishwick

2014). Afterward, several changes took place in the country; they included, among others, lifting its moratorium on the death penalty and authorizing military courts by a constitutional amendment. The army launched a country-wide operation called Operation *Raddul Fassad* that targeted these radicals.

Zia's Islamization and the Germination of Extremism

After seizing power from a democratic government, General Zia ul-Haq became the president of Pakistan, and in the name of restoring public order, suspended the promised elections to set the country on "an Islamic course." The Soviet invasion significantly fueled the realization of Zia's dream. Mohanty (2013, 68) maintains that the country, through waging a holy war (*Jihād*), nurtured the Saudi Arabian Wahabi school, in which the Saudi government financed several critical projects in Pakistan, alongside the insurgency in Afghanistan. During this enthusiastic engagement in the Afghan operation, according to Riedel (2011, 28), the USA remained inattentive to the other plans of General Zia, such as nurturing *Jihād* in Pakistan, that is, the flocking of volunteers from other countries to Pakistan to help the *Mujāhidīn*.

Riedel (2011) illustrates that Zia had already planned for the "next stage of *Jihād*," to wage wars with India and in Kashmir, since the inception of the Afghan war. In the early 1980s, Zia secretly met with Maulana Abdul Bari—a *Jamāt* leader and veteran *Jihādist* who fought in Operation Gibraltar in 1965 and promised that he would use the war against the Soviet invaders to build a support base for a Kashmiri insurgency (ibid., 25–6). To achieve this aim, Zia consulted the *Jamāt-i-Islamī* Party, whose founder Maulana Sayyid Abul A'ala Mawdudi, already advocated using force to make a Muslim state within India and opposed the secular vision of Jinnah and Jinnah's independence movement; later on, the party became the army's enthusiastic and active ally during the war against Bengali freedom in 1971.

Tariq Ali (1983, 164) notes that Ronald Reagan's winning of the US election in November 1980 occurred "as a sorely needed relief for military dictators" across the world, including Zia of Pakistan. As noted earlier, the Soviet invasion in December 1979 created an opportunity for both the USA and Pakistan to support each other against their rising enemies. During this time, Zia made substantial efforts to strengthen the influence of Islamic parties and the *Ulemā* (religious scholars) on the government and society with implicit American support for the formation and activities of militant extremist groups (Wynbrandt 2009, 215–16).

In his first address to the nation, Zia promised to make an exemplary Islamic society. He formed a government Sharia committee or religious law court for dealing with the cases according to the Holy *Qurān* and the Sunna.[4] The council was responsible for adjusting the legal statutes of the country, such as putting in place the Islamic ban on paying interest (literally: Riba), performing prayers five times daily, and avoiding food and drinks during Ramadan (ibid., 216).

Creation of a "real" Islamic society continued through introducing the Islamic Hadood (boundaries or limits) into the country's law to deal with "the drinking and manufacturing of alcohol, theft, adultery, false accusations of adultery, and highway robbery" (ibid., 216). General Zia passed this Hadood Ordinance in February 1979, to order punishments such as floggings, amputations, and death by stoning. Explicitly, the third ordinance adversely impacted women so that if a woman is raped and becomes pregnant as a result, she could be charged with adultery, and in that case, a testimony of two women together would invalidate the testimony of one man (ibid., 216).

Later, the *Zakāt* and *Ushr* Ordinance was passed and adopted in June 1980 to engage Islamic scholars to incorporate the Islamic principles and laws relating to finance and the economy. This ordinance introduced an annual deduction of 2.5% as *Zakāt*—a form of alms for the poor—from the bank accounts of all Muslims irrespective of a sect[5] that held more than PKR3,000 (almost $25) (Wynbrandt 2009). *Ushr* was implemented for the landowners and farmers in the form of a levy of 10% of the total produce. To oversee the distribution of the collected funds, *Zakāt* committees were constituted.

These significant changes continued with the implementation of the blasphemy law. As of 1986, if someone says something against the Prophet Muhammad, they risk life imprisonment or death. Islamic studies and the Arabic language became compulsory courses for numerous degree programs. The broadcasting of news in the Arabic language on television and radio started. Compulsory veiling was introduced for female newsreaders on television. Religious teachers were also promoted to the rank of commissioned officers in the army for the first time. Citizens protested against growing Islamization, but Zia manipulated the Soviet invasion to present it as an emerging threat to Islam from the infidel forces just across the border and called for the necessary Islamization to govern Pakistan based on Islamic ideals (ibid., 217).

For his position, Mohanty elucidates that the world praised "Zia for standing against the mighty Soviets and for giving shelter to three million refugees from war-torn Afghanistan" (Mohanty 2013, 89). As Casey's deputy for operations in Afghanistan would later recount, "Zia was a believer [and] without Zia, there would have been no Afghan war, and no Afghan victory" (Riedel 2011, 18).

The Soviet invasion provided Zia with an excellent opportunity to transform the country and alter the course of its future more than any other ruler since Jinnah—the country's founder. Zia can, therefore, rightly be called the grandfather of global Islamic *Jihād* (Riedel 2011, 20). Since he was an Islamist, he affiliated himself with *Jamāt-i-Islam*—a religious party in the country—and did as much as he could to Islamicize the country's army (Ibid., 20). Riedel (2011, 21) cites Shuja Nawaz—an expert on the Pakistani army—who says that "Islamization was the legacy [Zia] left Pakistan," but this was undoubtedly possible with external support.

Moreover, during Zia's transformation, Riedel (2011, 21) quotes Steve Coll, who counts the formation of Madrassa—of the Islamic schools—which multiplied from 900 to 8,000 official religious schools and 25,000 unregistered within 17 years from 1971 to 1988. Diplomas awarded by the Madrassas were made equivalent to university degrees. Needless to say, the series of external "events" provided Zia with the best chances to Islamicize the country, which caused internal chaos, as Pakistan's second-largest Islamic sect, that is, the Shia (in terms of number, the Shia are more than those who either practice other sects of Islam or other religions) came under attack as Zia attempted to use force against them after the Shia revolution in Iran (ibid., 22). More importantly, Nasar (1994) critically writes that—under Zia's support—the anti-Shia militant Sunni groups such as the *Sipāh-e-Sahābā* Pakistan (the Army of the Prophet's Companions) blossomed and attacked Shia mosques and religious festivities to intimidate the Shia community into quiescence.

During my upbringing in Pakistan, I observed how intense this chaos was. The Shia population came under attack. The Shia *Kafir* (Shia infidels) slogans loomed around the country: the hate speeches started; the slogans appeared in the form of chalk markings on walls. The targeted killings of Shia intellectuals and famous personalities commenced. Major Shia gatherings and processions were attacked, especially with suicide bombs. The repercussion included the Hazara community, who came to Europe, including Austria, for refuge during this decade owing to those historical events. Hundreds of Hazara, being the practitioners of Shia-Islam, were killed. These refugees are a result of the seed of Islamization that Zia germinated, and external forces watered to grow.

Moreover, there are different standpoints on the Soviet invasion event. On the one hand, the USA has been considered as "partly responsible for Pakistan's overreliance on the military, rather than civilian power, because it has provided so much assistance to the Ministry of Defense" (S.G. Jones and Fair 2010, xv). On the other hand, Mohanty (2013, 81) cites Ayaz Amir—a Pakistani freelance writer and politician—who bluntly writes: "These people [*Tāliban*] were certified as God's holy warriors by the White House itself. Now they have been transformed into the world's darkest villains. That is complicated. However, the opinion that Pakistan has no choice other than to fight these people is becoming stronger."[6]

Hence, the war against the invasion of the USSR in Afghanistan ended with what I call a great "leftover." For this involvement, Pakistan has to pay the "costs" in the form of "Kalashnikov culture"—especially the Soviet's Kalashnikov or AK-47 (Avtomat Kalashnikov 1947) and similar Eastern Bloc rifles that were used to drive the Soviet army—that people started using arms to settle any dispute. The easy availability of arms created a different set of attitudes and behaviors of using force.[7] Besides, Pakistan witnessed around four million Afghan refugees who entered Pakistan to escape war; thus, the war caused depopulation in Afghanistan (Riedel 2011, 24; Wynbrandt 2009, 218–19) and "over" population in Pakistan—an already overpopulated country.

In terms of Pakistan needing to pay the price of the leftover aspects, Wynbrandt (2009) mentions that an influx of Afghan refugees crossed the border and mainly settled into *Baluchistān* and Khyber Pakhtunkhwa (KPK) provinces. This influx aggravated the destabilization in an already unstable territory because both the regions became part of Pakistan in the name of economic benefit and Muslim solidarity (Wynbrandt 2009, 219). The federation's inequitable distribution and sharing of revenues and benefits from the provincial natural resources was one of the significant grievances of *Baluchistān*. Natural gas (Sui-northern-gas) discovered in *Baluchistān* in 1953 was available for the cities in *Punjāb* province by 1964. However, it did not reach Quetta—the *Baluchistān* capital—until 1986, except for gas supply to a military garrison in the province (ibid., 220).

Wynbrandt (2009) claims that the federal government foresaw "little need to placate" the population in *Baluchistān,* which was 5% of the country's population despite being a geographically bigger province that constitutes 40% of the whole country's land. With 45% Baloch and 38% Pashtun, the arrival of Afghan refugees to make up one-quarter of *Baluchistān* ignited a conflict between the Baloch and Pashtun. This is because refugees changed the ethnic composition in the province while making the Baloch less in number in their "homeland." Resultantly, the Baloch were devastated, and clashes started between these two social groups. In 1988, over disaffection with the federal government, Baloch hijacked a Pakistan International Airlines (PIA) aircraft to protest against the discrimination and "what they believed were planned tests of nuclear weapons" in their province (ibid., 221).

In contrast, similar agitation occurred in the KPK province in the Pashtun population who wanted to achieve more autonomy, since there were also some movements for an independent Pashtun nation, and the federal government's continuous negligence of the provinces aggravated the discontent. Therefore, the shift of refugees to KPK made the call for an independent Pashtun area more visible (ibid.).

Riedel (2011, 18) cites Robert Gates, who was a deputy director for intelligence and responsible for all intelligence analysis during William Casey's tenure (the CIA director), saying in 1996:

We examined ways to increase their [*Tālibān*] participation, perhaps in the form of some "international brigade," but nothing came of it. Years later, these fundamentalist fighters trained by the Mujahedin in Afghanistan would begin to show up around the world, from the Middle East to New York City, still fighting their Holy War—only now including the United States among their enemies.

Externally, the cost of being part of that holy war that Pakistan needs to pay includes the interventions which the Soviet Union and its Afghan Communist allies took "to destabilize Pakistan." Both countries hired agents to explode bombs in the refugee camps, assassinate *Mujāhidīn* leaders, and attack the ISI training facilities (ibid., 24–5).

Summing this historical sketch, the Reagan administration strengthened "the most revanchist elements inside the army, with a political short-sightedness that borders on suicide" (T. Ali 1983, 192–93). The current movements and the past "events" are directly connected, and "how much those events have affected, it seems difficult to answer with a clear certainty" (ibid., 190). Yet one can see their significant implications for the country, including its life-saving endeavor: the vaccination program.

The extremism often causes a "tug of war" between Pakistan and the USA. In 2017, the *Dawn* (2017) newspaper published, "Don't blame Pakistan, Haqqanis were your 'darlings' at one time: Asif tells [the] US[A]," while indicating to the USA, do not blame Pakistan for the Haqqanis (the Haqqani Network) and the Hafiz Saeeds (referring to the head of the banned Jamaatud Dawah). Twenty to 30 years ago, they were "your darlings," who were being "wined and dined in the White House, and now you say, go to hell Pakistanis because you are nurturing these people." The words used in the paper reveal the strength of opinion. Nonetheless, the same news report also contains the willingness of Pakistan to work with the USA for peace maintenance in Afghanistan.

Concluding Remarks

Significantly impacting the country, the critical events related to (geo)politics that I specified above, have shaped the general perceptions and practices that people in Pakistan hold and perform, including about vaccination. Consequently, they maintain their intransigent hostilities and positions against it. Historically, external problems and internal crises have gone hand in hand in Pakistan's short but critical history. External events have caused as well as aggravated the internal crises. The impact of colonization, as described by the renowned economist William Easterly (2006, 298), resulted in "the massacre during partition, four international wars, two genocides, six secessionist[s], and umpteen communal massacres later." The results of the aftermath still appear in one form or another.

Thereafter, I describe how during the USSR invasion, Pakistan became a vital ally of the USA in a massive covert program to raise and equip an army of Islamic fighters—*Mujāhidīn*—that caused global terrorism at the end of the century (Wynbrandt 2009, 202). Zia's impudent attempts to Islamize the country supported substantially by the external events, led toward a difficult-to-repair rift among the masses. These events are still creating further fractions in the country in diverse forms. Since then, the running of Pakistan, as Ian Talbot argues, never goes beyond the cliché of the three "As": *Allāh*, the Army, and America (Cohen 2004, 267).

The same *Mujāhidīn*, later on, called Pakistani *Tehrik-i-Tālibān* (TTP), has overwhelmingly challenged the country. In 2008, they took over the Swat region of Pakistan and executed several people. They also conducted numerous assaults on the vaccinators, and suicide bombings and assaults at public gatherings, mosques, shrines, airports, educational institutions, and army installations. During these assaults, over 100 vaccinators and their escorting security personnel have been killed. *Mujāhidīn* has openly opposed vaccination in the country. Studies have demonstrated that the poliovirus is highly prevalent in those areas of *Mujāhidīn*'s stronghold in the country.

Notes

1 That division received the name after Henry Mortimer Durand who was its architect and the foreign secretary for India.
2 To elucidate the rivalry between these two countries, Rudyard Kipling used the term "Great Game," for the first time in his novel *Kim* in 1901.
3 Charles Nesbitt Wilson (1933–2010)—a representative and naval officer and former 12-term Democratic US Representative from Texas—almost had "three dozen trips to the region, stopping in Cairo, Jerusalem, Riyadh, and Islamabad each time to get backing from America's key allies. Usually accompanied by a beautiful woman, Charlie flattered the allies, and they flattered him, even to the point of making him a secret field marshal in the Pakistani army" (Riedel 2011, 28). At the time of Zia's death in August 1988, "Wilson wept, telling Akhtar's successor, Hamid Gul, 'I have lost my Father on this day'" (George Crile III cited by Riedel, 2011, p. 28).
4 The book of conventions of the Prophet's axioms and deeds to follow Islamic law.
5 Here, it is essential to mention that the Shia sect has a different interpretation of Zakat. This implementation brought different forms of resentment across the country.
6 I have made a few changes to maintain the formatting such as from 'that's' to 'that is' or 'they've' to 'they have.'
7 On this impact of guns in Pakistan, the *Washington Post* (1996) published an interesting editorial.

9 National and Global Rituals of Containment

Controversies, Contestations, and Mistrust Surrounding Vaccination in Pakistan

Vaccinating Pakistan: The Beginning and the Current

Vaccination began in Pakistan in the 1970s. After the country signed the Charter with the United Nations (UN) for controlling and eliminating infectious diseases, the Expanded Programme of Immunization (EPI) began in Pakistan in 1976 on a pilot scale and then was expanded across the country in 1978 (Hasan, Bosan, and Bile 2010). In the beginning, the EPI aimed to protect children aged 0–11 months against six contagious diseases—childhood poliomyelitis, tuberculosis, diphtheria, tetanus, pertussis, and measles—to reduce child mortality and morbidity (WHO 2019a). However, over time, new vaccines were introduced, such as hepatitis B in 2002, Hemophilus influenza type b (Hib) in 2009, pneumococcal vaccine (PCV10) in 2012, and inactivated polio vaccine in 2015 (ibid.). Vaccination also immunizes pregnant women.

The WHO (2016b) mentions the specific objectives of this program: to interrupt poliovirus by 2012; eliminate neonatal tetanus and measles by 2015; reduce diphtheria, pertussis, and childhood tuberculosis to a minimum level so that they do not become a public health problem; control other infectious diseases by introducing new vaccines once they become available; and use EPI as a spearhead for promoting other primary healthcare activities, and integrate the EPI into primary healthcare.

The EPI follows a top-down approach: federal, provincial, district, subdistrict, and Basic Health Unit (BHU) levels. The vaccine transmission or delivery from province to district level occurs in a particular vehicle containing coolers so as to maintain the cold chain. The Executive District Officer (EDO) works as the district head and is responsible for receiving the vaccines. Also, there is an EPI focal person who is responsible for all duties from storage to distribution.

To ensure the administration of vaccines, the monitoring teams visit the field and interview the target group, for example, parents. The frequent questions asked include: (a) Does a vaccinator visit your village to vaccinate your children? (b) Could you please show us the vaccination card, if your child is immunized? (c) If the card is available, the vaccination status of that child

DOI: 10.4324/9781003253716-10

is written there. In the absence of the card, the BCG scar is monitored and considered as a proof that a vaccinator approached the child.

As a month starts, vaccinators of every BHU visit the district level office to receive vaccines according to the target population. A vaccinator maintains a stock register, which encompasses all daily records of a vaccine—the number of vaccines received, used, and remaining. The MO supervises the entire process. At a UC level, the vaccine is stored in the respective BHU at a controlled temperature and then distributed among vaccinators according to the due and defaulter list for the vaccination.

Despite the efforts of the government and the WHO's noteworthy partners, the country still has to meet the immunization indicators (WHO 2019a). The primary goals of eradicating polio, measles, and neonatal tetanus remain incomplete so far. Routine vaccination coverage is still not according to the standards for attaining the anticipated goals.

For instance, in September 2015, the *Dawn* newspaper published a report: "Over 75,000 children in Sindh never received polio vaccine" (Mansoor 2015b). According to this report, around 440,000 of the country's children never received a vaccine, and out of them, 56% are in *Baluchistān*, 17% in Sindh, 14% in the FATA, and 12% in KPK. It precisely demonstrates the state of vaccination in the country, though the figures are about polio vaccination. If polio vaccination is in such a critical state after receiving enormous attention from the government and global stakeholders, then one can predict something critical about the entire immunization program. Numerous outbreaks of measles, pertussis, diphtheria, and prevalence of polio in several parts of the country are evidence of the "poor" routine coverage.

Mushtaq and colleagues (2015) note that, from 2003 to 2006, polio was transmitted to approximately 24 polio-free countries, causing around 1,400 cases, most of which had originated from Pakistan. In 2007, Australia reported a poliovirus infection in a man who traveled from Pakistan (Stewardson et al. 2009). Likewise, the strains of the poliovirus in cases identified in China, Egypt, and Palestine during January 2012, December 2012, and March 2013, respectively, were also traced back to Pakistan (Luo et al. 2013; Ebrahim 2014).

Consequently, vaccination was made mandatory for Pakistani travelers to travel abroad, including to Saudi Arabia for the Hajj and Umrah (Mushtaq et al. 2015).[1] They were required to show a vaccine card at airports. Yet, how was the notion of receiving the vaccine before traveling put into practice? Sharing my fieldwork diary, which includes an anecdote illustrating this vaccination obligation, provides profound insight.

I was traveling to Austria for the second time after the completion of this fieldwork. Media regularly broadcasted about a travel ban without providing the "yellow card"—the evidence of vaccination—at Pakistan's airports along with the visa and passport. Because I was working on this project and considered it an urgent matter, I decided to receive the vaccine and a "yellow card." I talked to a friend[2] who was working in a health department at a district level, about it. While I was in *Islāmābād* to travel to Vienna, his suggestion was astounding: "You are too old to receive the vaccine, so please send me your details for the registration here. Then I will post you the card. After this WHO requirement, numerous people aspiring to travel abroad come to us and receive the cards without taking the vaccination." I declined the offer, which made my friend angry.

To receive the vaccination, I visited the NIH, where another aspiring traveler was already there for the vaccination. Interestingly, the unit head called us inside his office and asked about the countries we were planning to travel to and the purpose of our journeys. The interaction was a small interview. Subsequently, he reasoned with a smile, "See, my son! I have heard that people are not receiving the vaccine, but the cards. Therefore, I have decided to perform this duty with honesty and vaccinate people myself." He opened the vaccine's vial and gave each of us two drops of the vaccine. Although I have already received the hepatitis vaccine via injection, I received an oral vaccine for the first time in my life. After that, the person in charge provided us with yellow cards to show them at the airport. The most astonishing thing occurred at the airport when nobody inquired about the cards to prove the status of vaccination.

This personal experience shows a difference between theory about vaccination and practical initiatives: a gap between the proposed protocols and following them. This can be associated with the prevalence of infectious disease in the country. There are many reasons behind this gap: Why are the set objectives incomplete despite the efforts? This critical state compels questions to be posed to explore the underlying causes and consequences. Failure to achieve the anticipated results signifies that something is "wrong" or "missing" somewhere. This current study seeks to discover those causes.

Vaccination Programs as "Political Programs"

Vaccination, after a successful breakthrough of knowledge, has continuously refracted into multiple and successive transfigurations of meanings that carry certainties and uncertainties. Over time, vaccination has met with ambivalent attitudes and emerged as a complex and contested phenomenon. A vaccine as a "new technology"—connecting various stakeholders in diverse locations—has received a peculiar response across the globe (Feldman-Savelsberg, Ndonko, and Schmidt-Ehry 2000; Renne 2010; Blume 2017, 2006; Greenough, Holmberg, and Blume 2017; Colgrove 2006). Vaccination programs are also "political" in nature (Greenough, Blume, and Holmberg 2017, 1) as they contain politics happening at different levels around the world.

Anti-vaccination movements have occurred worldwide. For example, in Austria and the USA, some people refuse vaccines. In these two countries, the refusals have connections to an inherent potential of the body: the fact that it should work without intervention and, in the USA, the deep belief that vaccines can cause harm, including such diseases as autism, especially when too many are given at once, overwhelming the child's immune system. However, the refusals in Pakistan are distinguishable in multiple ways from those of other countries, which I will explore below. In Pakistan, there are also other factors related to economics and geopolitics that shape people's perceptions and practices of a vaccine. Controversies related to vaccination in Pakistan are comparable to some other countries, such as Cameroon (Feldman-Savelsberg, Ndonko, and Schmidt-Ehry 2000) and Nigeria (Renne 2010), where vaccination is under a spotlight and considered as a "Western plot" to "sterilize women." Mark Nichter (1995) finds a similar contestation in India, where Muslims and Hindus mistrusted the vaccination after linking it with some hidden political agendas: Muslims feared that Hindus might covertly want to reduce the Muslim population and justified the government's initiative to control the population. Nichter goes on to recount an encounter where a man revealed to him the perceived "real purpose of vaccination programs," interpreting vaccinations as an extension of Christian missionaries (ibid., 618). This resonates with what Fairhead and Leach (2007) term "vaccine anxieties" that reflect politico-economic concerns.

In Pakistan, people's narratives of vaccination are intertwined with geopolitics, international relations, and/or past and present "foreign affairs" and economic regimes. They suspect the subtle hegemonic forces at play and view vaccination not only as a material phenomenon but see a hidden ideology attributed to it. There is a link between the justifications of anti-vaccine sentiments and some other intertwined "critical events" that are happening now and have happened in the past, especially events related to geopolitics. These include colonization; the invasion of Afghanistan by the Union of Soviet Socialist Republics (USSR); and the creation and growth of the *Tālibān*, who cultivated extremism and suspicion in the country. These events happened in the 1980s when Pakistan agreed to produce the *Tālibān* to defeat the USSR. Recent events include a war on terrorism, drones, and the use of a "fake" vaccination drive to locate Osama bin Laden. Connecting global and local realities, forming new forms of knowledge and action, and rearranging social relations in significant ways, vaccination—an intervention to the individual physical body—indeed can be associated with the "body politic" and "social body" (Scheper-Hughes and Lock 1987). Vaccination in Pakistan, hence, is imbued with differing and widely varying dynamics. The anti-vaccination movements illuminate the complex connections among local, national, and global factors and stakeholders. They encompass intertwining shaped by sociocultural, economic, geopolitical, and historical factors. Mistrust has notably surfaced among parents and the government, local and global stakeholders, as well as national and global stakeholders. While these multiple links overlap, they cannot be simply reduced to one another.

The Vaccination–Reproduction Connection

Suspicions related to fertility control have a long history. Prior to industrialization, population growth was universally encouraged, because, in the absence of technological advancement, human power was the primary means to the production of wealth. Nonetheless, the Industrial Revolution in Western Europe also brought the so-called "demographic transition" of the late eighteenth century (Andrade and Hussain 2018). Cities attracted mass migration, and as technologies replaced human labor, overpopulation came to be a pressing concern (Bongaarts 2009).

About this overpopulation, Robert Malthus (1872) in his classic book, *An Essay on the Principle of Population,* argued that food resources grow at an arithmetic rate, while the population grows at an exponential rate. These different growth patterns would eventually lead populations to reduce their sizes through war, disease, and famine. He insisted on the need for abstinence rather than contraceptives for the sake of population control. Malthus opposed those laws and social programs that would give any assistance to the poor, because to him, these initiatives would encourage population growth (M. Rao 2004). Thereafter, the disciples of Social Darwinism manipulated Malthus's disapproval of welfare programs in the later nineteenth century (Rogers 1972). Their ruthless ambition to rid society of its "undesirable" population paved the way for conspiracy theories to point out a "New World Order"; namely that global efforts are underway to control population size through ulterior means (Andrade and Hussain 2018).

According to conspiracy theorist Leonard Horowitz (1997), the medical sector plays a pivotal role in that population control scheme. Horowitz claimed that new viruses and vaccines are produced by the medical industry to achieve population reduction. In this view, he suggests that these entities are intentionally involved in activities that would lead to a decrease in the global population. It's important to note that such claims lack scientific support and are widely considered unfounded and baseless by mainstream medical and scientific communities.

Likewise, in Pakistan, people harbored resentment toward vaccination after linking it with reproduction. This resentment most prominently surfaced after the introduction of the family planning system, when the country created the Family Planning Association of Pakistan (FPAP) in 1953 to ensure "the right population" (see Lock and Nguyen 2010). Afterward, controlling and managing the population became part of the country's five-year plans from 1965 to 1970 onward (see Chapter 7). Family planning, nevertheless, received immense resistance owing to specific sociocultural, economic, and political reasons (Hakim 2001; Robinson 1966). For Andrade and Hussain (2018, 1–7), the conspiracy theories related to reproduction have a Western origin.

Nevertheless, conspiracy mongering grows successfully in specific contexts such as the sociocultural and the political (Douglas, Sutton, and Cichocka 2017). First, family planning was perceived as contradicting the belief system: God controls and decides on the conception of a baby. Stopping conception or aborting a fetus are both *Harām* (prohibited) actions in Islam because, through them, one intervenes in the business of God. Every child brings *Rizq* (a source of survival) with birth through God's will; therefore, the number of children should not be a worry for the parents. Second, it is to interfere in what is locally considered people's most "private" matter—sex—on which an open discussion is wholly discouraged. According to my observations, many women are willing to adopt family planning interventions; however, shyness hinders them from discussing the precautionary measures. Third, Pakistan is an agrarian society; therefore, more reproduction means more economic production, as the underlying belief is that more hands guarantee higher production in the agricultural fields in the absence of technology. A famous proverb in Sindh province has it that *Jetrā Hath, Otro Fāido* (as the number of hands increases, so grow the rewards). Fourth, family planning is considered as a "Western plot" to decrease the Muslim population, as—according to belief—the West fears that Muslims may come to control their countries and pose a challenge to their sociocultural patterns. Laypeople believe that as many children as possible should be produced to spread the followers of the Holy Prophet, Muhammad. Fifth, family planning also has been strongly linked with colonialization, because, though the British came first for the sake of trade, later, they took advantage of their higher power to intervene in politics and to colonize the subcontinent to exploit its resources.

Resistance against family planning was not only in Pakistan but was also recorded in India and Bangladesh (see Nichter 1995). People perhaps had the stories and memories of colonialism in their minds, which ultimately led them toward resistance, fearing family planning as a new move to control them. I call this a "societal memory," which records and keeps fresh in people's minds the humiliating, horrific, unpleasant, and lingering experiences of the colonized. The memory, over time, may blur but does not entirely vanish. Resonant events or circumstances evoke societal memory. Analogous to the human body, society also develops antibodies and releases them when encountering happenings similar to those of the past. The memories of colonization are preserved in the societal memory. Several post-modern anthropologists trace the roots of violence to colonization (Otterbein 1999; Hinton 2002; Ferguson 2004; Scheper-Hughes and Bourgois 2004; Whitehead 2004).

Vaccines were locally perceived as a new move to control the population in Pakistan, as they were in Nigeria (Renne 2010). Various anthropologists have illustrated this point (e.g., Lock and Nguyen 2010; Feldman-Savelsberg, Ndonko, and Schmidt-Ehry 2000). These conspiracy theories give no meaning in a vacuum, but once connected, they paint a comprehensive picture that what is happening is entirely explicable (see Murakami et al. 2014; Andrade and Hussain 2018; Horowitz 1997).

Perception about Vaccination: Rumors and Conspiracy Theories

Our sociocultural history is full of narratives. We construct them to make sense of our lives—and, more importantly, to transfer knowledge and wisdom to the next generations. Rumors and conspiracy theories are critical, and many times untested facts. Rabo (2005, 163) considers them "tautological and self-referential" that "can be seen as a desperate expression of the weak." These are forms of narratives, social phenomena (Ali 2020g), which particularly emerge to make sense of extraordinary situations. Hence, these can be interpreted against the backdrop of sociocultural, economic, and geopolitical contexts, which are local and global in terms of scale, because they signify the connections between and among them.

Turner (1993) considers a rumor to be something beyond a symbolic phenomenon since rumors generate relationships between unequal social segments. Feldman-Savelsberg and colleagues (2000) discovered a rumor's ties to local, regional, and national contexts, which further are linked to global political movements in the case of anti-tetanus vaccination in Cameroon. Nancy Scheper-Hughes (1996), after exploring the organ-stealing rumors in the shantytowns of Brazil in the mid-1980s, contends that rumors can contain a global dimension. A rumor, hence, takes place in a specific social, cultural, economic, and political context as it indexes inequality and politics.

Similar rumors and conspiracy theories have surrounded vaccination in Pakistan, which mainly, as mentioned earlier, emerged during the family planning in the country in the 1960s (Ali 2020a). Rumors thereafter have continued in waves and never ended. Before going into detailed accounts of a rumor concerning vaccination and Osama bin Laden, here are a few words about how a rumor spreads in Sindh province. Although this event occurred in the district Khairpur (different than the locale of the study) of Sindh and is about an animal called a "honey badger" during 2016, it provides empirical evidence about the way rumors circulate. The event occurred in the recent past; thus, it helps us to comprehend how rumors and conspiracy theories emerge during a challenging situation. It illustrates how a rumor travels in the chosen area, and people start believing it as truth. This case would supply a context to understand various narratives related to vaccination. I learned about the event from my family and friends via mobile calls. The first time I heard about these narratives was from my family, as I usually made a phone call to them during my (post-fieldwork) stay in Vienna, Austria. One day, they shared stories, and then due to my curiosity, I followed it. Another day, I called one of my friends in my hometown who started telling the following story:

> During July and August 2016, word-of-mouth spread about a small animal. The rumor has it that a small animal appears and attacks people after sunset, especially with its paws that are highly poisonous. The animal is aggressive and dangerous, and no one knows its origin. It has the potential to kill an entire family at one time.

Consequently, the attacked person dies. There were two different narratives. First, the animal is an Indian conspiracy. Since the country's border is adjacent, someone set them free in Pakistan while importing them. An alternative version of it was that these animals were in a zoo in India, which had been deliberately broken to set them free to cause havoc in Pakistan. Secondly, the animal had just emerged from somewhere and was unknown to this area.

Fear grew larger and stronger as the rumor spread; villages started to ensure security by assigning duties to different individuals to provide 24-hour fool-proof security. People, especially children, were afraid to sleep. The male members stopped sleeping at an *Otāq* (men's guest house) or walking outside the house during the night, especially after sunset. People made frequent announcements about seeing the animal in this and that area. Such statements caused people to gather with their dogs and weapons such as sticks, rifles, pistols, and axes. These gatherings attracted the local media—print and electronic—that reached those sites and broadcast the news. A few deaths occurred, which were associated with the animal. The dead bodies contained "paw"-like marks. The dead bodies further added fear into an already chaotic situation. The terror of this rumor continued for over a month. On the other hand, some believed that the people who died were "thieves."

As I have shown at several places in this book, before May 2011, there was a perception in Pakistan about vaccination being a "Western plot" or a conspiracy. In essence, the theory goes that vaccination aims to sterilize Muslim women to decrease the population because the West feels threatened. This viewpoint became visible after launching the family planning program in the country (see earlier section). The program received considerable resistance. The reference point of 2011 does not mean that the perception is no longer there. However, the reshaping of it owes significantly to a critical event that happened in 2011, in which a "bogus" vaccination drive was conducted.

Vaccination started when family planning was receiving great resistance in the country. Hence, people perceived it in the same way as they perceived (and refused to accept) the contraceptives. Local people suspected that their refusal of contraceptives forced the officials to devise procedures to control the population by vaccinating children to make them infertile. It can be argued that the perception that vaccination was a replacement for contraceptives provided a basis for believing that vaccination was also a "Western plot" for sterilizing Muslims.

Yet the intensity of local perception of vaccination differs in the county. In the northern areas of Pakistan, people are resisting the vaccine, while in other parts, mostly, they are outright refusing it (Murakami et al. 2014; Andrade and Hussain 2018). The resistance primarily depends on the recent past's incident—the "fake" vaccination—while the latter one always has some historical roots. Some anthropologists have explored these connections between history and rumors (e.g., Ali 2020a; Sobo 2016; Biehl 2016; McGranahan 2016).

In 2015, the National Geographic Channel produced a series of articles with four parts (McGirk 2015b, 2015a; Mullaney and Hassan 2015; Motlagh 2015). Three of them mainly focused on Pakistan's immunization program while linking the vaccination and anti-vaccination sentiments with critical events shaped by global politics. The first article, entitled "How the Bin Laden Raid Put Vaccinators Under the Gun in Pakistan," contains eye-opener reasoning on the anti-vaccination movement that "some clerics claimed falsely that the vaccine was made of pig products, which are taboo for Muslims. Even more bizarre was a story, widely circulated after the US invasion of Afghanistan, that the vaccine contained urine from then President George W. Bush" (McGirk 2015a).

To produce such anti-vaccination sentiment in Pakistan, several clerics utilized the channels of the Friday Sermons and other platforms. The KPK province especially witnessed it in the form of sermons and distributions of pamphlets. The ideology—"stopping and aborting the children through artificial methods is intervening into the business of God"—played a pivotal role in spreading such views. These standpoints cultivated grounds for the clerics to propagate refusal of the vaccinations. On 13 June 2012, the *Express Tribune* (2012a) released a news report that a *Cleric declares Jihād [sic] against polio campaign* in *Punjāb* province while declaring it "un-Islamic." Eventually, the police tried to arrest him, but he escaped. The report reads:

> When the local cleric, Maulvi Ibrahim Chisti, found out about the campaign, he immediately went to the biggest mosque in the area and declared that polio drops are "poison" and against Islam. He added that if the polio team forced anybody to partake in the vaccination campaign, then *Jihād* [sic] was "the only option." As a result, the polio team returned to Muzaffargarh city without conducting immunisation activities and reported the matter to Muzaffargarh Health Executive District Officer (EDO), Dr. Aashiq Hussain, who in turn informed the Muzaffargarh District Coordination Officer (DCO), Tahir Khursheed. A police inquiry was ordered, after which a raid was carried out in the cleric's area. However, Chisti had already escaped by the time the police arrived. Residents said the cleric had tried to convince them that the polio campaign was a "Western conspiracy" to render the population impotent. After the police raid, the polio team returned to Khan Pur Bagga Sher to implement the polio immunisation campaign.

These news reports received global attention. These are broadcasted though not frequently. As in 2007, the *Guardian*—the UK leading daily—also reported, "Polio cases jump in Pakistan as clerics declare vaccination an

American plot" (Walsh 2007). The clerics' interpretation plays a massive role in creating anti-vaccination sentiment in the country (Warraich 2009).

The production and circulation of the abovementioned news reports signify a perception that continues to exist in Pakistan. The intensity in specific cases may be smaller or larger, but the prevalence of the reports itself speaks enough. The reports function as counternarratives against the biomedical standpoint on vaccination. The following section elucidates the conversion of that perception into reality.

"Vaccination Suicide": A Reality?

The previous description mentioned the details about vaccination based on events that occurred up to 2011. The current description is a post-2011 analysis, which describes some contemporary controversies related to vaccination. The anti-vaccination sentiment was further exacerbated after using the vaccination for a different purpose or with a "hidden agenda" as some claim. The American CIA administered a "fake" vaccination drive in Pakistan's northern areas in 2010, and then focused on Abbottabad city only to learn of the whereabouts of the most wanted person on the planet at the time: Osama bin Laden (McGirk 2015b, 2015a; Mullaney and Hassan 2015). The vaccination functioned as a means to an end: not to improve health but to find and kill bin Ladin.

Media across the globe reported this news of the "fake" vaccination campaign that the CIA started searching for Osama bin Laden in spring 2010 by hiring a local doctor, Dr. Shakeel Afridi, and nurses from Pakistan to implement a door-to-door vaccination drive against hepatitis B (J. Marszal 2016; Ahmed 2014; Fox News 2012; Online Mail 2012; S. Shah 2011). The sole purpose was to collect the DNA from syringes used to immunize the children living in that villa and make a connection to bin Laden.

As mentioned earlier, the National Geographic Channel produced four investigative reports, and three of them particularly focused on vaccination in Pakistan. The articles describe how vaccination was used as a cover to obtain information about Osama bin Laden and how that operation further affected the immunization program in the country. McGirk (2015a) writes:

> The Pakistani health official that [the] CIA operatives approached was Dr. Shakil Afridi. Tall and stout, with a cropped mustache that gave him a military bearing, Afridi had the right credentials from the CIA's perspective. He was a Pashtun and spoke the local language, Pashto. He had conducted a successful vaccination campaign near the Khyber Pass, in north-western Pakistan. He had lived in California for several months and had family in the United States. The doctor says that he never knew he was working for the CIA and that he was approached by a local representative of Save the Children, who asked him to run the vaccination campaign. (Save the Children denies having any connection with the

CIA or any intelligence agency, or having any role in the subterfuge.) Either way, the offer of the equivalent of $12,500 (US) to organize and administer the vaccinations came at a moment when the doctor was short on cash. Earlier, Afridi had been kidnapped and held for ransom by Lashkar-e-Islam, an extremist militia outlawed in Pakistan. The group's commander claimed that he'd heard rumors the doctor was overcharging patients in his private clinic. Afridi's family denied the allegations but paid a $10,000 ransom. According to Afridi's attorney, the Lashkar-e-Islam commander pocketed half and distributed the rest to the patients that Afridi allegedly had overcharged.

McGirk (2015a) further describes,

> When Afridi banged on the Abbottabad villa's colossal metal gate, a woman answered and refused to allow the children inside to be vaccinated. Stubbornly, Afridi demanded the cell phone number of the man of the house so that he could arrange for the children to be vaccinated at a later date. This cell phone number proved to be a vital piece of information to his handlers. It belonged to Ibrahim Saeed Ahmed, who turned out to be bin Ladin's guardian and messenger. The CIA knew of his existence but had never located him. Ahmed was the al Qaeda leader's sole link to the world outside the villa's 20-foot-high (six-meter) walls. Chasing down the lead from that phone number would lead to a major coup in the US-led war on terrorism, but it also would set back the war on polio.

Using vaccination in that specific case shows the strategic planning behind that particular "vaccination" campaign. The doctor looked like a strong Pathan who had, McGirk noted, "the right credentials from the CIA's perspective." The newspaper *Dawn* (2012) published that US Defense Secretary Leon Panetta, in his interview on 27 January 2012, also confirmed the CIA's launching of this "fake" campaign and praised Dr. Afridi for helping the agency. After that, the security agencies of Pakistan detained the doctor in custody "for launching the fake polio vaccination campaign and tipping the US government off about Osama." However, an alliance of about 200 US-based NGOs—many of them working in [actual] humanitarian operations in Pakistan—wrote a letter to the CIA director expressing deep concern over a vaccination campaign that may jeopardize the lives of their aid workers.

Consequently, this critical event changed the state of the vaccination program in Pakistan. The doubts regarding the Western, especially the US, involvement in the country with a "hidden agenda" turned into reality. McGirk (2015a) mentions the views of an international health worker: "After Abbottabad, these rumors became fact in the minds of many Pakistanis." The local people started to suspect vaccinators with doubts regarding their possible connection to the CIA. This perception became rather prominent in the northern areas of Pakistan, and the areas of Pathan settlements all over the country. Dr. Afridi was charged with "conspiracy against the state and high treason" on 6 October 2011 and is still in jail and awaiting trial (J. Ahmed 2014; Marszal 2016). In this regard, one of Pakistan's security analysts—Zaid Hamid—argued to Aljazeera television:

> What the government has done is they have committed a vaccination suicide themselves. The fact is that in Pakistan, there's a powerful perception which is backed by facts on [the] ground, that this vaccination campaign in Pakistan has been used by [the] CIA and foreign secret services for espionage and spying. When these facts were identified (...), the rage and anger in the nation were palpable (...) American CIA has committed the greatest disservice to humanity by using these humanitarian programs for spying and espionage against the state of Pakistan.

"Killing through Drones and Saving through Vaccines?"

Adding further to this sentiment, the USA also launched drone technology for targeting the strongholds of the *Tālibān* in Pakistan's northern areas. McGirk (2015a) cites the Bureau of Investigative Journalism, based in the United Kingdom, that between 2010 and 2014, around 400 strikes occurred, which killed "intended targets but also hundreds of Pakistani civilians" with a belief "that as many as two-hundred of the victims were children." The drones garnered proponents and opponents in the country. Nevertheless, there were news reports that drones also contributed to shaping anti-vaccination attitudes.

The effects of drones appear threefold. First includes the killing of the terrorists, which is, however, beyond my scope of discussion here (see Johnston 2016 on the matter). Second, they destroy the infrastructure that requires human and financial resources to rebuild. Third, the direct repercussions include the reactions related to violating a country's sovereignty and killing innocent people, considering that to be "collateral damage." Fair (2014) has described how drones create a sense of "second-class" citizenship, in which some citizens are considered as secondary or "objects," but not humans. This reaction then spreads to the rest of the country. How does it spread? I want to mention a case from my fieldwork in the following section that occurred during the Supplementary Immunization Activities (SIAs).

> In May 2014, the Sindh health department's 12-day SIAs, in collaboration with GAVI, activities to vaccinate 13.3 million children are already underway. Teams are scattered and working across the province. I am today with another TSV, who is in his fifties, in the *Sakhar* district, on his 70cc (cubic centimeter) motorbike (as it is locally called). He carries a register and a list of teams to know his field and locate them.

The hot wind is blowing. The day is warm, and warm wind burns our uncovered body parts, i.e., face, hands, and feet. Simultaneously, the wind functions as a dryer to dry our perspiration while riding on a bike. Despite that, our body feels the intensity of summer heat. We are keeping scarfs on our head to protect ourselves from heat. The marks of sweating are noticeable on our clothes, especially after drying up owing to the wind passing by due to bike speed. While following small busy streets, beeping the horn often, we are reaching mobile as well as fixed teams. Spending 15–30 minutes, we move to the next team. We keep searching for mobile teams since they are continuously moving. After visiting around eight teams, we reach a fixed team sitting in a hospital situated in the city center—this is the same hospital where children were brought during the measles outbreak in 2012–2013 by the ambulance from the selected village.

As soon as we reach this big hospital, which is full of people who are coming and going, we find the vaccination team sitting in a corner inside the hospital. The supervisor ensures that everything is according to the plans. I am also wondering whether the protocols are followed, such as vial labeling, and the procedures of vaccination. Of course, I am ensuring to be friendlier and avoid any "power" relationship and being treated as a "boss." However, the cases of refusals are among my prime focuses.

This team consists of two mobilizers, who are mobilizing people for the vaccination, and one vaccinator who is sitting on a chair with a table in front containing a vaccination brochure, vaccinator cooler, and register. Meanwhile, one mobilizer informs us of a case of refusal. The refusal in a city and especially in a fixed center increased curiosity significantly inside me as to why that person was refusing.

Accompanying the mobilizer, we go to a family that has come to receive some medication. The family consists of a man, woman, and two children less than five years of age. The man, let us call him Gul Khan, seems to be in his late forties and had a long, predominantly black beard, six feet tall, wearing an off-white *Shalwār-Qamīs* and glasses. The woman accompanying him is in a black burka (gown) that covers her whole body except her eyes and hands. The children, however, are wearing pants and shirts.[3]

I converse with the man to introduce myself and to be familiar with him: "*Aslam-o-Alikum,* brother, how are you?" I talk to him in the *Sindhī* language (the province's major language) while preceding this by offering my hand for a handshake. Although the mobilizer informs me that this person speaks Urdu, not *Sindhī,* I deliberately choose the *Sindhī* language to know his proficiency in the language of the area and decipher whether he is from Sindh.

"*Walikum-o-Aslam!*" he responds but does not answer the rest of my question. That shows whether he avoids speaking in *Sindhī* or knows nothing about the language. Lack of knowledge could help to infer that he had newly migrated to the area.

Given that, I switched from *Sindhī* to Urdu—using Urdu for a decade has changed my accent from most of *Sindhī*, who speak the language as their mother tongue. The accent gives him the impression that perhaps I am also not from this area. This impression makes him a bit more comfortable to communicate with us.

To my question, he states that basically, he is from the KPK province and has recently migrated here because of the poor law and order situation in that province.[4] He claimed, that there [in KPK] the situation of "terror" is prevailing, and imminent danger impends in the area. People are dying. Americans are targeting and killing people in the name of the war on terrorism. The army of the country and *"Tālibān"* are killing. Whether it is the USA, the Pak army, or the *Tālibān*, whoever is involved, *Baygunāh* (sinless, impeccable) people are targeted and being killed. Innocent children are killed. It is exactly a war-like situation. These recent activities together have wreaked havoc in the area. We did not have any other choice than being killed or migrating.

Furthermore, concerning the reasons for vaccination refusal, he claims: I know what the primary purpose of this vaccination is. It is not, indeed, for saving our children, but has some other ulterior motives. On the one hand, you [indicating toward the USA] are killing our people and children through drones and, on the other hand, showing great concern to save our children through vaccination. Is what you say not a huge contradiction? Is it not ethical, especially killing the innocents? Do you not see a prominent difference?

Better my children should remain unvaccinated; they will be healthy then. God will protect them from any illness. [In Urdu] *Allāh Mālik Hey* (God is the owner). [Secondly], many people now know how the vaccine was used in the KPK. It has not faded into oblivion. The media informed [us] that the mass campaign was a fake drive—it was a means to an end. The purpose of the vaccine, thus, is not literally to save the children but to safeguard some hidden interests. I cannot risk the lives of my children for the thing, which is neither suitable for them nor us but has something behind it.

He is quite assertive while uttering those words. Despite our continuous mobilization, he shows anger and resistance against getting his children vaccinated. He allowed nobody to immunize his children and left the hospital soon. Afterward, we both return to the site of immunization.

As usual, both children made it onto a list of refusals compiled by the concerned vaccination team—the list of "Metrix." Although this was a short encounter, Lal Khan's response elucidates the spread of anti-vaccination sentiment, his affiliation with his native province, and annoyance with global politics. This anti-vaccination sentiment and global geopolitics have cultivated suspicion among the people. The suspicion has led people to target the vaccination teams, which I discuss under the following heading.

Vaccination Teams under Attack

The "fake" vaccination campaign, as aforementioned, ignited the already existing anti-vaccination sentiment. The clerics began an anti-vaccination move in general and the *Tālibān* in particular distributed pamphlets for banning (especially polio) vaccination (Andrade and Hussain 2018). After that, attacks on the vaccinators started, killing and abducting them. The driving suspicion was that they collect some secret information and are "agents." The government employed police officers to escort vaccination teams, but attacks continued and are continuing despite that.

In 2016, the newspaper *Dawn* reported that militants had made 96 assaults on the teams and Law Enforcement Agencies (LEAs) since 2012 (Mansoor 2016a). According to this report, the geographical breakdown of attacks is as follows: 41 in KPK; 18 in FATA; 17 in *Baluchistān*; 13 in Sindh; and 5 in *Punjāb*. The attacks took the lives of 33 polio workers; out of those, 14 died in KPK, 7 in Sindh and 6 each in *Baluchistān* and FATA. However, the number of police officers and LEAs who died in these attacks is around 70 each in *Baluchistān* and FATA, 18 in KPK, and 10 in Sindh. Eight civilians lost their lives in attacks: 3 each in *Baluchistān* and FATA and 2 in KPK. Volunteers also died (11 in 2013 and 32 in 2014). Moreover, some 31 policemen and paramilitaries, 26 polio workers, and 20 civilians were injured too. Most of the attacks occurred in 2013–2014.

Lacking Exact Awareness of Vaccines

In addition to the vaccine–Western plot connection, another reason related to vaccine refusals is the lack of an accurate awareness about vaccines. A clear inequality of knowledge exists, as for most of the people living in rural areas, a vaccine is a *Teeko* (injection): a generic term used for every shot given for whatever reason. These inhabitants are given no knowledge about the specific properties of a particular vaccine to protect against one specific disease. During a campaign, vaccinators come and ask to give the vaccination. The narrative in a house or village runs that [in *Sindhī*] *Teekan Wāro Āyo Āhy* (a vaccinator has arrived), or *Furran Wāro Āyo Āhy* (the one who gives drops has arrived). The vaccination teams, in rural areas, call someone to inform them about the vaccination and ask them to bring children. Usually, people do not enquire about the vaccine, and a vaccinator does not inform them about which vaccine it is. The vaccine is given, marked "done", and the vaccinator is gone. This is how things often happen in the country.

In this regard, I would like to share two different encounters from my field diary. The first is based on my autoethnographic account:

I am sitting in my home. Meanwhile, children start shouting [in the *Serāikī* Language] *Tīkain Wāly Āy Hin, Teekain Wāly Āy Hin* (the vaccinator teams have arrived). After a few minutes, I see a girl who seems in her twenties, in my house. To my query, my mother responds that she is a vaccinator. She is the one who always comes here and gives *Tīkay* (literally: injections) to our children. The matter interests me, thus, I talk to her about why she is here and what she is doing. She replies, "I am a mobilizer for bringing children to the vaccinator." And, in my family, no one knows that she is a mobilizer indeed. My casual dress—*Goadd or Lungī* (a piece of cloth that is wrapped around the waist and worn in place of trousers, especially by men from South Asia) and *Qamīs* (loose shirt)—does not provide any indications that I am doing my Ph.D. abroad. This dress pattern gives her the flexibility to communicate with me. For this, I keep questioning. She starts telling me that they vaccinate children to protect them against various diseases. I ask which vaccine it is. She replies that the present dose contains vitamins and a vaccine against measles. Simultaneously, she seems in a hurry and apologizes that they have to cover a wide geographical area, so we should facilitate her by bringing all the children as soon as possible.

Following her request, we come to the main entrance of our house, where a vaccinator is eagerly waiting while holding a small cooler and a register. After looking at him, I recalled my childhood memories and realized that he was a dispenser. I recognize him, but he does not recognize me as I have been away from my village for more than a decade. To vaccinate the children, he opens the cooler to take a vial of the vaccine and fill an injection. He also asks one of the children to move her arm forwards. The baby girl follows the instructions and keeps her eyes closed due to expected pain. The mobilizer moves forward to support the vaccinator to hold the right arm of the baby girl after folding the sleeves of the child. The dispenser administers the injection but follows no prescribed protocols: he does not give the vaccine subcutaneously. I am aware of the protocols after working on this present thesis and know that there is a prescribed way to give a subcutaneous measles vaccine. I ask him, "Is there not a specific way to administer this vaccine? It seems you have not followed the given recommendations." To my queries, he is stunned. He replies: "Yes, there is a specific way and how I have administered is the right way. I have been following it for many years." His answer, then, astonishes me. He asks me who am I. After that, I give them a brief introduction, including of my project, and explain that I am exploring this arena for my PhD research and follow a 12-day campaign of Supplementary Immunization Activities (SIAs). Through this, I learned about the specific protocols to follow. It further enhances his worries. Afterward, he tries to follow the protocols and departs for another part of the village.

The second experience is of a "fixed vaccination team" that also comes from my field diary. As mentioned earlier, there are two types of vaccination teams: fixed and mobile. Briefly, fixed teams sit in one place such as a bus station and at a hospital to immunize the children. Mobile teams visit each house in a city or village to vaccinate the children.

> I see a fixed team that is vaccinating in *Islāmābād*. The team has one female and one male team member. The female is sitting on a chair with a small table in front of her containing a vaccination banner and a vaccine cooler, a register, and a pen. The male member is, however, wandering around to see families with children to mobilize them and bring them to the vaccination spot. Both are wearing a cap like a base-ball cap with an EPI logo. The team is sitting under a newly constructed overpass near a bus station, where pieces of paper and plastic are visible here and there.
>
> I go to talk to them. After receiving their consent, we start a discussion about the vaccination program in the country. The team shows a willingness to share their experiences. About the mobilization, the team replies: "We ask people to let us give them the vaccination. If a person insists on us telling them about the benefits of vaccination, we suggest that they consult a doctor. Further to this, if they resist the vaccination and consider it bad, unnecessary, harmful, or refer to any economic or political or religious contexts, we then do not insist much, but report the case to our higher authorities."
>
> Furthermore, explaining the mentioned contexts, they share, "Some people refer to the 'fake' vaccination, 'Western plot,' or economic motives behind vaccination. To them, vaccination encompasses some secret agendas and intentions. Knowing the situation, we, therefore, avoid insisting too much on them. The insistence can be harmful to us, as there are many cases of killing vaccinators. We feel scared, as well."

Such occurrences are not limited to a few vaccination teams. Indeed, one can discern various levels upon which these phenomena occur and operate, providing opportunities for nuanced observation and detailed elaboration. In urban settlements, linking vaccination to political interests is higher compared to rural settings. Nonetheless, other links that a vaccine is a harmful substance injected into the body and immunization is a "Western plot" to control the population are common. The capacity of vaccination teams also significantly differs between rural and urban areas due to several reasons. Some of them could be the quality of education, lack of exposure, lack of training, and the geographical spread of the area.

The Body Needs No Intrusions

Another form of refusing vaccines is related to perceptions of the body. Many believe that the body has a powerful internal mechanism and needs no external support. In the selected villages, the body is not perceived as a "machine," but rather more holistically, as something that sees no separation between body, mind, and soul. Although no one knows where the soul resides in the body, it receives significant attention during daily discussions. The body's internal mechanism is quite strong and capable of countering any external threat or a foreign invasion. To maintain the potential of a body, one needs to follow the given sociocultural directions, mentioned in Chapter 5, about a food regimen and physical, psychological, and spiritual exercises. In that way, the body is rendered potent to grow internally (Kumar 1997).

According to a *Hakīm*, that the body lacks mechanism to digest all the substances put into vaccines. A vaccine is, therefore, harmful to the body. It makes the body dependent on further medication. It disturbs the natural mechanism of the body, especially for children, whose bodies are not yet fully developed but in a state of development. Vaccines often have side-effects, which quickly appear in the form of fever and pain. That shows a resistance of the body against this external substance. In this regard, a male interlocutor from the village of *Rāmpur*, in his fifties, says:

> We survived without any vaccine. Our parents taught us what was beneficial and harmful for our bodies like food, *Ibādat* (worship, prayer), speaking the truth, avoiding excessive sex, and physical work. They taught us to stay happy and not to worry about anything. We have an expression: *Khushī Jehrrī Khorāk Konhy, Gham Jehrrī Bemāri Konhy* (no food nourishes as well as happiness (for health), and similarly being worried has no parallel illness). That means we need to stay happy and avoid apprehension, as both impacts on health profoundly. These expressions convey meanings based on wisdom and experience(s) of our previous generations. During our childhood, we consumed butter, fresh fruit, and milk, which strengthened our body. We had our homegrown food, for example, chicken, eggs, vegetables, and wheat. Everything was pure, but not now. We use chemicals, herbicide and pesticide to produce crops, which ultimately, come into us when we eat that food. No food, presently, is without any chemicals.
>
> Consequently, these chemicals have brought various illnesses such as *Sai* (hepatitis) and cancer, which were unknown to us. People are dying due to them. The chemicals have destroyed our livers. To avoid such illnesses, you need further medicines like vaccines. You are healthy, but you still need such medication. That is like becoming ill through consuming chemicals in the food and then taking medicine to recover. We have been continuously fooled. We were happy in our childhood.

Our parents were delighted while plowing in the field, then consuming pure food.

This statement signifies a holistic and comprehensive view of life. People do not see any separation among sociocultural, psychological, spiritual, and environmental factors. The passage describes the production of an illness and the need to cure it or them. This tale tells the story of what I call the "economy of illnesses," which has been increasing with time. The intention to serve humanity or the purpose of medicine to cure human suffering has been blurred with profit-oriented business. The increased use of chemicals has lessened the potential of the body and made it vulnerable to further attacks. Hence, we need vaccines. There is nothing wrong with declaring that if "pure" food is consumed, then there are fewer chances of getting an illness.

Mistrust in Vaccines

The current discussion may reiterate some of the earlier discussions and explanations, yet that is worth doing. As mentioned earlier, mistrust of vaccines is not exclusive to Pakistan, but can also be found across the globe with higher or lower rates depending on the country or region (Tafuri et al. 2014). Stuart Blume (2006) discusses the anti-vaccination movements in Britain and the Netherlands. Some studies have specifically linked the measles–mumps–rubella (MMR) vaccine with autism or shown that vaccines cause reactions and allergies. The controversy was instigated with the publication of Wakefield and colleagues (1999), then followed by various studies refuting the claims of Wakefield and colleagues that there was a link between MMR and autism (Wakefield et al. 1999; T.S. Rao and Andrade 2011). Yet, in actuality, Wakefield and his colleagues never claimed such a link; they simply suggested that further research was needed to find out if there was. Nevertheless, their article was retracted by the *Lancet*, and Wakefield lost his medical license as a result of extreme pressure by vaccine advocates and Big Pharma, as he describes in his book *Callous Disregard: Autism and Vaccines—the Truth Behind a Tragedy* (Wakefield 2010). Although he himself claims not to be an "anti-vaxxer" but rather an advocate of one vaccine at a time, he is still regarded as a culture hero for the anti-vaccine movement in the USA and around the world.

This negotiation of a vaccine is comparable to other areas of science. Some studies elaborate on a relationship between vaccines and autism, and others reject these claims. This contest has generated questions about knowledge production: What counts as truth? What is evidence, and how it is produced? Who should we trust, if not the scientists? What happens when scientists disagree? The contestation highlights a term that as I coin, an "economy of knowledge production." Many resources are invested to generate the desired results and claims about a phenomenon, and it is true that vaccines are a big business.

Suspicion of vaccines has two levels: mistrust in the ingredients in a vaccine and mistrust in its actual ability to immunize. However, in Pakistan, vaccination suspicion is more about the running, making, and implementation of the vaccination program—about the intentions of the stakeholders, national and global. In other words, the first form of mistrust asks what is a vaccine, while the second form of mistrust is about why is an expensive vaccine free of charge?

This section deals with people's perceptions of the substance of a vaccine: its ingredients. From the beginning of the EPI program, the perception of the "Western plot" to sterilize Muslim women has been prevailing in the country. Since then, one could observe waves of this suspicion. The suspicion is a result of colonization that is part of societal memory, which transfers from generation to generation through the process of enculturation. People doubted the substance of contraceptives, injections, and vaccines, considering that they significantly disturb and change body functions. Consequently, a female body never conceives—the vaccine interferes with God's business, which is a big sin. I have already discussed the "vaccination–reproduction connection." Some of the other significant reasons for the increase in this suspicion include lack of efforts to mobilize people, insufficient resources, a dearth of required awareness, education, and an increase in "extremism."

Furthermore, as discussed in Chapters 4 and 5, owing to practicing *Unānī-Tib* and Ayurvedic medical systems, people perceive a body as a combination of individual elements and humors. The balance among them guarantees "health" and imbalance causes illness, and so specific guidelines and regimens exist to ensure this balance. People, for instance, use food as a medicine, but not "medicine as a food." On these grounds, people question the substance or the ingredient of a vaccine while referring to their life histories and their folk wisdom. They believe that elements of a vaccine significantly affect the internal functions of a body. For them, a vaccine is a shortcut, and ultimately, in the long run, it makes the body weaker and more vulnerable to various other illnesses. The substance artificially causes an interruption in the processes of "natural" mechanisms that make the body healthy. This belief was further strengthened by reports of measles vaccines causing morbidity and mortality. The news circulates quickly due to accessible media, contrary to the past. People listen, quote, and claim that "we were right to believe vaccines are not safe for our children. Vaccines do not save people any longer." People suspect a vaccine that may cause deaths. The reactions against vaccines, especially the reported deaths of children linked to vaccines, in any case, require a systematic and objective analysis exploring the reasons. Lay people tend to believe in cultural narratives. The government established several committees in the country to unearth the explanations. With unbiased and researched results, one can construct a counternarrative and convey the benefits of a vaccine to people. These reactions to the vaccines have increased the "vaccine hesitancy" of people: their likelihood of refusing or resisting a vaccine.

Mistrust in the Government: Vaccine Good for the Government or People?

In Pakistan, the bond between the citizens and the government has never matured. The causes are numerous: historical, political, and "ethnic." This relationship is reflected in various frequent terms like "puppets," "corrupt," "irresponsible," "uneducated politicians," "filling their own pockets." Mistrust of a vaccine is highly related to mistrust in the government. Let me present another anecdote from the field:

> On a sweltering day of summer in May 2014, when the heat of the sun is burning, the body is perspiring and often needing water, the supplementary immunization activities (SIAs) are underway in the Sindh province. The district headquarters is engaged in allocating resources, distributing teams, receiving records while sitting in an air-conditioned control room. These officials are also supervising the vaccination teams in air-conditioned vehicles with escorting police vehicles. I am with a *Talukā* superintendent vaccination (TSV) on his bike to inspect fixed and mobile teams. Our journey starts by visiting a fixed center in a hospital of *Sakhar* city. TSV checks the entire process of vaccination, accurately the record and vaccine, in order to ensure that everything is going according to the designed plans. The team replies that everything is "normal" and working. The "inspection" continues, and cases of refusals are recorded in a list. We keep moving from one team to another. After a few hours, we reach the premises of the city.
>
> He calls a mobile team using his mobile phone. "Although this is not an easy task, as you need to locate the teams, to encounter a harsh environment, to handle any [undesired] situation—whatsoever, you must do it. Thus, let us go to that mobile team," he informs me. From constant noise pollution of rickshaws and vehicles, we turn to an unpaved street with dust enough to make us dusty. Nonetheless, there are big trees on both sides, giving an impression of an avenue and reducing the effect of summer heat.
>
> We take almost half an hour to reach the team. One team member, who vaccinates, is sitting on a chair with a vaccination banner with a white background and red highlighters to highlight the text.[5] The banner reads [in *Sindhī*]: "*Ur'rrī Jay Khātmy Lai Muham*" (a movement for measles elimination). In black, the text further reads: "*Izāfī Tuko*" (additional vaccine); "*Cha Mahīnan Khān Ddah Sāl Jay Har Bbār Lāi Zarurī*" (necessary for every six-month-old to ten-year-old child). Moreover: "*Hifāztī Tuko Aj Hī Waijhi Sarkārī Isptāl Yā Sehat Jay Markaz Khān Muft Laggrāyo*" (Get preventive injection [vaccination] from any hospital or a health center free of charge). The banner furthermore contains cartoons about two babies holding a smiling syringe in their hands. There are two words below this figure, which

reads as "*Tundrast Pakistan*" (Healthy Pakistan). At the bottom of the poster, there are icons and names of the following organizations: (1), Expanded Programme on Immunization, Government of Pakistan; (2) Ministry of National Health Services Regulations and Coordination; (3) the WHO; (4) UNICEF; and (5) GAVI.

Around 20 people, including children, surround the said vaccinator. The remaining two team members (one male and one female) knock at each door and ask people to bring their children for the vaccination. The children receiving the vaccine are crying loudly. Some of them are crying even before the inoculation. The cries are "infectious." The supervisor reviews all proceedings, inspects the record and vaccine. He is checking the record, and I am observing the entire event while talking to people standing around. Meantime, the female team member reports about a woman who does not allow her children to be vaccinated. As always, I take a considerable interest in the matter. The supervisor, the team member, and I go to that house—a house with one room and a broken main gate. The female mobilizer calls the woman and asks her to please come outside for a moment. Although the woman responds after a while, she arrives. She seems to be in her 40s and is wearing old clothes with a small piece of cloth on her head. Let us call her *Māī Karmā*. Her hands contain wheat flour, as she perhaps is busy preparing lunch. *Māī Karmā* comes without washing her hands, maybe owing to our constant shouts. Her appearance shows that she, in terms of economic resources, is a poor woman.

After that, the mobilizer introduces us to *Māī Karmā*. We ask her to let us know the reasons for her reluctance to vaccinate her two children—one boy and one girl. She completely ignores us and wants to go back to prepare her lunch. However, our continuous insistence stops her, and she responds with questions: "Why should I vaccinate my children? What has the government done for me, even though I am a [in terms of economic resources] poor woman and go for work daily? My husband does not live with me, so two children are my responsibility. I am performing all these duties as a single parent. With what I earn, I buy things for basic needs such as food and clothes. It is a tough life. Despite that, the government does not think about us. At my neighbors, the government distributed the *Benazīr* Income Support Program (BISP) cards but did not issue one to me.[6] I am also a needy and deserving person. You can look at my situation. And, now vaccination, why? If the government does not care about us, then why should we?

Furthermore, after getting children vaccinated, the children also get fever and pain. To heal them, we do not have any medicine. We cannot buy from a [medical] store, as we lack money. When we go to these people [indicating toward the vaccinators], they neither respect us nor give us *Dawā* (medicine). To look after our children, we need to stay at home to warm clay for massaging the injected place, so that they can get some rest. Consequently, the entire day passes by, and we cannot go to work. If we do not work, then, how should we manage to buy food and eat? We need to stay hungry or leave the children crying and suffering from fever and pain."

At a very surface level, the reasoning of *Māī Karmā* is so sound and well thought out, and shows that vaccination programs should be accompanied by food vouchers or money to buy food for those who really need it, or medicines for the kids to help with the fever and pain. With a critical look, this excerpt unpacks various levels of mistrust. First, *Māī Karmā* bargains with the government indirectly through these vaccinators, considering them as (officials of) the government. She does not trust the government, believing that the vaccination is good for the government, not for her children. Although she is unaware of funds and guidelines recommended to the government by global stakeholders such as the WHO, she indicates this indirectly. She understands that there are some benefits for the government if she allows the vaccination of her children. She sees no good for her children, only "fever and pain." She instead forecasts "suffering" and problems in the form of wasting her time and not earning. As a result, her children will suffer from both the direct consequences of fever and pain and the indirect consequence of hunger.

The second level is the trust deficit between the people and the medical practitioners. This can be seen when *Māī Karmā* complains that she is neither treated with due respect nor receives medicines she needs.[7] She thinks that these officials are powerful, and if they are dominant in the hospitals, then, in her house, it is she who has the authority to accept or reject something, including vaccination.

Analysis of this "refusal" shows that there is an invisible discourse beyond this apparent refusal. The refusal carries importance for officials and the government. Her one refusal increases the rate of unvaccinated children that leads other children (not merely of the country but the world) to vulnerability. A single refusal can cause an outbreak and wastage of resources. In other words, her refusal pushes the government into a critical situation in terms of the obstacles it creates in following the received guidelines of the global stakeholders. The government is responsible for meeting objectives and implementing the protocols. Ultimately, the global stakeholders would state that "there is a lack of commitment at the government level" (a WHO official expressed these views during our discussion).

Again, a single refusal encompasses enormous importance. It significantly affects policies and translations of those policies. Although invisible, *Māī Karmā* is an equal stakeholder in the making of such a program. There is no doubt about her absence in the meetings, which take place in an air-conditioned environment, but her "refusal" is there and functions as an active "actor" in the light of Latour's concept of network theory (Latour 2005). Her refusal is visible in the form of numbers. It compels powerful stakeholders to hold meetings to deal with the situation and devise "satisfactory" plans. It forces these stakeholders to show a high level of "optimism," as Closser (2010) finds in her work on polio. The optimism never ends between the government and the WHO officials. The WHO also is responsible for completing the translation of the promised objectives of the "donors" such as the Bill and Melinda Gates Foundation. This is how a single refusal, together with others, affects policymaking. Although she is unfamiliar with the names of the big cities and hotels where those decisions are made, an economically and politically poor local woman pivots decision making at a global level.

The cycle of negotiation continues. Refusals (can) cause further outbreaks. The continuation of dealing with the refusals, therefore, requires more planning and vaccination movements. During the vaccination campaign, refusals occur again. The cycle repeats. The power of these local people has gone unnoticed in discussions considering the "less powerful." Although some works discuss refusals (Sobo 2016; McGranahan 2016; Blume 2006; Fairhead and Leach 2007), these have received less attention.

In other words, the mistrust between the citizens and the government is quite visible in the vaccination programs. That mistrust leads to further "critical events," quoting Veena Das (1995), as some of these events can be meetings, outbreaks, and travel bans. The refusal based on mistrust shapes further instances of mistrust. It makes the bargaining and negotiation visible. A refusal hints at a "breaking of promises" and challenges the power and the network of relations running between various stakeholders.

Furthermore, *Māī Karmā*'s views illustrate that she comprehends that although she has difficulties in getting food to fulfill her and her children's basic needs, the government offers a vaccine but not sufficient food. That means she faces problems in the present while the government talks about future problems. She understands "first things first." Dealing with "secondary" things creates suspicion in her mind that there is something behind the vaccine. No one tells her about the obscure underlying objective, but she reads between the lines. *Māī Karmā* knows that her children would suffer enormously if not given food but can recover from measles—after seven days—with home-based measures, as she recovered during her childhood. In simple words, she knows that vaccination has an alternative, but food does not.

In the end, the vaccinator and supervisor assure her that she would receive respect and be offered medicine when she visits the hospital. Afterward, she brings her daughter to get vaccinated. The girl was crying before vaccination and continues after, too. Out of fear, her son hides somewhere in the house. *Māī Karmā* says, "I could not bring him as he was crying loudly and was scared. I have already done you favor to bring one child." That means she has done what she could do. She does not bring her son, and we return while mentioning an "unvaccinated" child in our booklets.[8] Let us now move further to the final form of mistrust that is in the global stakeholders and has links to geopolitics.

Mistrust in the Global Stakeholders

Current mistrust has significant links to the British colonization. The impacts that colonizers caused still prevail. People remember the *Lut Mār* (occupying and taking away the resources in a violent way) of *Gory* (White people, which became a part of "societal memory" after British colonizers) and are still suspicious about their presence in the country. I remember that during workshops in Pakistan in the late 2000s, a female colleague asked the officials of USAID, "Why does the US want the welfare of Pakistan? What is the interest lying beneath this?" The official became numb. "She twisted the answer but did not hit the point directly. She has not told the truth," the colleague commented afterward in our informal gathering.

Mostly such suspicions are unquestioned; nonetheless, their presence is undeniable. During the vaccination campaign, a case of mistrust in the global stakeholders occurred; such mistrust is dominant in the KPK province and the Pashtun community in particular. Journalists and public health researchers have produced a stream of work on it (Mushtaq et al. 2015; Hussain, Nagaraja, and Menezes 2015; S.O. Ahmad et al. 2016; L. Roberts 2019); nonetheless, this stream flows in one direction because of the lenses of their disciplines. During the SIAs, I observed several refusals.

Different levels of mistrust regarding the vaccination campaigns signify the interconnections, interplays, and intertwinement of the local, the national, and the global, all of which influence each other (see the section on "vaccination suicide"). The interconnections, at times, are visible as well as subtle. These refusals and mistrusts differentiate between "us" and "them." They strengthen and indicate a strong sense of unity among "us." Annika Rabo (2005, 163) rightly argues that these comparisons allow to manifest and create a political order of inclusion and exclusion, and these "boundaries of 'us' and 'them' are contextually fixed." This has been discussed in terms of the roles that refusals and mistrust play (McGranahan 2016; Sobo 2016).

Concluding Remarks

Pakistan commenced the rituals of containment after becoming a signatory of the UN to eliminate infectious diseases. Yet several infectious diseases, such as polio and measles, prevail, and controversies surround vaccination, which has put the country in the spotlight worldwide. Many people view vaccination as a "Western plot" or a conspiracy against Muslims. Some explanations are related to sociocultural factors, economic aspects, and geopolitical whys and wherefores. The weavings are inseparable, as there are significant interlinkages among them. On these grounds, family planning was considered a "Western plot," "un-Islamic," and *Harām* (something forbidden in Islam) in Pakistan that cultivated grounds to be suspicious of the immunization program, too. Because of the politics and controversies surrounding vaccination, the vaccination teams have faced assaults, in which over 100 of them have died.

Local people linked vaccination with reproduction due to colonization, and then supported this argument with the "fake" vaccination drive in 2011 that was termed as a "vaccination suicide." Due to these several crucial factors, the engaged stakeholders have been negotiating vaccination.

I demonstrated that refusals and showing resistance against vaccination is not a cause, but instead an effect of something. Implementers of vaccination campaigns seem highly focused on dealing with the effects but not the causes. In essence, the causes are ultimately cultivating an environment of anti-vaccination sentiment. Dealing solely with the effects is an apparatus of neo-liberals to advocate "the dominance of a competition-driven market model" for governing "the nobodies" (Galeano 1991).

Moreover, there are substantial issues in cold chain maintenance, lack of skilled vaccinators, and weaknesses in the catchment areas in terms of distance and their geographical location. These factors, including the perception, significantly affect the vaccine uptake. The country has been considered responsible for transmitting polio to many countries, which made vaccination mandatory for Pakistani travelers who would like to travel abroad to show a vaccine card at airports. However, I presented my anecdote to show a gap that exists between the theory and practice of vaccination, as no one checked my "yellow (vaccination) card" at the airports—either in Pakistan or in Austria.

Addressing the low-vaccination uptake and prevalence of infectious disease requires a thorough understanding of responsible reasons. Such perspectives should be apprehended in the context of several interconnected heterogeneous domains: the social, economic, geopolitical, and historical background. Considering the outlined qualitative aspects of vaccination would significantly help to create an effective vaccination program in the country. Summing up, I want to suggest that vaccination should be separated from (geo)politics.

Notes

1 Hajj and Umrah are holy pilgrimages for Muslims, during which they travel to Makkah and Medina cities of Saudi Arabia to visit the holy *Qabā* and the shrine of the Prophet Muhammad.
2 Due to ethical reasons, I am not disclosing the name of my friend, as otherwise, there could be severe consequences, such as him losing a job.
3 The dress pattern is signifying a cultural "mosaic." The parents' dress seems purely "Islamic" while the children are wearing "Western" dress. A contradiction appears that "Western" dress code is acceptable (for the children), but not the "Western" vaccine. This tension compels me to ask what is the parameter to differentiate between "us" and "them"? How do people make sense of a phenomenon: What is the dividing line?
4 Apart from it, thousands of Pashtu-speaking people migrated to Sindh province from Afghanistan and KPK province. Now, they are settled in the city of Karachi

as well as in the towns and villages of the province. Those who are living in the villages have learnt the Sindhi language. They are mostly engaged in transport like driving buses in Karachi, and trucks and tractor-trolleys in the towns and villages. In the towns and villages, most of them are doing work in the mountains—crushing stones and supplying them, as they have trucks. In Karachi, clashes have erupted many times among *"Muhājir"* (a term used for those who migrated to Pakistan after the Indo-Pak separation in 1947), Pashtun and *Sindhī*. In the towns, these Pashtun "immigrants" have been incorporated into local life. They attend marriage and death ceremonies of the "native" people (Gayer 2003; John 2003; Gayer 2014; Yusuf 2012; T. Ahmad 2014).

5 The colors of the banner also reflect some meaning. Red is simultaneously a sign of both life and danger. An expression of "[a] movement for the elimination of measles" is highlighted with red. The "additional injection" is written with black, perhaps indicating the "darkness" of incompletion of the aims. "Healthy Pakistan" is written in yellow and green, respectively. That means health signifies a "noble" phase and bringing health to the country would make it prosper (green).

6 According to the BISP website (2019a, [italic in original]), in July 2008, BISP was inaugurated as the National Cash Transfer Programme (NCTP) "as *the premier safety net institution.*" BISP originated at the time of precipitous food price inflation, as prices of food, grain, and fuel became highest, comparing data from the last 30 years. The situation of already vulnerable households was further exacerbated by the global economic downturn in 2009. The BISP focused on the poor women by providing unconditional cash transfers with an objective to protect them from the adverse consequences of decelerated economic growth. During fieldwork, I witnessed the BISP deliveries. These women have a card to withdraw money from Automated Teller Machines (ATMs). The locations of the ATMs, during the days of cash delivery, are full of women. Most of the women do not know how to operate the cards. They need someone to help them withdraw the money. This has created a different kind of dependency, and "malpractices." Many people working as "mediators" and "facilitators" get some "commission" or "token."

7 This signifies the genre of literature produced in the arena of the "doctor–patient" relationship (Becker and Nachtigall 1991; Pappas 1990; Fainzang 2002), indicating the power and authority of the medical professional.

8 After my fieldwork, I did not follow whether she was given any medicine for her daughter when she visited a biomedical facility again.

10 Measles Vaccine
From General to Particular

Measles Medication: The Beginning

Measles has been challenging humankind from almost the sixth century BCE (Düx et al. 2020). The term "measles" is believed to have roots in the Latin word *misellus,* which means "miserable" (World Health Organization 2007b). It also has links to the Latin word *miser,* which also means miserable. According to Peter Strebel and colleagues (2012, 352), this meaning signals the suffering caused by the rashes and sores that occur during measles.

In the past, several scholars worked on measles to find its causes. In the third century, a Chinese alchemist, named Ko Hung, distinguished between smallpox and measles; and similarly, in AD 622 Ahrun, a Christian priest, worked on measles in Egypt (Fenner et al. 1988). In the seventh century, a Hebrew physician called Al Yehudi recognized measles (Strebel et al. 2012). Some scholars, however, see the earliest truly elaborative work on measles as happening during the tenth to eleventh centuries (Furuse, Suzuki, and Oshitani 2010). In 910, the elaboration of Muhammad ibn Zakariya ar-Razi (865–923) or Rhazes—a Persian philosopher and physician—concerning measles is considered as a ground-breaking diagnosis, because after differentiating measles and smallpox, he declared measles as more dreaded and lethal than smallpox in his famous book *Kitab Fi al-Jadari wa-al-Hasbah* (Hamborsky, Kroger, and Wolfe 2015; Rāzī 1848; Mead 1748; Fenner et al. 1988). That differentiation won him the title of the first physician or "*Hakīm*" in history (Kaadan 2000; Modanlou 2008).

Early Asian and North-African physicians deemed measles similar or close to smallpox. Furthermore, although many studies recognize Rhazes' contribution, he left the transmittable potential of measles undiscussed (Strebel et al. 2012). Subsequently, further research addressed whether measles was an infectious disease. According to Strebel and colleagues (2012), the current scientific opinion on measles evolved in the Middle East after discussion of the possibility that measles was transmitted from animals since the virus causing it was analogous to rinderpest, which infected cattle. Further developments commenced from the beginning of the seventeenth century and after.

Thomas Sydenham, known as "the English Hippocrates," provided a clinical description at the beginning of the seventeenth century while defining

DOI: 10.4324/9781003253716-11

the characteristics of measles and hinting about its infectious nature (Strebel et al. 2012; Low 1999). In 1757, Francis Home—a Scottish physician—sufficiently studied and explained the contagiousness of measles and affirmed the presence of an infectious agent in the blood of a patient as the cause of the disease (Strebel et al. 2012). Furthermore, Peter Panum—a Danish physician—conducted "the classical investigation" of a measles epidemic in 1846 that transpired in the Faroe Islands, which furthered comprehension regarding the epidemiology of measles (ibid., 352). Afterward, the work of Joseph Goldberger and John Anderson—two American physicians—advanced understanding by transmitting an infected substance into a monkey. This experiment revealed the presence of an "agent," causing measles and helped in creating techniques for isolating and culturing the agent (ibid.). In 1954, John Enders and Thomas Peebles—an American biomedical scientist and an American physician, respectively—segregated it in humans and monkeys in a continuation of this development to isolate the virus causing measles (ibid., 2012). This final work provided the base to produce the MV.

Developing a Measles Vaccine: The Biomedical Perspective

The unrelenting investigations to discover the causes of measles never ceased until Peebles, who shared the lab with John. F. Enders, visited a suburban school in Boston, America, where an outbreak of measles occurred (Enders et al. 1957). The team collected specimens from throat swabs and blood and brought them to the laboratory for experiments in 1954. Enders used "sacrificed kidneys," crumbling and trypsinizing[1] them to develop the required cell cultures with nutrient media that led to the successful cultivation of the measles virus in these cells, which was then passaged or subcultured further (Katz 2009, 4–5).[2]

That experiment in the same year proved a "breakthrough," as Enders and Peebles positively isolated the measles virus from David Edmonston—an infected 11-year-old boy of that school. The strain of that virus was named after Edmonston. This cultivated virus, later, was inoculated into measles-susceptible monkeys, which first developed fever, rash, viremia, and then "measles-specific-antibodies." Afterward, Enders harvested these yielded cells in the human amnion cell, where their replication occurred effectively, then he inoculated the virus into pathogen-free chicken eggs via an intra-amniotic method. The trial of the cultivated fluid further proceeded while putting it into the human amnion cells, where the virus multiplied. After six passages in the fertile eggs, Enders and his colleagues prepared a cell culture from the chick embryo and incubated it in test tubes. This experiment showed "visible cytopathology" and "demonstrable replication" (Katz, Milovanovic, and Enders 1958).

To compare it with the "early kidney-cell-propagated," 13-times passaged or subcultured chicken cell material was inoculated for a second time into the measles-susceptible monkey, which that time showed no measles symptoms, such as no rashes or detectable viremia, but instead complemented the "fixing and virus-neutralizing antibodies" (Enders et al. 1957). The experiment ended by inserting the virulent human kidney cell virus into the immunized monkeys, who maintained full resistance against measles.

After testing this live-attenuated vaccine on animals, the first-time vaccine was applied to immunize humans in an "institution of physically and intellectually challenged youngsters" in the USA, where outbreaks triggered morbidity and mortality every second or third year. Katz and colleagues (1960, 6) describe how it was evaluated in humans:

> Following discussions with the institutional director, we were able to meet with the parents of several dozen children who had not yet suffered measles. After explaining to them the background of our potential vaccine and our plans for a clinical trial, most of them agreed to have their children participate. Using the same materials with which we had inoculated one another in the laboratory, we proceeded to inject a dozen susceptible children subcutaneously with the vaccine and several with sterile tissue culture fluid as a placebo. We examined them daily, obtained nasopharyngeal cultures and venous blood samples on alternate days and followed them carefully over the next three weeks. Five to eight days after inoculation, many of them developed fevers that persisted for several days and were then followed by an evanescent rash. Throughout this time, they nevertheless remained well and went about their normal activities. No virus was recovered from the throat cultures or blood, but within two weeks all had detectable measles virus-neutralizing and complement-fixing antibodies in their sera.

The vaccine developers did not aim "to patent the virus or to seek monetary return," but soon after, numerous universities and pharmaceutical firms in the USA jumped in to produce the Edmonston measles virus vaccine (Katz 2009), turning it into a lucrative business. Some investigators and firms produced "for-malign-inactivated, alum-precipitated measles vaccines" with comparatively low temperatures and increased passages, but the Enders team continued working on the live-attenuated one (ibid., 7–8).

On 21 March 1963, both vaccines were licensed in America. The subsequent vaccine showed no "enduring immunity" among the recipients against their exposure to "wild-measles," who "developed a severe measles infection with high fever, unusual rashes on the extremities, pneumonia and some central nervous system obtundation" (Fulginiti et al. 1967; Annunziato et al. 1982). Owing to these reasons, the inactivated vaccine was withdrawn in 1967 (Katz 2009; Hamborsky, Kroger, and Wolfe 2015). In 1969, "the responsibility of wild measles virus for subacute sclerosing panencephalitis (SSPE) was discovered" (Katz 2009, 8). Katz further mentions that by then, millions of children received this vaccine of live-attenuated measles virus that led to reducing the annual measles cases by over 90%. Also, he mentions that by 1993 transmission of measles was halted in the USA and, by 2002, in the entire Western hemisphere.

Afterward, David Morley, a British pediatrician, was in constant contact with Enders and colleagues and informed them about measles-caused mortality in Nigeria, where 125 children out of 555 died in his clinic. Enders ensured the effectiveness of a vaccine, for which "premature studies would be regarded as taking advantage of human guinea pigs rather than as a humane medical mission" (Enders et al. 1957). However, Katz moved to Nigeria in 1960 with the Edmonston vaccine, produced by Merk, which was in "commercial production" (Katz 2009, 8). The local mothers desperately brought their children knowing about the mortality and morbidity caused by measles. Although these children were also suffering from malaria, protein malnutrition, and intestinal nematode infestations, their response to the vaccine was encouraging, and they developed antibodies in due course (Katz, Morley, and Krugman 1962).

Katz writes that their Nigerian experience led to the MV being considered on a global scale and then added to the Expanded Programme on Immunization (EPI). Despite that, millions of children were still dying each year due to no international effort for measles, while polio received global attention (Katz 2005). Nevertheless, in 2002 the American Red Cross, International Red Cross, and Red Crescent Societies, joined by the CDC, UNICEF, the UN, and the WHO, formed the Measles Partnership (Measles and Rubella Initiative) with its goal to reduce measles mortality from 873,000 annually (WHO figures for 1999) to half in the next five years (Katz 2009).

Consequently, the Measles and Rubella Initiative (M&RI) was inaugurated as a global partnership to ensure coordination against measles and rubella to eliminate them.[3] Considering it to be a problem, the Initiative (2019) has a catchy slogan—"Measles and Rubella Move Fast. We Must Move Faster"—to indicate the rapid escalation of both viruses that need extravagations to contain them. It further reads, "The Measles [and] Rubella Initiative is committed to ensuring that no child dies from measles or is born with congenital rubella syndrome. We help countries to plan, fund, and measure efforts to stop measles and rubella for good" (ibid.).

The initiative follows in the footsteps of the Global Vaccine Action Plan as the latter helps countries to raise vaccination coverage against all diseases—including measles and rubella—and to fund, plan, implement, and monitor the quality of supplementary campaigns. The M&RI supports the investigation of outbreaks and provides the technical and financial support required for dealing with measles effectively. To strengthen the immunization system, it proposes solutions and supports a global network for measles and rubella. It focuses on reducing measles-caused mortality worldwide by 95% by 2015 and eliminating both the diseases in at least five of the six WHO regions by 2020. The initiative has assisted 80 countries since 2001 by providing two billion doses of MV, to increase the coverage to 85% globally and reducing measles-caused deaths by 79% as per the then-Millennium Development Goals (MDGs).[4] Following the mentioned objectives, 29 countries received support—bundled vaccines, operational costs, or technical assistance—to reach more than 221 million children during 2014. Thus far, this partnership has invested more than USD 1.2 billion in such activities.

The principal supporters of this global initiative are countries affected by measles, rubella, and congenital rubella syndrome. The M&RI appreciates its several individual private donors and supporters and is content that "together we move faster." A total of 24 key members support this initiative.[5] After offering this brief overview of the history of measles vaccination, I now describe its situation in Pakistan.

Measles Vaccine in Pakistan: Suspected "Reaction" and Deaths

As noted above, the MV is part of Pakistan's EPI program. Earlier in Pakistan, a single dose of MV—called "measles 1"—was compulsory to be given to nine-month-old infants. Over time, the EPI introduced a booster dose—"measles 2"—to be given during the 15th month (Tariq 2003).

Nonetheless, growing concerns have been emerging regarding this vaccine, especially at a local level, and on its effectiveness and suspected reactions in the country. On the effectiveness of the MV, Khan and colleagues (2015) found in their study in Peshawar that measles has occurred in those who received the MV. On the suspected reactions, the media have repeatedly reported concerning suspected reactions in children and about local people, who are suspicious about the side effects of the vaccination: the reaction can result in deaths of the children. Besides its purpose to immunize bodies against attacks of external forces (e.g., bacteria, viruses), vaccine reactions in those bodies have also been seen. The reactions to this vaccine are not merely limited to fever and pain but have been linked to children's deaths in Pakistan.

In other words, the vaccine substance is questioned and contested. First, despite receiving an MV, one remains susceptible to contracting the virus. Second, it does not solely kill the external forces, but in some cases, it may cause the death of the vaccinated body. Thus, the MV carries risks. Vaccine reactions, therefore, are another strong reason to refuse the vaccine.

Predominantly surfacing in the media, these occurrences and concerns were reported from across Pakistan when the MV caused a suspected reaction and some deaths. In particular, the reports came during a nationwide vaccination campaign of the Ministry of National Health Services in 2014 against measles to celebrate the World Immunization Week Campaign for vaccinating children less than ten years of age. On 22 May 2014, the Pakistani English newspaper *Express Tribune* (2014b; 2014a) published two reports related to reactions: (a) *A normal reaction?: Six more children faint during measles drive* and (b) *30 children fall sick in Swat upon receiving measles vaccinations*. The reports generated a debate in the country, in which various competing narratives emerged, especially in the print, electronic, and social media.

The online version of these stories received numerous comments showing contestation. Although the first news did not receive a single comment, the second story received 12 comments, in which people critiqued, supported, or held a neutral position concerning vaccination (Express Tribune 2014a). One can question the underlying purpose of comments, as these may be willingly and strategically written. Yet the commentators' ability to read and write in English is important since it distinguishes them from the rest of the inhabitants of Pakistan. The knowledge of English may help to assume that these people are "educated" and take an "interest" in politics nationally as well as globally. These comments would help to make sense of the competing narratives told around the case of vaccination. I mention such comments to show why and how many people contest the MV, along with the cultural reasons I explained in previous chapters.[6]

While criticizing the news report, some commentators satirically criticized the media for false reporting and transmitting disinformation on the side effects of vaccines, which would encourage people to not get immunized. For some, the media should "refrain from such headlines and stop giving a tool in the hands of extremists," as immunization-caused "sickness" is "very normal." A vaccine like any medicine could cause allergic reactions, and the risks involved in the MV are minimal; hence, the better option is to receive a vaccine rather than contract measles. Yet some critiqued people who reported reactions because it is abnormal to develop side effects. There were suggestions that the concerned authorities need to explain the misconceptions related to vaccination that is already making it tough to vaccinate children (Express Tribune 2014a).

Moreover, other groups discussed the vaccine itself, noting that it might have expired in the absence of the required facilities to maintain the cold chain, which is complicated. In a country like Pakistan, where power cuts and low-voltage electricity are chronic problems, appropriate maintenance of vaccines can be problematic. Falling unconscious is not a side effect of the MV. The hospitalization of 30 children is a clear sign that something fundamental went wrong with the given vaccine. There are chances that the vaccine was modified and thus became ineffective. Immunization should be temporarily halted until the vaccine is re-examined in order not to waste efforts being put into this vaccination drive and leave people unprotected (ibid.).

Furthermore, commentators linked the higher rates of unexplained vaccine side effects to corruption at the governmental level. As one commentator writes, some government officials possibly bought expired vaccines at a lower price and "pocketed the rest of the sanctioned money" (Express Tribune 2014a). Others mentioned that since the vaccination is spreading diseases rather than protecting against them, an ordinary person should be aware of the "Western conspiracy" against the Muslims and Pakistan.

One thought-provoking comment was from an American person named Jay, as mentioned on the website.[7] His interest in following vaccine-related news from Pakistan and adding his perception to create an impression was astonishing. Jay criticizes the multi-million dollar pharmaceutical companies that are injecting chemicals into children. To give a better idea, I reiterate his comment with minor corrections related to punctuation:

> Hello. I was surfing the [Inter]net, and this article got the better of my curiosity. They usually give the MM&R [Measles, Mumps, and Rubella] vaccine here in the states. I read some responses on other pages from citizens here, and so many had the same story. I don't know if I got the shot in my school days or not, so I cannot refer to my own experience for you, but there are many people out [t]here that said they got sick after the vaccine (some immediately, some precisely one week later). Many of them said they were so violently sick, they had to go to the hospital. Yet, in story after story that I read, all the "professionals" told them the sickness, while cause unknown, was definitely not related to the vaccine—and when you read about the vaccine, they keep researching and changing it because it does not even seem to be effective, or (...) not promising enough to overcome the effects caused by it.
>
> I love my country and stand behind its citizens, but these multimillion-dollar companies injecting our children with harsh chemicals does not seem right to me. They require them to have the Hepatitis C vaccine. How many small children are really in jeopardy of Hepatitis C (but they do not need for Hepatitis A/B, shingles, smallpox, Pneumonia). My grandma refused to let her kids have the Polio vaccine back in the 50s, and she was right not to as it was causing Polio.
>
> (Express Tribune 2014a).

Analogously, the newspaper *Dawn* (2014b) published a report, *Two More Children Killed Due to Anti-Measles Vaccine in Charsadda* district of KPK. The newspaper *Express Tribune* published another story: *Alarming Situation: Four Children Reportedly Die*. These reports stimulated dialogue on the website and similarly received numerous comments. I call it an online dialogue or a virtual group discussion and describe it below. The dialogue unfolded as a platform for diverse opinions and reactions. Users engaged in the digital space, expressing criticisms directed at the government, raising suspicions regarding the vaccine, and offering validations for the reported stories. This virtual exchange of ideas and perspectives mirrored a dynamic and interactive discourse, where individuals shared their thoughts, concerns, and assessments in response to the published reports. The online environment thus became a catalyst for a multifaceted discussion, illustrating the power of digital media in shaping public discourse and opinions on the reported incidents.

Engaging in the Digital Space: An Online Dialogue

One news report, *Two More Children Killed due to Anti-Measles Vaccine*, received 40 comments.[8] In the commentary, several subjects were brought up: the greater good and acceptable risk, health officials, the governance and political parties, vaccine and autism, rumors and conspiracy theories, and the criticism in the media. Although categories overlap, I have classified them for a better understanding of the negotiation processes. The dialogue starts when a commentator, who calls him/herself *Citizen*, asks: "If vaccination kills people, then how could they believe that vaccination is good?"

The Greater Good and an Acceptable Risk

While these commentators strive to maintain a balanced perspective on the perceived reactions, urging society to reflect on the concept of an "acceptable risk," they perceive the reactions as an inherent "loss" that can be rationalized in pursuit of a broader "good." In essence, they advocate for a nuanced consideration of potential adverse effects in the context of achieving greater societal benefits. The underlying notion is that, in certain situations, accepting certain risks might be justifiable when weighed against the potential overall good or positive outcomes.

Tom asserts that while it may not offer great comfort to the parents of the deceased children, the reality is that in the absence of vaccination, a more significant number of children could succumb to or be disabled by a measles epidemic. The same principle applies to polio vaccination, as no medical procedure is entirely without potential risk. Thus, society is tasked with determining what serves the common good and what level of acceptable risk is tolerable for the overall benefits obtained. Tonya asks, "[H]ow many people in that country died from measles? Vaccines kill only a few, where the disease kills millions. I have a father that suffered from polio; he will testify that vaccines save [lives]."

Imran Ali, writes, "the Institute of Medicine in its 1994 report states that the risk of death from vaccines is extraordinarily low." He emphasizes that deaths from a particular area may not necessarily be attributed to a vaccine but rather to sudden infant death syndrome (SIDS). Consequently, he advocates for a thorough and appropriate investigation into incidents of vaccine reactions to accurately discern the cause.

Criticizing Health Officials

A few other commentators focus on a probable agency of deaths. Considering the deaths that occurred due to the carelessness of in-charge officials, Ahmad argues, "The health minister should be held responsible for these deaths, and immediate action is necessary for those officials who are involved in this process." Jungraiz opines, "This is so troubling. Why is this happening, [perhaps due to an] expired vaccine?" Yet Ishrat Salim claims that deaths occur due to untrained vaccinators, using the same syringe, not using vaccines according to the protocols. Lazy and untrained vaccinators tend to use the same vaccine and syringes to save time and quickly do the job. Saleem thinks, "They [the officials] are using a '*Do* Number' (of poor quality: the expression is used for the things, which are not genuine, pure, but a copy of the original)." Moreover, Ali Ahmed, another commentator shares his experience working as a registrar in a *Karāchī* hospital:

> When I was doing [a] residency and [working] as registrar in [a] big hospital in *Karāchī*, I used [to] see many children dying from measles, tetanus neonatorum and T.B meningitis (...) and after [the] EPI [the expanded program on immunization] programme I really saw children dying from measles, no case of tetanus in newborn and BCG [Bacillus Calmette–Guérin] prevented T.B. meningitis. The case of death may be [a] faulty vaccine not meeting the standard or due to some other cause, so we should not blame [the] vaccination programme.

Moreover, Mobeen from New York shared that he has been vaccinating children of all ages for the past 25 years, and no child has ever died from the vaccines. He questioned what might be wrong with Pakistani vaccines, raising concerns about their purity or the possibility of them being mixed with something or administered intravenously.

Issues in Governance

Mahmood expresses concern about the significant impact of such reactions, stating that they will "kill all the efforts to convince people to vaccinate children." He deems it poor governance. Similarly, Salman remarks that such incidents are occurring during Pakistan *Tehrīk-i-Insāf* (PTI), calling it a "Poor [governmental] show" and describing it as abysmal.[9] Dr. Ain-ul-Momina criticizes, "Imran [the then Prime Minister], Nawaz Shareef [the previous Prime Minister] took the vaccine before going to India. So much for KPK [Khyber Pakhtunkhwa] government (PTI) busy blaming others with no time take stock of its own doings." A person who uses initials of his/her name, K.C., views that it is a result of "a bribe." Zaim also criticizes, urging Imran Khan (the PM) to stop criticizing the Federal and *Punjāb* governments, claiming that his own governance in KPK should be examined. Zubair criticizes PTI in the following way:

> So much for *Sehat ka Insaf* [Justice for Health]. Had it been not for an ill-planned and poorly executed vaccination campaign, these children would have been alive and those suffering would not have suffered. Anyways "who" is worried about a handful of children getting sick or dying. We have greater problems at hand [such as] stopping NATO [the North Atlantic Treaty Organization] supply, *Dharnas* [protests] and staging rallies against election rigging to deal with. Welcome to *Naya* [New]* Pakistan.[10]

Lubna expresses her skepticism, remarking, "What a joke! The government must be using expired vaccines donated by the WHO for the poor Pakistanis." In an indirect context, Lubna questions the integrity of the government's vaccination efforts, suggesting a possibility of using expired vaccines that were donated by the WHO, specifically for the disadvantaged population in Pakistan. Her statement reflects a blend of sarcasm and suspicion regarding the quality and source of the vaccines being administered.

Vaccination and Autism

The dialogue further discusses the relationship between vaccination and autism. Some propose that the vaccine causes autism, and others reject it. One commentator, named Imran, argues:

> There is ample proof that vaccination causes auto-immune diseases, asthma, autism, and other allergies. Vaccinations weaken the immune system. No research has been done on vaccination because it is a very lucrative business for [the] pharmaceutical industry in North America. The only research was done [by] a doctor [named] Andrew Jeremy Wakefield, and he was later ridiculed instead of finding the link between measles vaccination and autism. After his research, no one is allowed to do independent research in North America on vaccination. Pharmaceutical industries only sponsor all research; not even the government can sponsor such research. I will not travel to Pakistan at any cost, and I am sure a lot of other people think the same. This [lack of tourism] will bring the economy of the country down ... I hope PM [Prime Minister] Nawaz Shareef also has to take the vaccination on his next trip abroad, and it will be a headline about what happens to him next. Side effects of vaccination are death.

A few people object to Imran. *Jamāl* views, "Imran, you are ill-informed and your assertions wrong. Vaccines have saved countless millions. Deaths are extremely rare in a properly administered program. If the vaccine is prepared carelessly and has many contaminants, this [reaction] will happen. Teams must be trained to treat such reactions!" Furthermore, Ali Ahmed says:

> Imran, because signs of autism may appear around the same time children receive the MMR [measles, mumps, and rubella] vaccine, some parents may worry that the vaccine causes autism. Vaccine safety experts, including experts at CDC [Centers for Disease Control and Prevention] and the American Academy of Paediatrics (AAP), agree that the MMR vaccine is not responsible for recent increases in the number of children with autism. In 2004, a report by the Institute of Medicine (IOM) concluded that there is no link between autism and the

MMR vaccine, and that there is no link between autism and vaccines that contain thimerosal as a preservative.

Sajjad also makes a counterargument:

> Imran, unfortunately, every statement you made is completely false. "Ample evidence?" there is not even scant evidence, only conjectures and half-baked theories. On the other hand, evidence supporting [the] safety and efficacy of vaccines is overwhelming. A study in Denmark reviewed half a million children (537,000) and found zero links between vaccination and autism. There is no grand conspiracy to hide the side effects of vaccines. In fact, in 1999, a new vaccine Rotashield, was banned and withdrawn from the market upon discovery of a previously unknown side effect. As for Mr Wakefield & his so-called study, it has been conclusively proven that he took a bribe from the largest medical malpractice law firm in [the] UK to falsify the data in his study in an attempt to create medical malpractice business for his clients. Reports of deaths from Measles vaccination in Pakistan are most troubling. There is something criminal going on here, intentionally or unintentionally. Millions upon millions have been vaccinated against Measles in [the] USA without a single death!

Another commentator, who uses initials of his/her name, S.Y. responds, "Imran, there has actually been a good deal of research after the example you listed supporting Dr. Wakefield's theory, but it is never widely publicized even though the studies are published in several medical journals. There is also ample evidence of the neurotoxicity of several ingredients present in vaccines, especially detrimental to infants because of their size and still developing systems."

Furthermore, Dr. Saqib Sardar views, "All vaccines, and all medicines have benefit and potential for adverse reactions. Please also report the hundreds of children who die because they have not taken the vaccine." Dr. Sardar emphasizes the dual nature of vaccines, acknowledging both their benefits and the potential for adverse reactions. He urges for a balanced perspective by considering the fatalities among children who haven't received the vaccine. Tricia responds that children in the USA rarely die from measles. One can check the mortality chart from the Centers for Disease Control and Prevention (CDC). Tricia's response implies a skepticism about the severity of the measles threat in the States and encourages fact checking through reliable sources like the CDC.

S.Y. mentions:

> Just so you know, the American court system ruled back in the 80s that vaccines were "Unavoidably Unsafe" and then exempted the vaccine manufacturers and physicians from liability due to vaccine-related

adverse reactions and death. Now there is a tax on all vaccines which goes into a fund to pay out to those injured people who go to the Vaccine Injury Court, which has paid out several billion dollars over the years. Including cases involving autism.

Abrar argues, "After years of research, no correlation between vaccines and autism has been found. Please do us all a favor and get your information from [the] latest reputable sources rather than spew out what you discussed with your buddies over a cup of tea last evening. Most medical journals are not funded by big pharma." Abrar emphasizes the lack of evidence supporting a connection between vaccines and autism after extensive research. He urges individuals to seek information from current and reliable sources, cautioning against spreading unfounded opinions based on informal discussions. Additionally, he challenges the assumption that most medical journals are influenced by large pharmaceutical companies, advocating for a more informed and evidence-based discourse on vaccine-related matters.

Rumors, Conspiracy Theories, and Vaccines

Some commentators refer to rumors and conspiracy theories. For instance, Coupe (pseudonym) asks that who decided to import the faulty vaccine from Bharat [India], and can the government figure this issue out? "Can we please permanently ban any import of medicines from Bharat." Adi responds to Coupe, "Perfect, stop getting medicines from Bharat, [and] ask China, let me know how you make out with that." This exchange reflects concerns about the source and quality of imported medicines, with Coupe proposing a solution and Adi offering a somewhat ironic alternative. It highlights the complexity of decisions related to vaccine and medicine imports, involving considerations of safety, reliability, and international relations. Naseem Altaf also questions Coupe, "What made you think that it was from Bharat." Altaf suggests that the manufacturer must be brought to book: it is essential to disclose the name and details of the manufacturer for knowing whether it was the manufacturer's fault, or there was something wrong in the system, or in the procedures of vaccinators. One commentator, named Unbelievable, states:

The rest of the World uses Measles vaccine without a problem—so what is up with Pakistan. Enough with the ignorant conspiracy theory nonsense so typical with Pakistan. The E.T. [*Express Tribune*] article indicates that 40 percent of the people providing vaccinations are not properly trained—that's fixable. Further—chronic power outages might contribute to inappropriate vaccine storage, and someone needs to be in charge of certifying that the vaccines have been properly stored/handled. Time to step up to the plate and join the 21st century.

Moiz Omar argues, "Our local vaccination supply may not be good or they [vaccinators] are incorrectly vaccinating [the children]. The equipment may possibly be unsterilized. Please, anti-vaccination conspiracy theorists, do not start now." The last two commentators suggest improvement in training, infrastructure, and healthcare practices to ensure effective and safe vaccination procedures in Pakistan. They emphasize a rational and evidence-based discourse, discouraging the spread of unfounded conspiracy theories related to vaccinations.

Criticizing the Media

There were two comments which criticized the role of media. Mansoor Naqvi contends that the media coverage lacks responsibility. He acknowledges the existence of diverse views on vaccination, asserting that vaccines are generally safe unless scientifically proven otherwise. Naqvi places the responsibility on journalists to either thoroughly investigate and report the actual cause or provide evidence that the vaccines are the cause. Alternatively, he suggests reporting the truth if the deaths are attributed to medical negligence unrelated to vaccines. Similarly, Shahid questions the omission of statements from KPK's doctors, including the Director General, who reportedly see no link between measles and the deaths discussed in the article. Shahid highlights the broader issue of infant mortality in the country and suggests that people's cynicism about vaccinations may lead them to attribute any infant deaths shortly after vaccination to the vaccine. Shahid alludes to societal beliefs in phenomena like "*Kala Jadoo*" (black magic) and "*Nazar*" (evil eye) as alternative explanations for infant deaths. Both comments criticize the media for what they perceive as irresponsible reporting, emphasizing the importance of balanced and evidence-based journalism in the context of vaccination-related deaths. They highlight the need for thorough investigation and contextual reporting to avoid contributing to misconceptions and public skepticism about vaccinations.

"Alarming Situation: Four Children Reportedly Die"

On this news report of the *Express Tribune* (2014b), there were a total of 11 comments from readers. In an effort to enhance readability and organization, I have categorized these comments for easier reference and analysis. The categorization allows for a systematic examination of the varied perspectives and opinions expressed by individuals in response to the news report. This approach facilitates a more structured and comprehensive understanding of the public discourse surrounding the reported events.[11]

The Firsthand View of "Reactions"

In terms of the situation caused by the vaccine, a person named Zakir states that in his children's school, two buses full of students were shifted on an emergency basis to a hospital, which is run by the Worker Welfare Board. He offers a "firsthand" view of the situation and tries to validate the news report that it is not false.

Analyzing Zakir's contribution, it becomes evident that his testimony serves as a corroborating piece of evidence supporting the authenticity of the news report. The mention of emergency measures and the use of a hospital managed by the Worker Welfare Board underlines the seriousness of the situation. Zakir's willingness to share this information implies a sense of concern or urgency, further emphasizing the gravity of the vaccine-related events. This individual account, when considered in conjunction with the news report, contributes to a more comprehensive and nuanced understanding of the impact of the vaccine situation on the local community.

Issues of Governance

Anam satirically questions, "So much for Sehat Kā Insāf." She points out that the PTI's initiative of "Justice for health" in the KPK province shows no progress, though the political party claimed to improve things after power. The party has not done anything extraordinary.[12] Although the party made significant pledges, it could not deliver as the party was ruling the KPK province after winning the general elections in 2013. Anam holds a skeptical view of the PTI's performance in the health sector. The reference to the party's failure to fulfill its promises indicates a perceived gap between political rhetoric and actual achievements. Anam suggests that, despite being in power in the KPK province following the general elections in 2013, the PTI has not implemented any noteworthy initiatives to improve healthcare, undermining the credibility of their commitments.

The Role of Media and Vaccination

As in the previous case of news reports, some commentators criticized the media. Shahid criticizes publishing the news because it would generate anti-vaccination sentiments in the country. He questions that when doctors and other health officials have clarified "that the measles vaccine is safe and *not* causing these deaths," why is the newspaper justifying "stooping so low and publishing this misleading headline"? Shahid further argues that the paper did not realize the potential effects of the report that may "lead to more people refusing vaccination and resulting in more deaths from measles," as "measles causes almost *one million* deaths" in the country annually.[13]

Nonetheless, Jeff Mountain counterargues to Shahid that needless to say, doctors and health officials declare vaccines safe. Yet a healthy child becomes immediately sick, and eventually dies after being given the vaccine. Hence, did that sound safe to him [Shahid]? Mountain further argues that health officials have a career, and mostly, they need to "protect" additional income, for example, "payoffs by pharmaceutical companies." Given that, he questions

Shahid, "What would you expect [from them]? You have a brain. Use it. Do your research."

A few other commentators also criticize Shahid for his claims. Dee responds to Shahid, "Wow, a million [deaths], that is quite a trick considering there were only 14,000 cases in 2012. Sadly, 306 died with measles, not necessarily, from measles." Megan Lane also criticizes Shahid that according to the WHO, in 2011, Pakistan reported fewer than 5,000 infections; hence, where exactly did Shahid find that number of one million. Taking on Shahid, Kari also argues that the global deaths associated with measles are not even a million: according to the WHO, there are around 122,000 deaths per year. Therefore, Kari suggests it is better not to "assume that the doctors are right; adverse reactions to the vaccine are not uncommon."

Another person with the name "Me" also takes on Shahid: "The latest figures from the WHO show the number of measles cases in Pakistan has increased from 4,000 in 2011 to 14,000 in 2012. Of those, 306 died last year—up from 64 deaths in 2011. One million deaths, eh?"

In this regard, two more commentators question vaccines. First, based on his/her vaccination experience from the USA, Treacy claims that vaccines are unsafe, as her/his son had "a serious vaccine injury." For these "injuries," the USA has set a special fund for paying compensation to these affected families. Furthermore, Treacy claims that the CDC website contains a list of side effects caused by the measles vaccine. Given that, how can one consider "mercury, [and] formaldehyde squalene, which are toxic to the body, are good for" one's health? Therefore, "Educate yourself. It is better [to have] sanitation, clean water, and nutritious foods that combat disease."

Second, Dean contends, "Vaccines are a lethal scam. Do not vaccinate if you love your kids. Agenda 21 of the UN [United Nations] wants to reduce the population. So, does the agenda of the New World Order." Moreover, Christina Waldman questions, "I do not find the information as to which measles vaccine and who manufactured the measles vaccine given to the children who died after receiving it, in the article."

In the subsequent section, I present a specific anecdote that illustrates this phenomenon. In this particular instance, my interlocutor approached me, seeking my opinion on the matter as he contemplated whether or not to have his son vaccinated. This narrative provides a firsthand glimpse into the local impact of vaccine-related concerns, showcasing the intricate dynamics at play as individuals grapple with the decision-making process amidst uncertainties and perceived risks.

Consequences of Suspected Side Effects: An Anecdote from my Field Diary

After this last incident of the vaccine reactions in which four children died, Mr. *Bādal*—one of my interlocutors from the village of *Rahīmpur*—sought my opinion about the vaccination: should he vaccinate his baby boy? The following description is from the field diary:

He and his family had been longing to have a son for years, as he had daughters, but no son. It is important to mention that patriarchy is dominant in Pakistan, where the line of succession runs through a male ego. Therefore, *Bādal, Samrīn*—his wife—and their respective families were eagerly desiring and making vows for a male baby. Ms. *Samrīn* suffered enormously in that way, as her-in-laws usually, directly, and indirectly, indicated that she had not given them a son. She was always considering herself significantly inferior and more misfortunate than the women with sons. Mr. *Bādal* was also highly worried about having a son. The couple, including the mother of *Samrīn*, made significant efforts to have a baby boy in terms of vows at various shrines, offerings, prayers, supplications, and food regimens.

After four daughters, during conception, Mr. *Bādal* used to bring *Samrīn* for an x-ray to ensure whether it was a male or female baby. After two confirmations that it seemed to be a female baby, he opted for abortion. The first time *Samrīn* agreed. However, after experiencing the pain of abortion, next time, she utterly refused to do so, but an enforced abortion happened. She could not resist, as in most cases, a male dominates decisions at a household level. This enforcement made *Samrīn* ill; she suffered psychologically, emotionally, and physically. Her treatment continued for a couple of months until she fully recovered.

Moreover, her daughters, especially the elder one, often asked them to have a brother. The daughters prayed to God for a brother. The daughters, particularly when looking at someone else's brother, used to mention that they also wanted a brother for their parents. The situation further changed for *Samrīn*, when *Bādal*'s brother's wife gave birth to a son. Everyone was indirectly taunting her. She, while pretending to be brave enough, patiently waited for her turn, and continued to pray.

Meanwhile, she conceived and refused an x-ray. *Samrīn* and *Bādal* had a severe fight, including a physical assault. She, even then, refused and went to her parents' home for a few months until the phase of abortion was gone. Indeed, *Samrīn* stayed there until her delivery. Fortuitously, this time, she gave birth to a son in a maternity home. It brought great happiness for them, for their daughters and family members. The birth of a son relieved her extreme pressure and shut the mouths of in-laws.

This story of longing to have a son illustrates everyday experiences to comprehend the subtle connections and contexts. This longingness put me in a state of worry. The *Samrīn–Bādal* story quite resonates with the tale of Hussain mentioned earlier, who died—as her mother claimed—due to vaccination in the *Benazīrābād* district. The single child counts as an individual considering quantified models that Adam (2016a) calls Metrics, which are applied in global health projects worldwide. Nonetheless, a child, irrespective of gender, simultaneously counts as equal to the world for parents, especially for the mother. The hankering to have a child, especially a male baby, further adds importance for the parents.

Thus, on the one hand, I was thinking about them, about their son, and their longing for a son. On the other hand, the making of a vaccination program was sufficiently visible to me after researching this arena for years. Most of the grey areas, such as issues in maintaining the cold chain, were no longer hidden. Indeed, I am not an opponent of vaccination, but I adopt a rational position for sure. The vaccine itself, if administered according to the required protocols such as cold chain maintenance of vaccine and proper injecting into the body, is undoubtedly helpful. However, if there are lapses in the rules, then the vaccine provides no protection but puts the receivers in a precarious position. Knowing all that, I felt numb and could not give a good suggestion despite my intentions. I could only make things more complex and put the responsibility on his shoulders to decide. Although the fact that I did not provide this valuable suggestion made me feel exceedingly bad, there was no other suitable option available except complicating the answer.

Analyzing the Dialogue

The aforementioned commentaries form an ongoing virtual group discussion and offer insights into a wide range of perspectives on vaccines that extend beyond immediate concerns. While the language barrier of English newspapers may limit their readership, these comments vividly capture the depth of the ongoing dialogue within the country. Participants in this virtual discourse actively negotiate ideas and practices related to vaccines and vaccination, engaging in a dynamic exchange.

Critiques within the commentaries are multifaceted, encompassing the vaccine itself, the vaccination process, the role of the media, national politics, the government's actions, and the involvement of global stakeholders, such as the WHO. To fully comprehend these commentaries, it is crucial to contextualize them within broader national and global economic and geopolitical landscapes. These online comments not only signify an ongoing contestation but also point to a social conflict surrounding Pakistan's vaccination program. Fundamental questions arise, such as the safety of the vaccine and the reasons behind adverse outcomes following vaccination. These inquiries highlight concerns about the overall design and implementation of vaccination programs, revealing a perception that something in the vaccination process may be amiss.

Some comments, although brief, are rich in allusions. For example, one comment hints at a conspiracy theory suggesting the formation of a New World Order through vaccination. This resonates with the earlier discussion in this chapter concerning the connection between vaccines and reproduction. These subtle references add layers to the discourse, demonstrating the complexity and depth of the ongoing conversation surrounding vaccination in Pakistan.

Needless to say, we cannot generalize the sentiments expressed by such commentators to the rest of the country. Nonetheless, the analysis of these comments yields exciting insights about the controversies and points of view about what is going on in the country and how vaccination in Pakistan is dynamic and distinctive from other countries. The question about what is normal and abnormal in the domain of immunization has received plenty of attention from these commentators. These comments reveal how people are negotiating vaccination by finding a "scapegoat." People often need somewhere to go with their anger and confusion and blaming and shaming serve that purpose and make the people doing it feel powerful. Many commentators have anonymized their personal threats yet made their points simply and vividly. Unquestionably, the methodology of these or similar comments can be questioned due to their accuracy, agency, and obscuration: Who is behind them? As some comments can be "funded" to deliberately phrase from a specific angle or perspective. Nonetheless, this "paid-comment/content" phenomenon also signifies playing politics via conspiracy theories—this world of politics occurs on a grand global scale.

Furthermore, the suspected adverse reactions to the vaccine not only have implications on an individual level but also ripple through the local community. The apprehensions generated by these reactions prompt parents to reconsider the decision to vaccinate their children. Faced with anxiety, parents often turn to their peers for guidance, seeking support to navigate through their concerns and arrive at a reasoned decision.

Precisely, all these news stories and the firsthand story of my informant illustrate several aspects of the vaccination program in Pakistan. The claimed deaths resulting from vaccine reactions consequently spread fear and cause anxiety among parents, which ultimately led toward resistance to and refusals of entire vaccination programs. The question of my interlocutor mentioned above is a vivid example of this fear and anxiety. These reports do have profound effects. Apparently, they have compelled people to think about vaccination and its potential consequences. This situation of parents being anxious and critical is not merely limited to the vaccine itself, but the practice of immunization. To say it more clearly, people are fearful of improper administration of vaccines.

Food—Not Measles Vaccine

Certain instances of vaccine refusals stem from an established association between the MV and potential side effects such as fever and body pain. These perceived associations understandably instill anxiety in parents, creating a hesitancy to proceed with the vaccination for fear of subjecting their children to discomfort. In the course of fieldwork, numerous parents voiced their concerns, noting that their children did not receive adequate attention or treatment for the anticipated side effects of the vaccine. This hesitation arises from the common understanding that vaccines can often induce fever and discomfort in children. The parental complaints shed light on a broader issue where the fear of adverse reactions becomes a significant factor influencing vaccination decisions. The need for effective communication and support to address these concerns is underscored, emphasizing the importance of comprehensive healthcare strategies that address not only the vaccination process but also the aftermath and potential side effects perceived by parents.

In the previous chapter under the heading "mistrust in the government," *Māī Karmā*, mother of two children, separated from her husband, complained,

> After receiving the vaccine, our children became sick. They got a fever and cried. This sickness bothers us, as the healing, the effects of the vaccine consumed our time. When we go to these people (indicating toward the vaccinators) at their hospitals, they do not give us medicine for it. We, then, make some efforts such as warming clay in the fire and then placing it on the scar of injection (vaccination). We are poor people, work on a daily wage. What should we do then, sit with the children or go and earn something? We need to eat. Work brings us food, not the vaccine. For us, food is essential, not the vaccine.

This statement specifically addresses the context of measles vaccination, distinct from the broader immunization program in progress within the country. It delves into a nuanced debate surrounding needs and wants, drawing a parallel between the fundamental necessity of food and the perceived nature of vaccines as a want. From this perspective, the vignette emphasizes the immediacy of food as a basic and essential need for the present, contrasting it with the perceived future-oriented importance of vaccines. The consideration here is that while food sustains the current well-being, vaccines play a crucial role in safeguarding future health. The notion of foreseeing a future where diseases might occur, and children might suffer, introduces an element of uncertainty and risk assessment. Local expressions, such as the *Sindhī* saying "*Pait Wārī Lāi Kach Warī Khay Na Mārjy*" (do not kill the one in your lap for the one in your belly), are brought into the discussion. This expression illuminates the prioritization of immediate needs over potential future concerns. The woman views "the child" as one in the belly, while she and other family members are considered grown and, in the lap, capable of contributing to the household. These everyday expressions and experiences are critical elements to consider when understanding decision-making processes. They offer insight into the contextual factors that shape choices, shedding light on how individuals navigate between immediate necessities and future considerations in the complex landscape of healthcare decisions.

Concluding Remarks

Tracing the general history of the MV, this chapter highlighted various perspectives and rationales woven around MV in Pakistan. The weavings reveal scales and types of mistrust. As argued in an earlier chapter, a deeper comprehension of these explanations can be achieved by examining the continuous interplay among sociocultural, economic, and geopolitical factors. People suspect the "substance" of the vaccine as well as those who administer and advocate the vaccination. This suspicious perception is highly interlinked with the general perception of vaccination, for example, a "Western plot." In this chapter, I also demonstrated how people negotiated the MV during an online dialogue on media websites. Based on different orientations, standpoints, and experience, they brought different claims and counterarguments that either the vaccine is safe or unsafe. These people criticized the media, the government, the vaccine and its use, and global stakeholders. These online sites have emerged as vibrant platforms to contextualize the phenomena of infectious diseases, including vaccination.

Notes

1 Trypsinization is the method of dissociating cells using trypsin, a proteolytic enzyme that breaks down proteins for dissociating adherent cells from the vessel in which they are cultured.
2 Often known as a "passage" or a subculture: a passage number is the number of times a cell culture was subcultured, and a number of passages will make or break an experiment.
3 Rubella is a contagious viral infection best known for its distinctive red rash, also called German measles or three-day measles. In terms of viruses, measles and rubella are distinct, allowing rubella to be less contagious and as serious as measles. According to M&RI (2019), rubella can have severe consequences for pregnant women while giving birth to a baby with Congenital Rubella Syndrome (CRS).
4 Now they are called "Sustainable Development Goals (SDGs)."
5 (1) Anne Ray Charitable Trust; (2) American Academy of Pediatrics; (3) the Bill and Melinda Gates Foundation; (4) the Canadian International Development Agency (CIDA); (5) the Church of Jesus Christ of Latter-day Saints; (6) the GAVI Alliance; (7) Global Payments, Inc.; (8) Herman and Katherine Peters Foundation; (9) International Federation of Pharmaceutical Manufacturers Association; (10) International Federation of Red Cross and Red Crescent Societies; (11) the International Pediatric Association; (12) Izumi Foundation; (13) Jeppesen; (14) the Lions Clubs International Foundation; (15) Japanese Agency for Development Cooperation (JICA); (16) Merck Co. Foundation; (17) Norwegian Ministry of Foreign Affairs; (18) ONE Campaign; (19) Sabin Vaccine Institute; (20) Task Force for Global Health; (21) United Kingdom Department for International Development (DFID); (22) the Vodafone Foundation; (23) the World Bank; and (24) the Women's National Basketball Association (WNBA).
6 I have not translated these comments, except modifying, correcting the spellings or editing errors, since commentators used the English language. However, I have changed the order of comments to maintain coherence.
7 Jay is a name used for the male gender, so I have used a masculine pronoun.

8 The comments have been corrected, e.g., "Childer" to "children" or inserting articles and rearranging to maintain coherence among them to show an online dialogue. Some commentators have used pseudonyms, and some names seem real. Moreover, I have left out two comments because both seemed an advertisement.

9 As noted earlier, the PTI is a political party that continuously protested against the ruling party—at the federal level for corruption, and probable rigging in the general elections held on 11 May 2013—the Pakistan Muslim League (Nawaz) (PML-N) that won the elections. For the first time, in 2018's general elections, the PTI won and became a ruling party at the federal level.

10 *Nayā* Pakistan was a slogan used by the PTI government.

11 I have corrected the comments for clarification. For example, its = it is; that's = that is, or correction of spelling, editing of errors.

12 The party ruled the KPK province after winning the general elections at a provincial level for the first time in 2013.

13 The commentator, to give an emphasis, has used the uppercase and I have just changed the words from uppercase to lowercase and then italicised them to retain the emphasis.

11 Creating the Anthropology of Vaccination

Most people desire to live a long and healthy life. Thus, human-made immunization/vaccination was heralded as a breakthrough and bulwark against many infectious diseases that caused disability and premature death. Covid-19 has highlighted the importance of effective vaccines (Ali 2020c); people around the world had been longing for vaccination against this disease, which pharmaceutical companies had been actively engaged in preparing. Politicians had repetitively been announcing its coming and global philanthropists had invested in it. Hence, vaccination has once again emerged on the world stage as a critical intervention and apparatus of global health.

Connecting the local and global worlds, vaccination has garnered both proponents and opponents located in diverse locations. Vaccination involves several micro- and macro-processes and what I am metaphorizing is a *ship of relations* carrying multiple stakeholders onboard, ranging from the local to the global level. These stakeholders include international organizations, governments, medical practitioners, scientists, health goods providers, donors (local and international), nongovernmental organizations (NGOs), policymakers, philanthropists, pharmacists, vaccinators, vaccine recipients, and the media.

As a medical invention, I argue that vaccination has become concurrently a (geo-)political, economic, and sociocultural problem, as it is often heavily contested in various countries, including Pakistan and the USA, which both have a large "anti-vaxx" movement, as it is called in the USA. Such contestations require full qualitative attention to address the politics as well as the knowledge and economic gaps they represent. These negotiations and contestations make vaccination and its related phenomena promising subject matter for anthropology. Particularly, anthropology can study the controversies and politics revolving around vaccination and the varying reasons for them. Employing vaccination as an analytical concept, anthropology can paint the intricate relationships among the diverse stakeholders on board that metaphorical ship: individuals, institutions, and countries.

Precisely, considering characterizations of anthropology *as the most scientific of the humanities, the most humanistic of the sciences* and vaccination *as a scientific invention with a plethora of sociocultural, economic, and (geo-) political, weavings*, each carries significant importance for the other. In this

DOI: 10.4324/9781003253716-12

chapter, after presenting the negotiations and contestations surrounding vaccination in Italy, the USA, and Pakistan, I ask for the allocation of a focus toward a new anthropological field—*the anthropology of vaccination*—demonstrating why vaccination can be an intriguing analytical entry point for anthropology, and what anthropology can contribute to the field of vaccination. In the following sections, after describing materials and methods, I offer an overview of vaccination and its ongoing contestations; present three brief case studies; and then bring the main question to center stage: What can vaccination and anthropology offer to each other?

Modern Vaccination and Its Roots in Traditional Folk Medicine

Vaccination draws on the triumphant story of smallpox eradication, which took more than 180 years. Historically, the "variolation technique" (smallpox is also known as "variola") was used by various ancient civilizations, such as in India and Tibet; it was based on the subcutaneous inoculation of attenuated pustule material. The method was brought to Anatolia by the Seljuks (also spelled Seljuq), who were a ruling military family of the Oğuz (Ghuzz) Turkic tribes throughout the Caucasus (Dinc and Ulman 2007). This inoculation of small amounts of pus from smallpox (or maybe even cowpox) was in practice in Turkey as part of traditional folk medicine for an unknown amount of time. It was first detected by foreigners from the West in 1717. Starting then, the West learned of this method mostly through the writings of Greek physician Emanuel Timoni and of Lady Mary Wortley Montagu (Dinc and Ulman 2007). Lady Mary, the wife of the then-British consul in Turkey and a well-known poet of her time, wrote letters explaining this method, and actively worked to introduce it in Europe (Weiss and Esparza 2015; Dinc and Ulman 2007). She had suffered from smallpox and noticed that unlike in Europe, in Turkey, there were almost no pock-marked people. She discovered that every September, people were gathering to get inoculated by older women who repeatedly pricked them with a needle dipped with material taken from person infected with smallpox or a recently variolated individual. In her letter of 1 April 1717, Lady Mary mentions:

> The small-pox, so fatal, and so general amongst us, is here entirely harmless by the invention of ingrafting, which is the term they give it. There is a set of old women who make it their business to perform the operation every autumn, in the month of September, when the great heat is abated ... the old woman comes with a nut-shell full of the matter of the best sort of small-pox, and asks what vein you please to have opened. She immediately rips open what you offer to her with a large needle (which gives you no more pain than a common scratch), and puts into the vein as much matter as can lye upon the head of her needle, and after that binds up the little wound with a hollow bit of shell.
>
> (Sinclair 2016)

Lady Mary let her five-year-old daughter be inoculated as well and popularized the procedure in Europe. Frederick the Great of Prussia, Empress Maria Theresa, Catherine the Great of Russia, and many others followed her example. By the end of the eighteenth century, the procedure had spread to the public when Edward Jenner detected that a safer procedure using pus from cowpox has the same effect and announced the probability of smallpox eradication. Jenner replaced this variolation with what is now called vaccination (Dinc and Ulman 2007). In Bavaria, smallpox vaccination was made compulsory in 1807, and the number of deaths there from smallpox declined from c.7500 to zero by 1810. Global smallpox vaccination lasted until 1977 after the last case of smallpox in Somalia during that year, and on 8 May 1980, the WHO declared the world smallpox-free (Fenner 1982; Strassburg 1982; Hopkins 1983).

Even after this worldwide success, vaccination nonetheless steadily confronted enormous controversy. Nowadays, vaccination often makes headlines in the media and is a major topic on social media, where debates occur between those who are pro- and anti-vaccination. Examples include news reports about banning children with no proof of vaccination from schools in Italy; and from libraries, gyms, supermarkets, or any public place in Rockland County in the US state of New York; and banning of "misinformation" about vaccination on social media in the UK (Rampton 2019; Mandel 2019; Edwards 2019). Analogously, the much-awaited Covid-19 vaccine has revealed the same visibility, as mainstream and social media are currently full of stories that show contestations.

The Continual Contestations Surrounding Vaccines

As mentioned previously, over the years, vaccination has garnered multiple proponents, many successes, and there are internationally funded vaccination programs continuously at work in almost all countries, as some nation-states lack the required abilities, skills, and platforms to manage their own vaccination programs. Yet a growing number of antagonists are refusing and resisting vaccines (Burki 2020). Their resistance is quite analogous to public resistance to other scientific and technological inventions and advancements (Blume 2017; Hughes 2006). They rationalize their decisions to avoid, refuse, and resent vaccination (Durbach 2000; Wolfe and Sharp 2002; Fairhead and Leach 2012; Blume 2017; Bulled 2017; Stöckl and Smajdor 2017; Ali 2020c) in ways that vary according to geographical region and local cultures and subcultures. In some countries, parents refuse vaccines for their children, believing that vaccines have harmful effects on the body (Roberts and Mitchell 2017). Many in the USA believe that the MMR (measles, mumps, and rubella) vaccine, or the cluster of 25 vaccines given to US children in their first two years of life, can cause autism. Although multiple studies have shown no link between vaccines and autism (Offit and Coffin 2003; Jick and Kaye 2003), there are some studies revealing a possible link (Madsen et al.

2002). In some cases, people go beyond such logic and believe in "hidden" links between vaccination and "vested interests" (Davidson 2017; Ali 2020b, a). People can resist a vaccine due to religious ideology, mistrust of biomedicine, doubt about a vaccine's efficacy, or as an unwanted contravention of individual liberty (Bulled 2017). At present, in some countries, vaccination refusal has become a public health emergency as some people link vaccines to autism while others consider it a "Western plot"—as I will further discuss below. These varying rationales beg the anthropological investigation of vaccination in terms of cultural and subcultural beliefs, power dynamics, local and global perspectives, and the impacts of vaccine refusal, especially as a Covid-19 vaccine is on its way around the world.

Will people accept this vaccine or refuse it? How will their reasons for refusal differ among countries and cultures, and what will be the impacts of that refusal? For example, a recent poll has shown that only 53% of US citizens will accept the Covid-19 vaccine, leaving the disease free to spread among the other half and necessitating the continued use of PPE for all (Zoellner 2020). Due to the reasons mentioned above and further described below, many Pakistanis are quite likely to refuse it as well. Thus, vaccination has appeared as a new anthropological problem that needs to be critically and thoroughly studied and analyzed. The global circulation of vaccines and vaccination—and the varied forms of resistance to it—shape and transform various worlds. Vaccines and resistance to them entail a global assemblage (Collier and Ong 2005)—my metaphorical ship—of thoughts, things, and representations, as they connect micro- and macro-level structures and institutions.

Three Distinctive and Contrasting Cases: A Brief Overview

To demonstrate the politics and constant negotiations surrounding vaccination, I concisely present cases from Italy, the USA, and Pakistan: two are similar in their anti-vaccine perspectives, while the other is distinctively different. In both Italy and the USA, parents denying vaccination for their children draw significantly on the work of Andrew Wakefield—the recognized leader of the anti-vaxx movement in the USA and other countries—although the scientific community considers his work to be fraudulent (Wakefield 1999; Godlee, Smith, and Marcovitch 2011). Nevertheless, Wakefield considers his work to be valid, and has continued it. He is also an opponent of the Covid-19 vaccine and even a denier of Covid as a dangerous disease, along with Robert F. Kennedy Jr., with whom Wakefield has been working (Jamison 2020). Some in the USA also believe in the conspiracy theory that "the virus may have been designed and released in order to benefit vaccine makers" (Jamison 2020). In contrast, in Pakistan, vaccination is refused for different reasons; rumors and other conspiracy theories abound and are linked to current and past sociocultural, economic, and geopolitical inequalities that are encoded in "societal memory" (Ali 2020b, a).

The Italian Case

Due to the measles outbreak of 2017 in Italy that accounted for 34% of the number of measles cases in Europe, in 2019, the Italian government made measles vaccination mandatory (European Centre for Disease Prevention and Control (ECDC) 2018; Siani 2019). Afterward, Beatrice Lorenzin—then Italy's health minister—got a law passed, named the "Lorenzin Law" to make ten vaccines compulsory, in order to meet the WHO's target of ensuring a 95% children's vaccination rate in every country. Not providing proof of vaccination could ban unvaccinated children from attending school or compel parents to pay a fine of €500. Lorenzin stated: "No vaccination, no school" (Rampton 2019).

Consequently, unvaccinated children under the age of six years were ultimately denied school admission, while those from six to 16 years of age had a chance not to be banned, but parents needed to pay the fine in the absence of proof of vaccination. Yet the law received significant opposition. In 2017, protests occurred in Rome against the obligatory vaccination. To avoid the vaccine mandate, around 100 Italian families planned to seek asylum in Austria. Again, in 2018, the political opposition to the law was strong, and Italian Interior Minister Matteo Salvini even argued that vaccines "are useless and in many cases dangerous, if not harmful"; therefore, "I confirm the commitment to allow all children to go to school. The priority is that they don't get expelled from the classes" (Mezzofiore 2018).

Accordingly, we see that vaccination in Italy, as in the USA, is not free from contestation. Laypeople do suspect it, and "vaccine hesitancy" has emerged in the case of the Covid-19 vaccine. Not many Italians seem willing to accept this vaccine, and studies have shown this Italian mistrust in research on vaccines (Palamenghi et al. 2020; Barello et al. 2020). Consequently, these studies conclude that it may not be possible to effectively contain Covid-19 in Italy despite vaccine availability there.

The US Case

Before the measles vaccine was introduced in the USA in the early 1960s, measles caused critical epidemics among school-aged children that occurred almost every second or third year (Hotez 2016). Usual hospitalizations during measles outbreaks were of around 50,000 children, including 500 deaths and 4,000 cases of measles encephalitis, leading to permanent neurologic complications, deafness, or both (Strebel et al. 2013). With improved control of measles throughout Central and South America, the disease was declared eliminated from the USA in 2000 and from the WHO region of the Americas in 2002 (Parker Fiebelkorn et al. 2010). Yet, recent measles outbreaks test the status of "elimination" in the USA, which may lead the WHO to take the USA off the list of measles-free countries.

Between 2010 and 2020, infectious diseases such as measles have caused severe outbreaks in the USA. For instance, in 2019 there was a measles outbreak in New York among unvaccinated children (Patel et al. 2019; Benecke and DeYoung 2019; Phadke et al. 2016). As noted earlier, this outbreak led to banning children with no proof of vaccination from libraries, gyms, supermarkets, or any public place in Rockland County, New York (Mandel 2019). The New York parents who refuse to vaccinate their children are part of the large "anti-vaxx" movement in the USA—these "anti-vaxxers" believe in a link between vaccines, autism, and other diseases (Benecke and DeYoung 2019). Measles vaccination coverage in some Texas counties is critically dropping below the 95% coverage rate required for ensuring herd immunity and preventing measles outbreaks (Hotez 2016). The US anti-vaxx movement has been associated with political elements such as people who believe that measles is "imported" from other countries (Parker Fiebelkorn et al. 2010) and is based on a dangerous mix of "pseudoscience and conspiracy theories" (ibid.).

Some older Americans who grew up in the 1950s also refuse the measles vaccine for their children due to their experience. A US colleague recalls that her and other parents in her community in the Northwest considered measles and chicken pox to be "no big deal" and just "a normal part of childhood," so they often held measles or chicken pox parties so that other kids could get those diseases and get them over with. This colleague said that, long before Andrew Wakefield was even heard of, when she was raising her kids in the 1980s, she chose not to vaccinate them because of the mercury in the vaccines (which has since been removed). In order to get them into school, she got an official-looking vaccination card from her doctor's office, and just lied on it! And she was by no means alone in doing so, while other anti-vaxx parents claimed an exemption for religious reasons, which was allowed.

The Pakistani Case

Akin to Italy and the USA, a plethora of weavings around vaccination prevails in Pakistan. On the one hand, the government is making efforts to organize vaccination drives to meet the goal of more than 95% of vaccination coverage to fulfill the recommendations charted by global stakeholders such as the WHO. On the other hand, anti-vaccination movements in Pakistan are strong. Yet the underlying rationales in Pakistan are different from those in Italy, where the underlying rationales seem to match those in the USA. Vaccination as a generic category in Pakistan is not merely refused based on its purported harms to the body, but also due to the circulation of certain rumors and conspiracy theories that imagine vaccination as a "Western plot" to sterilize the Muslim population (Ali 2020b, a)—which people have reason to believe as they tend to be aware that many in "the West" do not want more Brown and Muslim people to come pouring into their countries. People's suspicion that vaccination programs are an apparatus of bio-geo-politics became a reality in 2011 when the US CIA used a "fake" vaccination campaign to identify the location of Osama bin Laden (McGirk 2015;

Hussain et al. 2016). This "critical event" (Das 1995), which Pakistani analysts called "vaccination suicide," significantly and adversely affected vaccine uptake in the country, and continues to do so (Ali 2020d, b, a).

As a result, low vaccination uptake has become a public health emergency in Pakistan. During the decade of 2010–2020, many thousands of children were unvaccinated, and there was a declaration of *jihad* against vaccination by extremists such as religious leaders and the Taliban in some parts of the country. Since the fake campaign that discovered bin Laden, at least 100 vaccinators and their escorting security personnel have been assaulted or killed. The government has retaliated by arresting parents who refuse vaccinations. Yet during that decade, the Pakistani media also reported some children's reactions to measles and polio vaccines, which have caused complications and side effects in a few hundred children, including the deaths of approximately ten (Yusufzai 2014; Ali 2020b, a). (Especially in rural areas, many children in Pakistan are stunted and have weak immune systems due to malnourishment.) Therefore, many local people suspect both vaccines and vaccinators and then attack the vaccination teams. Regarding these killings and assaults, the government has issued statements saying, for instance, "They [the vaccinators] laid down their lives to secure the country's future" so it is "sacrifice that will not go to waste" (Raza 2016).

Despite these challenges, global stakeholders use, in the terminology of Closser (Closser 2010), a "culture of optimism" to seek more funds for vaccination programs that often fail. I see this culture of optimism as political; therefore, I call it the *politics of optimism*, as these stakeholders, such as the WHO, assure their funders that, although things have not significantly changed, "we are doing our best to improve them." In addition, they quantify these politics, as has been done in dealing with Covid-19 (Ali, unpublished). Lower numbers reflect a success story of the government—"the proper management"—of the outbreak. For instance, fewer deaths recorded means greater success; thus, it is suspected that the government is "cooking" its statistics on Covid-related deaths (Ali, unpublished). This "valuation" and quantification of loss is highly prominent in political circles as well as among governmental and nongovernmental health officials. The Pakistani case is analogous to the polio vaccine resistance in Nigeria, which stems from sociocultural, political, and historical factors (Renne 2010) and to the case of Cameroon, in which schoolgirls jumped from windows to flee vaccination teams while linking them to colonization and corrupt government (Feldman-Savelsberg, Ndonko, and Schmidt-Ehry 2000; Feldman-Savelsberg, Ndonko, and Yang 2017). Hence, vaccination in Pakistan involves a negotiation process that often revolves around numbers (discussed in the section below).

As far as the Covid-19 vaccine is concerned, it is still unclear whether Pakistanis will accept it since no vaccine is yet available in the country, which is currently planning to buy vaccines from China. During my discussion with a Pakistani health official, I learned that many people refused to participate in vaccine trials despite the offer of payment. Again, in some parts of the country—most especially in rural regions—laypeople have refused routine vaccines after linking them and Covid-19 to "Western" or "Jewish" plots (Ali et al., in press). Based on these preliminary observations, it can be claimed that, as with other vaccines, once it arrives, the Covid-19 vaccine will confront severe challenges in Pakistan.

What Can Vaccination Offer to Anthropology?

There are fears and predictions about the emergence of new pathogens beyond Covid-19, and the reemergence of old ones, such as polio and measles. On the other hand, dealing with them, such as vaccination, face profound challenges, as I have shown. The three cases—Italian, USA, and Pakistani—described briefly herein demonstrate some of the relationships among states (global) organizations, society, and culture, illustrating the entanglements of science, politics, and culture.

In vaccination, using numbers is a quite prominent practice, for example, the number of vaccinated children and reports of 95% vaccination coverage to create success stories to receive further funding and continue projects. The engaged stakeholders, such as the vaccinators, the government, and the WHO, understand the importance of numbers and "craft" them accordingly. If reporting greater numbers of vaccine refusals has an advantage, then high numbers are communicated, or the other way around. For instance, the reported number of measles-infected children, unvaccinated children, and refusals would demonstrate the efforts of a vaccinator to the federal level health officials, governments, and the WHO. A lower number of such infected children is better for a vaccinator, as it would show that s/he is effectively performing the required tasks. In contrast, as stated earlier, if the number of unvaccinated children and refusals is high, then stakeholders, such as the government and the WHO, play politics by practicing the "culture of optimism." In other words, even if the numbers of unvaccinated children are significant, there is still great hope to substantially minimize them in future projects.

I argue that the use of numbers reveals an "optimism bias" (Ali 2020a): good "numbers" are relative phenomena. To put it differently: good (higher or lower) numbers make success stories while weak numbers are used to show how much further effort is required to run global health projects. Either the project fails or is successful; the numbers determine further interventions as success stories rationalize similar interventions in other villages, towns, countries, or continents for the same or similar diseases.

A deliberate fabrication of data has started, primarily in development projects, to receive aid at local and global levels. For example, Biruk (2018) finds a "cooking" of data in development projects in Africa, in which the African researchers fabricate the data to gain more funding. Stakeholders use numbers for manipulation. For instance, Adams (2016b, 189–90) argues that stakeholders like the Bill and Melinda Gates Foundation and the Global

Fund can engineer profit-making to "tether neoliberal forms of profit-seeking to global health by making 'scalability' the primary measure of efficacy." Depending on the circumstances, such organizations seek to generate good numbers and minimize negative numbers such as those related to casualties.

For example, current studies on Covid-19 from the USA reveal that reported Covid-19 infections and deaths "do not represent the full SARS-CoV-2 disease burden" (Angulo, Finelli, and Swerdlow 2021, 4–5). According to one study in the USA, during November 2020, approximately 35% of Covid-19 deaths were not reported (Woolf et al. 2020). Based on these studies, one may hypothesize that governments have "cooked" these numbers to make it appear that fewer people have been infected and died in their countries in order to show that they are doing a good job of viral containment, which then carries a severely negative ripple effect as people become less afraid of Covid based on supposedly low numbers of deaths compared to numbers of infections. Therefore, the issue is how much one should (mis)trust such numbers. Clearly, false or "cooked" numbers can be extremely misleading, as they speak for actual humans and can point our thinking in the wrong direction.

Like other public health interventions, vaccination exhibits intricate connections among people and institutions at local, national, and global scales. Illustrating the negotiation of technology between "technoconservatives" and "technoprogressives" (Hughes 2006), vaccination offers a window to the world of the ongoing politics between these two segments of society. The three case studies presented above highlight numerous relationships: between society and science; between an individual living in a village and a global institution (e.g., the WHO or the UN); between citizens and their governments; among countries (e.g., diplomacy) (Kaufmann and Feldbaum 2009); between a country's government and global stakeholders; and between non-governmental organizations (e.g., the WHO) and the donor organizations (e.g., the Bill and Melinda Gates Foundation). Revealing tensions and profound disagreements, these scales and stakeholders sometimes reinforce and sometimes compete with each other (Bulled 2017). All of these are on board my metaphorical vaccination ship, where they quarrel with one another over drinks on deck about contesting narratives, behaviors, and attitudes. Many on board report and repeat rumors, conspiracy theories, refusals, resistance, fear, and anxiety. Others present advocacy, acceptance, favorable scientific evidence, and strong resentment against vaccine opponents whose failure to vaccinate their children leaves many countries vulnerable to infectious disease outbreaks that could be entirely prevented by universal vaccine uptake. Existing at the nexus of bio-geo-politics, vaccination today is made far more salient on the world stage by the advent of the Covid-19 vaccine and its potential refusals, which highlight both new and old tensions among national and international stakeholders and the public.

Theoretically speaking, anthropological studies of vaccination can significantly corroborate the deliberations initiated to theorize refusal and hesitancy (Ortner 1995; Sobo 2016; McGranahan 2016). Medical anthropologists have already paid significant attention to vaccination and its challenges and debates (Feldman-Savelsberg, Ndonko, and Schmidt-Ehry 2000; Fairhead and Leach 2012; Closser et al. 2016; Feldman-Savelsberg, Ndonko, and Yang 2017; Roberts and Mitchell 2017; Ali 2020b, a). Yet there is a need for further explorations, and that is why *this chapter constitutes a call for the development of an official anthropology of vaccination.* Studies can focus on the "social life" (Kopytoff 1986; Appadurai 1988; Geest, Whyte, and Hardon 1996) of vaccines to illustrate the forms of rationalities and logic used to negotiate vaccination. Likewise, forms of trust and mistrust occurring at various levels can be an appealing endeavor to be explored and examined. The creation of optimistic evidence to seek funding from donors to continue projects (Closser 2010; Adams 2016a; Biruk 2018) shows the *politics of quantification,* (Ali, unpublished), which is also an attractive endeavor to be studied. Anthropologists can research competing narratives—rumors and conspiracy theories—surrounding vaccination to understand their underlying cultural rationales and to reveal (geo-)politics and biopolitics. Focusing on the creations of vaccination programs, the discipline can inquire about the local-level politics between vaccinators and laypeople and between vaccinators and the (sub-)district health officials. More importantly, anthropology can study the relationships between institutionalized forms of disparities and vaccination uptake. For instance, although their work is critical and vaccinators may face tremendous logistical difficulties and even threats to their lives, their salaries in low-resource countries are very low compared to those of their official supervisors, who do not face such threats. Also, the power dynamics surrounding vaccination at various levels constitute a promising subject to be explored.

Studying vaccination can help us understand the relationships between and among local, national, and global stakeholders. Not only is studying vaccination an endeavor for medical anthropology, but is also an exciting feast for other subdisciplines, such as economic anthropology, political anthropology, the anthropology of development, and the anthropology of migration. Focusing on vaccination can add to critical discussions related to the "individual body," the "social body," the "body politic" (Scheper-Hughes and Lock 1987), and the "ethical turn" (Fassin 2014; Faubion 2014).

What Can Anthropology Offer to Vaccination?

Anthropological accounts would be significantly useful for stakeholders such as policymakers and implementors. Since anthropological studies and analyses dig deeper to reveal invisible factors shaping vaccine refusal and resentment, findings can exhibit the qualitative aspects of vaccination, especially social tensions surrounding it. For instance, in public health, significant attention has been directed to vaccine hesitancy (Schuster, Eskola, and Duclos 2015; MacDonald 2015; Roberts et al. 2015; Karafillakis et al.

2016; McClure, Cataldi, and O'Leary 2017), yet with a different angle and focus. Thus, anthropology can enormously add to the "vaccine hesitancy continuum" developed by the WHO's Strategic Advisory Group of Experts (SAGE) on vaccination (MacDonald 2015). In this model, McDonald claims that *"complacency, convenience, and confidence"* create vaccine hesitancy (italics in original) (2015, 4163). Yet this is not always the case, as in some countries such as Pakistan, people not only refuse vaccination but are also deeply resentful of vaccination programs, believing such programs to be part of larger geopolitical forces acting against them—a topic not covered in the studies listed above (Feldman-Savelsberg, Ndonko, and Schmidt-Ehry 2000; Feldman-Savelsberg, Ndonko, and Yang 2017; Ali 2020b, a).

Thus, anthropological scholarship offers a critical and necessary perspective to search underneath this continuum of accepting and refusing a vaccine—or accepting or refusing some vaccines but not others. The discipline can inquire and demonstrate how one parent's vaccine refusal can impact decision making at the global level and how global-level decisions, such as the fake vaccination campaign in Pakistan, can spur anti-vaccination movements. Anthropological accounts of vaccinations can reveal the impacts of sociocultural, economic, and political particularities concerning the acceptance and rejection of a vaccine. Just as Lock and Kaufert (2001) find "local biologies" at play in the case of menopause, there are what I call local sociologies, anthropologies, geographies, and economies at play in vaccination. For instance, there could be a significant difference between a Pakistani body and an Italian body. In the former country, as previously noted, malnourishment and stunting of children are significant problems (Ali and Ali 2020; Ali 2020a). This difference puts Pakistani children at a significant risk compared to Italian or Usonian children for vaccine reactions and for contracting infectious diseases. Therefore, vaccine refusal and vaccination itself can have vastly different consequences in these three countries.

In this regard, anthropology has a meaningful and indispensable perspective to contribute to global health, including vaccination. Panter-Brick and Eggerman (2018) have showcased four central characteristics of medical anthropology—critically reflective, cross-cultural, people-centered, and transdisciplinary—to study the interrelationships between health and society. Keeping in view these four characteristics, (1) vaccination appears to be an excellent critical entry point to study sociocultural viewpoints, lived experiences, and contested social worlds by studying and interpreting vaccination programs from conception, implementation, and strategies to approaches. (2) Since vaccination receives multiple local and global understandings, it is an intriguing entry point from which to conduct cross-cultural inquiries, for example, comparing societies and countries by using concepts of local biologies, anthropologies, sociologies, geographies, and economies. (3) Demonstrating local perceptions, concerns, and particularities to be incorporated into the vaccination programs, vaccination offers a platform to record people-centered views of the world in the form of their lived experiences, their structural vulnerabilities, and their social agency (or lack thereof). (4) Vaccination is a great endeavor to design multidisciplinary research agendas to study and analyze "the nexus of cultures, societies, biologies, and health" (see Panter-Brick and Eggerman 2018, 233). Anthropological studies of vaccination can present conversations on the body, mind, person, community, environment, prevention, and therapy: for example, devising a joint project that engages epidemiologists, public health specialists, and medical anthropologists to study and improve vaccination in a given society simultaneously.

Concluding Remarks

Providing three brief case studies—of Italy, the USA, and Pakistan—in this chapter, I have highlighted some of the ongoing contestations and negotiations around vaccination. Given that these phenomena hold immense value for future anthropological explorations and theoretical vistas, I have proposed that vaccination demands profound anthropological attention. Other disciplines, especially public health, have invested laudable efforts, but with a different lens. Public health studies of vaccination primarily center on finding solutions while drawing mainly on the administration and monitoring side for an increase in vaccination coverage. Although there are some recent claims that the reasons responsible for people's refusal and resistance to vaccination "are, unfortunately, all too well known" (Turner 2019), these phenomena are actually not well enough understood and considered. These claims seem the result of this discipline's theoretical and methodological interests, orientations, and limitations. I argue that public health studies of vaccination do not delve deeply enough into the reasons behind people's vaccine refusals and resentments and the cultural and subcultural variations among them. The deeper understandings of these anthropologists can provide *and aid public health programs by guiding them in how to overcome such refusals via culturally appropriate educational programs.* Before vaccine uptake can be heightened, vaccine refusal must be reduced. I believe that anthropologists can aid greatly in that endeavor by sharing their findings with public health vaccination program designers and helping them develop locally effective vaccine education. This kind of culturally informed education has enormous potential to increase vaccine uptake and thereby to decrease people's suffering from preventable infectious diseases. I conclude by again arguing for the official establishment of an anthropology of vaccination, for all the reasons outlined above.

Conclusions

Interrelations between Measles' Sacredness and Systematic Disparities

Microorganisms causing infectious diseases have been challenging human-kind at the latest since we began to live in close quarters as agriculturalists around 10,000–12,000 years ago. The 2020 Covid-19 pandemic—that overwhelmed the entire world for more than two years—is a convincing example of those extraordinary challenges. By the middle of August 2020, when I was completing my thesis that is the basis of the current monograph, the pandemic was still unfolding while infecting around 22.5 million people and had caused 783,000 deaths globally. These figures were constantly changing, as by mid-August 2022, as I am finishing this book, the virus has infected 590 million and 6.43 million deaths. As the pandemic progressed, we gradually learn from diverse sources and our firsthand experiences that its velocity of ethical, sociocultural, and politico-economic implications is significant yet differs considerably at diverse locations. It has substantially affected economies worldwide, disrupted lives, exposed the existing forms of institutionalized inequalities, and highlighted the politics of care.

Considering this difference in impacts that also occurred during the outbreaks of measles around the globe, this book focused on two measles outbreaks that occurred in 2012 and 2013 and challenged Pakistan, mainly Sindh province. Thousands of children contracted the virus and a few hundred passed away. With a focus on these types of unequal unfolding of outbreaks, this long-term ethnographic project explored the following central questions. Why does measles still cause outbreaks in the province, especially in rural areas? How do different stakeholders, ranging from local people to global-level institutions, perceive and deal with measles? Why are vaccination programs not more effective? And in which ways can anthropology help us understand the occurrence of measles through its unique perspective? These questions were chosen to understand the world in which various forms of structured inequalities are appropriated—these disparities create fertile ground for several infectious diseases, including measles, to overwhelm specific populations. To address the research questions, I utilized a range of anthropological theories, processes, and methods. Employing the interpretive and the critical approaches in medical anthropology as the major theoretical frameworks, I have also significantly borrowed and benefited from several other theoretical frameworks for conducting this project and analyzing

DOI: 10.4324/9781003253716-13

its results (see Chapter 1). Those theoretical concepts helped me to develop the central thesis of this project, which is that geopolitical and economic regimes have cleverly and subtly carved out diverse local and global inequalities, which then lead to various health crises, including the measles outbreaks in Pakistan. The existence and specific shape of measles in Sindh province is a result of this unequal distribution of resources, lack and shortcomings of healthcare institutions, as well as a dearth of adequate facilities, and the lack of education of lay people about health and effective healthcare, in particular about the benefits and importance of vaccination. Drawing on these concepts, I developed new theoretical concepts such as "societal memory," "local colonization," and "optimism bias."

Trying to become innovative, I provide personal anecdotes to explain data collection processes that I called a *Researchlogue*. I introduce a new method called *Kachaharī*. Although this method exists in the local culture of Sindh (and across South Asia), it can be termed as a novel method because no social scientist prior to me has used it. It is crucial to mention that I have not used *Kachaharī*, which has colonial roots, but the one that is rooted in the sociocultural patterns, especially of Sindh. *Kachaharī* primarily consists of informal and voluntary social gatherings where individuals engage in discussions, sharing insights on various aspects of life, including personal, collective, sociocultural, economic, political, religious, and current affairs. Unlike traditional focus groups, *Kachaharī* differentiates itself by putting participants in the role of discussion leaders rather than relying on anthropologists to guide the conversation. This distinctive method integrates local knowledge and wisdom to provide a unique lens for the anthropological tool-kit. I am confident that by challenging established methods, such as Western-derived focus group discussions, and embracing the *Kachaharī*, we can contribute to an anthropological turn or decolonizing theory and method.

Driven by various considerations, I adopted a "multi-sited" approach and employed the extended case method. Two specific villages, *Rahīmpur* and *Rāmpur*, situated in *Sakhar* and *Tharpārkar* districts, respectively, within Pakistan's Sindh province, served as the central field sites. These villages experienced severe measles outbreaks. *Rahīmpur* in northern Sindh, predominantly Muslim, was contrasted with *Rāmpur* in the south, where Hindus were predominant. This intentional diversity allowed exploring how religion shapes perceptions of measles, its treatment, and attitudes toward vaccination. Despite *Rahīmpur*'s Muslims calling it "*Ur'rrī*" and *Rāmpur*'s residents terming it "*Ourhī*," both villages share the view that measles is an extraordinary, necessary, and sacred event. In *Rahīmpur*, Muslims do not name a specific manifestation of *Mātā*, while in *Rāmpur*, Hindus refer to it as *Sitālā Mātā*. Muslims in *Rāmpur* observe measles rituals but skip daily worship, whereas Hindus conduct fortnightly *Thadrrī* worships to invoke *Mātā* (refer to Chapter 6). This selection was pivotal in highlighting diverse perspectives within and across the chosen villages.

Medical pluralism prevails in Pakistan. These healthcare sectors include *Unānī-Tib*, homeopathy, home-based remedies, shrine behaviors, and bio-medicine. Each system reflects distinct bodies of knowledge and practices related to conceptualizing, sustaining, and restoring health. Despite differences in etiology, diagnostics, and therapeutic practices, the overarching goal of all these systems is to alleviate illness-related suffering and restore health. People seek health measures by consulting a specific medical system, which are greatly shaped by factors such as beliefs, perceptions, economic situation, education, the ill person's gender, and the geographical area and accessibility to a medical system.

Moreover, the legal integration of Indigenous medical systems into the healthcare system is acknowledged, with established colleges offering education and degrees in these fields. However, the government's predominant focus is on the biomedical healthcare system, which was introduced during British rule and has significantly impacted folk healthcare practices. Despite this attention, critical issues prevail within the biomedical system that include a lack of health facilities, doctor unemployment, low motivation among medical staff (especially in rural areas), pharmaceutical company monopolies, profit-centric approaches, and, notably, inadequate access to clean water and sanitation. There is a "class-bias" as well as "urban-bias" in the healthcare system, perpetuating institutionalized inequalities and violence, particularly affecting those with less economic and political power. While Pakistan faces significant healthcare challenges, there is a persistent lack of adequate resource allocation. The average percentage of GDP spent on healthcare from 2000–2001 to 2019–2020 has never surpassed 1%, except for the last two budgets, which saw slightly higher percentages. Insufficient expenditures hinder the construction of effective healthcare facilities, addressing logistical issues in vaccination, improving hygiene, overcoming illiteracy, and enhancing public knowledge. The government attributes healthcare system deficiencies to rapid population growth, citing factors such as uneven distribution of health professionals, a deficient workforce, insufficient funding, and limited access to quality healthcare services. While some in the government acknowledge these issues, the overall response appears inadequate.

Measles reveals multiple competing narratives and rituals of containment. From the local standpoint, measles—as a necessary sacred illness—needs to be handled by observing the ritual of *Chandā*, in which a child is kept under a *Chillā* (quarantine), and certain stringent "dos" and "don'ts" are carefully observed by an elderly woman. During this time, *Lorī* or *Bhajjan* (lullaby) is played, and specific people are allowed to see the child. For these ideas and practices, government officials and doctors blame local people—and yet there is some wisdom in such practices, most notably in the quarantining of the ill. It is a fact that most children recover from measles, so, often, the best that parents can do is keep others from becoming infected as they care for their sick child. These people avoid biomedical treatment while believing that it displeases *Mātā*.

This negotiation process became prominent during the measles outbreaks of 2012 and 2013. Local politicians paid money and supplied an ambulance to the local people for bringing their sick children to biomedical hospitals. They also wrote letters to the federal government concerning measles, which initiated a debate in the Senate. Consequently, the *Wafaqi-Mohtasib* (Federal Ombudsman) formed a committee to explore the reasons for these outbreaks. The committee consulted several stakeholders, including the governmental institutions (about health and economy), and global stakeholders, such as the WHO. The Federal Ombudsman's report concludes that the most crucial cause of the measles outbreak was a "failure" of the EPI system, which is further deteriorating. A district official participating in a *Kachaharī* with me attributed the outbreak to the lack of sincerity, commitment, and ownership among health officials at the service delivery level. Further challenges include persistent load-shedding and insufficient investment in the EPI infrastructure at the provincial level. Almost all trained human resources were shifted to polio, considering it a more pressing issue—the focus results in a lack of attention to other diseases such as measles.

Geopolitical regimes fuel rumors, conspiracy theories, and resistance, fostering socioeconomic and political disparities impacting health, causing infectious disease outbreaks, and opposing vaccination programs. The "extremist" segment, like the *Tālibān*, links vaccination to geopolitics. Government officials blame "extremists" for low vaccination rates and violence against vaccinators, overlooking broader geopolitical and economic factors nurturing extremism. Over its 70-year history as an independent state, Pakistan has grappled with the intertwined challenges of external problems and internal crises. British colonization led to enduring consequences such as the partition massacre, four international wars, two genocides, six secessionist movements, and numerous communal massacres, leaving a lasting impact. In the 1980s, the USSR's invasion of Afghanistan made Pakistan a crucial ally of the USA, supporting the covert creation of the *Mujāhidīn*, who later turned against the USA, contributing significantly to global terrorism. Rooted in the 1980s, extremism emerged as Zia-ul-Haq attempted transformation supported by external events, deepening societal divisions. Critical events like the *Mujāhidīn*'s formation had a lasting impact, leading to the emergence of the Pakistani *Tehrīk-i-Tālibān* (TTP) in 2008, seizing Swat and perpetrating violence. They targeted vaccinators, conducted suicide bombings, and attacked public spaces, mosques, shrines, airports, educational institutions, and army installations. These historical and contemporary events significantly influenced perceptions and behaviors in Pakistan, particularly regarding vaccination, resulting in conflicting narratives. Extremists persist in their uncompromising hostility and opposition to immunization programs.

The immunization program has been facing multiple challenges in the form of controversies and tensions. Rooted in critical events, there was a perception that vaccination is a "Western plot" or a conspiracy against Muslims, so it holds some "hidden interests." This perception became a reality in 2011 when the American CIA used a fake hepatitis vaccination drive as a cover in *Abbotābād* city for discovering the location of Osama bin Laden. The agency hired a local doctor named Dr. *Shakīl Afrīdī*, who is still in jail on charges of treason against the country. This campaign was termed a "vaccination suicide" in Pakistan. Afterward, the vaccination teams came under attack, and extremists killed more than 100 vaccinators and their escorting security personnel. Evidently, ideas woven around vaccination have roots not only in rumors but also in realities.

These perceptions and practices have challenged the elimination of communicable diseases such as polio and measles. There is a growing number of parents who refuse a vaccine as well as resent vaccination. These perceptions result in children with no vaccination. Owing to these events, the country has remained under the spotlight at the global level. At the beginning of the 2000s, the country was criticized due to transmitting polio to approximately 24 formerly polio-free countries, as most of those cases had originated in Pakistan. Consequently, vaccination was made mandatory for Pakistani travelers to travel abroad.

Vaccination remains a contested phenomenon. Following a vaccination drive in the country, rumors and conspiracy theories emerged about suspected side effects related to vaccination. Such news reports generated an online dialogue, in which people negotiate vaccination while criticizing the government, media, and the global stakeholders. These weavings demonstrate scales and types of trust and mistrust, as explanations relate to sociocultural factors, economic aspects, and geo-bio-political connections. Yet the weavings are inseparable, as there are significant interlinkages and entanglements among them.

As a medical invention, I argue that vaccination has become concurrently a geopolitical, economic, and sociocultural problem, as it is often heavily contested in various countries. Such contestations require full qualitative attention to address the politics as well as the knowledge and economic gaps they represent. These negotiations and contestations make vaccination and its related phenomena a promising subject matter for anthropology. Particularly, anthropology can study the controversies and politics revolving around vaccination and the varying reasons for them. Employing vaccination as an analytical concept, anthropology can paint the intricate relationships among the diverse stakeholders. Considering characterizations of anthropology *as the most scientific of the humanities, the most humanistic of the sciences* and vaccination *as a scientific invention with a plethora of sociocultural, economic, and geopolitical weavings*, each carries significant importance for the other. I ask for creating *an anthropology of vaccination*.

Two Perspectives on Measles: Summing Up

I examined measles from two perspectives—as a disease and as an analytical window to the world. From the first perspective, I demonstrated that the occurrence of measles outbreaks is related to structured disparities that are, in turn, related to sociocultural, political, and economic factors that occur at local, national, and global levels. These factors can be individual or collective. From the second perspective, measles as a window has substantially helped me to understand the interplays among these factors. Understanding forms of institutionalized vulnerabilities and inequalities has assisted me in reaching that macro-level where policies are formulated, and decisions are taken, which afterward can produce certain forms of "structural violence" at national and local levels. Put simply, I elucidated that measles offers a platform to observe and analyze the links between micro- and macro-levels, local and global scale, and the particular and general: how these different worlds are interconnected, which seem different yet significantly affecting each other. Through measles, it has become possible to study and understand various forms of social negotiations, tensions, and contestations. One can see the currents of trust and mistrust that occur between and among them.

Measles outbreaks are effects of continuous sociocultural, economic, and political (local and global as well as present and past) processes. Hence, the outbreaks can best be understood against a broader and historical spectrum of economic and (geo)political inequalities, which are enormous and prominent, persistent, and deepening.

In short, I argued that contemporary inequalities are the result of disproportionally distributed wealth. First, these inequalities provide a fertile ground for diseases, such as measles, to cause an outbreak due to inappropriate vaccination. Second, disparities shape who will contract the virus and be significantly affected. Third, these variations affect local people's perception of whether or not to view the disease as a problem severe enough to bring the infected child to a biomedical center. Fourth, because they are economically poor, local people do not want to give up their daily wages to take the time to visit a hospital. Fifth, there are not enough healthcare facilities and providers to deal with measles, often rendering moot the question of whether to go to a hospital or not, thereby creating a sort of "Catch 22" situation. These interwoven factors make their implications challenging to understand; thus, the Pakistani government finds it easier to "blame the victims" and blame population growth than to effectively deal with the problem.

Appendix: Practical Suggestions and Recommendations

I will present my practical suggestions after making two points, one theoretical and one practical.

Theoretically, much attention has been paid to the critical medical anthropology school of thought, but issues in applying critical frameworks to low-income countries have received insufficient attention. Insufficient attention has been drawn to the risks and precarity that may emerge for specific anthropologists after employing a critical framework. Every researcher—especially those who come from low-income countries where several (geo)political risks already prevail—cannot analyze a phenomenon from a critical perspective without inviting serious risks and dangers. Although work on this direction has already started, there is a vast gap available documenting and exploring these experiences by conducting critical (auto-)ethnographies of the scholars at risk.

Practically, global stakeholders, such as the USA, should refrain from policies and practices that have disturbing ethical and political implications. It can include withholding foreign aid or granting it for political reasons, for example, gaining power in a particular region. Such policies adversely affect the lives of millions of people. These stakeholders should not misuse lifesaving endeavors like vaccination programs. Since life cannot be separated from politics, in my view, the solution cannot be to ban politics from health but to install the right politics (such as allotting more than 1% GDP to the health sector). Yet I suggest geopolitics and vaccination should be separated to the extent that one may not misuse the lifesaving project.

The Government of Pakistan should provide people with the required infrastructure (including clean water and adequate sanitation), education, and healthcare facilities. The perception and practice of measles as a sacred illness are stronger in the rural areas than the urban areas, in part due to local culture and in part to unavailability and inaccessibility of the said facilities or mistreatment upon arrival there. Regarding this local dealing with measles as irrational and superstitious makes it easy for the government to blame the victims instead of itself for low vaccine uptake and measles outbreaks.

The government should build the capacity of vaccinators who should significantly focus on the necessary information: what the vaccination is and why it is necessary. Many vaccinators are unaware of the advantages of immunizing children and are therefore unable to explain them to reluctant parents. Nor do they know the ingredients of vaccines, leaving more unanswered questions. The second area of training should be the roles and responsibilities of the vaccinator. Some of them lack awareness about the geographical boundaries of their field and their responsibilities therein. The health of a nation can significantly depend on them.

Thus, the vaccinator should be provided with practical transport to reach distant areas, and with better pay. Given that federal level supervising teams travel in air-conditioned vehicles and are well-paid, it is necessary to significantly raise the salaries of vaccinators and provide equally comfortable transport for them, as they are the ones on the ground facing severe challenges such as harsh weather and threats against their lives.

The government should also better maintain the cold chain system. In areas where electricity is unavailable, the government should find viable means, such as solar-powered batteries, to maintain the required temperature of vaccines. These measures are particularly necessary at the bottom level, that is, the Basic Health Units (BHUs).

Additionally, the functioning of the biomedical healthcare system should be improved. The staff should be trained in how to politely and ethically deal with people in respectful and culturally sensitive ways. Their improper dealings with locals also contribute to anti-biomedical and anti-government sentiments. Lay people see these healthcare providers as the faces of the bio-medical system and the government. For effective capacity building, the government may engage specialists like anthropologists, who are well-positioned to bring the otherwise unheard perspectives of local people to the attention of health officials, including the government.

The government should engage social scientists, including anthropologists, not only in the making of the vaccination program at the policy level but also at the delivery level. These scientists can help to address the areas related to misinformation and mistrust. The government must understand that health is not the domain of medicine only but has multiple aspects that require a multidisciplinary approach.

Besides, there is a need to sensitize the media about reporting on outbreaks of infectious diseases, especially on the suspected reactions to vaccines. The media should publish well-researched news reports on such critical themes, engaging social scientists in their reporting process.

It is also necessary that the government revisit its relationship with its citizens. To build a trustworthy relationship, the government should eliminate all forms of corruption that are occurring at the federal to the Union Council (UC) level.

The government should revisit the "development" budget as related to infrastructure, education, and health. Right from the independence of the country, the health budget has hardly crossed 1% of the country's GDP, except for the last two years (2018–2019). In contrast, the country has spent too much on the defense sector. It is highly suggested that the government should significantly revise its budget and allocate enough resources to infrastructure, education, and health.

There is a dire need to inaugurate more healthcare facilities and produce more healthcare providers. As suggested above, revisiting the health budget would allow the government to increase facilities and produce sufficient providers.

Moreover, it is indispensable that the government utilize the research conducted by social scientists, including anthropologists, as well as allocate enough resources to facilitate further research. The decisions should be based on thoroughly researched evidence.

Rumors and conspiracy theories are social phenomena. These also emerge and spread from person to person under specific circumstances like viruses (Ali 2020d, g); thus, the government and the vaccination planners should pay close attention to what I call *epidemiology* of rumors and conspiracy theories.

Many of my suggestions seem idealistic, yet I believe that with sufficient effort and will, they can be achieved.

Bibliography

Acemoglu, Daron, and James A. Robinson. 2012. *Why Nations Fail: The Origins of Power, Prosperity, and Poverty.* London: Profile Books.

Adams, Tony E., and Andrew F. Herrmann. 2020. "Expanding Our Autoethnographic Future." *Journal of Autoethnography* 1 (1): 1–8. https://doi.org/10.1525/joae.2020.1.1.1.

Adams, Vincanne, ed. 2016a. *Metrics: What Counts in Global Health.* Durham: Duke University Press.

———. 2016b. "What Is Critical Global Health." *Medicine Anthropology Theory* 3 (2): 187–97. https://doi.org/10.17157/mat.3.2.429.

Adams, Vincanne, Nancy J. Burke, and Ian Whitmarsh. 2014. "Slow Research: Thoughts for a Movement in Global Health." *Medical Anthropology* 33 (3): 179–97. https://doi.org/10.1080/01459740.2013.858335.

Adams, Vincanne, Thomas E. Novotny, and Hannah Leslie. 2008. "Global Health Diplomacy." *Medical Anthropology* 27 (4): 315–23. https://doi.org/10.1080/01459740802427067.

Adelson, Naomi. 2008. "Discourses of Stress, Social Inequities, and the Everyday Worlds of First Nations Women in a Remote Northern Canadian Community." *Ethos* 36 (3): 316–33. https://doi.org/10.1111/j.1548-1352.2008.00017.x.

Agence France-Presse (AFP). 2018. "Un: Measles Cases Rise 30 Percent Worldwide." *The Independent*, 30 November 2018. Accessed 27 August 2019. https://www.timesofisrael.com/un-measles-cases-rise-30-percent-worldwide/.

———. 2019. "Austrian City Suspends Bus Services over Measles Case." *The Local*, 10 April 2019. Accessed 23 April 2019. https://www.thelocal.at/20190410/austrian-city-suspends-bus-services-over-measles-case.

Ahmad, Habib, Ghulam Raza Bhatti, and Abdul Latif. 2006. "Medicinal Flora of the Thar Desert: An Overview of Problems and Their Feasible Solutions." *Zonas Áridas* 8 (1): 73–84.

Ahmad, Khabir, Tazeen H. Jafar, and Nish Chaturvedi. 2005. "Self-Rated Health in Pakistan: Results of a National Health Survey." *BMC Public Health* 5 (1): 51. https://doi.org/10.1186/1471-2458-5-51.

Ahmad, Syed Osama, Fouad Yousuf, Ahmed S. Bux, and Ahmed Abu-Zaid. 2016. "Pakistan: The Final Frontier for Global Polio Eradication." *Journal of Epidemiology Community Health* 70 (2): 109–10. https://doi.org/dx.doi.org/10.1136/jech-2015-205530.

Ahmad, Tania. 2014. "Socialities of Indignation: Denouncing Party Politics in Karachi." *Cultural Anthropology* 29 (2): 411–32. https://doi.org/10.14506/ca29.2.12.

Ahmed, Jibran. 2014. "Shakil Afridi, Pakistani Doctor Who Helped U.S. Find Bin Laden, Charged with Murder." *Huffington Post*, 25 January 2014. Accessed 12 January 2016. http://www.huffingtonpost.com/2013/11/22/shakil-afridi-charged _n_4322432.html.

Akhtar, Jamāl, and M. Khalid Siddiqui. 2008. "Utility of Cupping Therapy Hijamat in Unani Medicine." *Indian Journal of Traditional Knowledge* 7 (4): 572–4. http://nopr .niscair.res.in/bitstream/123456789/2380/1/IJTK%207%284%29%20572-574.pdf.

Alex, Gabriele. 2009. "Folk Healing and the Negotiation of Shifting Social Identities in Tamil Nadu, India." *Max Planck Institute for the Study of Religious and Ethnic Diversity.*

Ali, Imran. 2002. "The Historical Lineages of Poverty and Exclusion in Pakistan." *South Asia: Journal of South Asian Studies* 25 (2): 33–60. https://doi.org/10.1080 /00856400208723474.

Ali, Inayat. 2011. "Cultural Construction of Health and Illness: The Case Study of a Potohari Village." M.Phil Qualitative, Department of Anthropology, Quaid-i-Azam University.

———. 2019a. "Paradigms to Investigate the HIV Epidemic." *Daily Times*, 16 May. Accessed 17 May 2019. https://dailytimes.com.pk/395401/paradigms-to-investigate -the-hiv-epidemic/.

———. 2019b. "Viral Hepatitis Is Sindh's Silent Killer." *Daily Times*, 10 May 2019. https://dailytimes.com.pk/391391/viral-hepatitis-is-sindhs-silent-killer/.

———. 2019c. "The Aftermath of HIV Surge in Sindh." *Daily Times*, 4 June. Accessed 5 June 2019. https://dailytimes.com.pk/407280/the-aftermath-of-hiv -surge-in-sindh/.

———. 2020a. "The COVID-19 Pandemic: Making Sense of Rumor and Fear." *Medical Anthropology* 40 (3). https://doi.org/10.1080/01459740.2020.1745481.

———. 2020b. "Covid-19: Are We Ready for the Second Wave?" *Disaster Medicine and Public Health Preparedness*: 1–3. https://doi.org/10.1017/dmp.2020.149.

———. 2020c. "Impact of COVID-19 on Vaccination Programs: Adverse or Positive?" *Human Vaccine and Immunotherapeutics* 17 (1): 2594–600.

———. 2020d. "Anthropology in Emergencies: The Roles of Anthropologists During the COVID-19 Pandemic." *Practicing Anthropology* 42 (3): 16–22.

———. 2020e. "Anthropology in Emergencies: The Roles of Anthropologists during the COVID-19 Pandemic By Inayat Ali." *Practicinganthropologyblog* (blog), The Society for Applied Anthropology (SfAA), 20 June. https://practicinganthropology .sfaa.net/2020/06/20/anthropology-in-emergencies-the-roles-of-anthropologists -during-the-covid-19-pandemic-by-inayat-ali/.

———. 2020f. "Goethe Wears a Mask against COVID-19." *Co-existing with Covid-19: Moving into the Post-pandemic World with the Social Sciences* (blog), Medical Anthropology Department, University College London, 1 June. https://medanthucl .com/2020/06/01/goethe-wears-a-mask-against-covid-19/.

———. 2020g. "COVID-19 Amid Rumours and Conspiracy Theories: The Interplay between Local and Global Worlds." In *Coronavirus Disease (Covid-19), Advances in Experimental Medicine and Biology (AEMB)*, edited by Nima Rezaei, 673–86. New York: Springer.

———. 2021. "Rituals of Containment: Many Pandemics, Body Politics, and Social Dramas during COVID-19 in Pakistan." *Frontiers in Sociology* 6. https://doi.org /10.3389/fsoc.2021.648149.

Ali, Inayat, and Robbie Davis-Floyd. 2020. "The Interplay of Words and Politics during COVID-19: Contextualising the Universal Pandemic Vocabulary." *Practicing Anthropology* 42 (4): 20–24.

Ali, Inayat, Salma Sadique, and Shahbaz Ali. 2021. "Doctors Dealing with COVID-19 in Pakistan: Experiences, Perceptions, Fear, and Responsibility." *Frontiers in Public Health* 9: 647543.

Ali, Inayat, Salma Sadique, Shahbaz Ali, and Robbie Davis-Floyd. 2021. "Birthing between the 'Traditional' and the 'Modern': Dāī Practices and Childbearing Women's Choices during COVID-19 in Pakistan." *Frontiers in Sociology* 6: 622223.

Ali, Inayat, and Shahbaz Ali. 2022. "Why May COVID-19 Overwhelm Low-Income Countries Like Pakistan?." *Disaster Medicine and Public Health Preparedness* 16 (1): 316–20.

Ali, Mumtaz. 2003. "Illnesses as Representation of Social Problems and the Role of Healers in Resolving the Socio Medical Problems." M.Sc, Department of Anthropology, Quaid-i-Azam University (414/M.sc).

Ali, Syed Asad, et al. 2009. "Hepatitis B and Hepatitis C in Pakistan: Prevalence and Risk Factors." *International Journal of Infectious Diseases* 13 (1): 9–19. https://doi.org/10.1016/j.ijid.2008.06.019.

Ali, Tariq. 1983. *Can Pakistan Survive?: The Death of a State*. Harmondsworth: Penguin Books.

AlJazeera. 2013. "Pakistan: Battling Measles and Mistrust." Doha, Qatar: AlJazeera. Accessed 20 June. https://www.aljazeera.com/programmes/insidestory/2013/01/20131375914693905.html.

Anderson, Warwick. 2014. "Making Global Health History: The Postcolonial Worldliness of Biomedicine." *Social History of Medicine* 27 (2): 372–84. https://doi.org/10.1093/shm/hkt126.

Andrade, Gabriel E., and Azhar Hussain. 2018. "Polio in Pakistan: Political, Sociological, and Epidemiological Factors." *Cureus* 10 (10): 1–7. https://doi.org/10.7759/cureus.3502.

Angulo, Frederick J., Lyn Finelli, and David L. Swerdlow. 2021. "Estimation of US SARS-CoV-2 Infections, Symptomatic Infections, Hospitalizations, and Deaths Using Seroprevalence Surveys." *JAMA Network Open* 4 (1): e2033706. https://doi.org/10.1001/jamanetworkopen.2020.33706.

Anjum, Saira. 2000. "Health Seeking Behaviour from Traditional to Modern in the Village Jhugian." M.Sc, Department of Anthropology, Quaid-i-Azam University (317/M.sc).

Annunziato, David, et al. 1982. "Atypical Measles Syndrome: Pathologic and Serologic Findings." *Pediatrics* 70 (2): 203–9.

Appadurai, Arjun, ed. 1988. *The Social Life of Things: Commodities in Cultural Perspective*. Cambridge: Cambridge University Press.

Aristotle. 1984. "On Interpretation." In *The Complete Works of Aristotle: The Revised Oxford Translation*, edited by Jonathan Barnes, 53–89. Princeton: Princeton University Press.

Asad, Talal. 1995. *Anthropology & the Colonial Encounter*. Amherst, NY: Humanity Books.

Ashraf, Masooma. 1994. "Ethnomedicine and Women's Health in Rural Potohar: A Study in Village Sadqal in District Attock." M.Sc, Department of Anthropology, Quaid-i-Azam University (203/M.sc).

Ashraf, Sadia, and Aftab Ahmad. 2015. "Viral Hepatitis in Pakistan: Challenges and Priorities." *Asian Pacific Journal of Tropical Biomedicine* 5 (3): 190–1. https://doi .org/10.1016/S2221-1691(15)30004-6.

Associated Press of Pakistan (APP). 2017. "Don't Blame Pakistan, Haqqanis Were Your 'Darlings' at One Time: Asif Tells Us." *Dawn*, 27 September 2017, 1. Accessed 27 September 2017. https://www.dawn.com/news/1360368/dont-blame -pakistan-haqqanis-were-your-darlings-at-one-time-asif-tells-us.

Attewell, Guy. 2013. "Yunani Tibb and Foundationalism in Early Twentieth-Century India." In *The Body in Balance: Humoral Medicines in Practice*, edited by Elisabeth Hsu Peregrine Horden, 129–48. London: Berghahn Books.

Azeem, Muhammad. 2013. "Most Measles Deaths Took Place in Sindh: WHO." *Dawn*, 17 March 2013. Accessed 27 August 2019. https://www.dawn.com/news /795831/most-measles-deaths-took-place-in-sindh-who.

Baer, Hans A. 1982. "On the Political Economy of Health." *Medical Anthropology Newsletter* 14 (1): 1–17.

———. 1989. "Towards a Critical Medical Anthropology of Health-Related Issues in Socialist-Oriented Societies." *Medical Anthropology* 11 (2): 181–94. https://doi .org/10.1080/01459740.1989.9965991.

———. 1996. "Bringing Political Ecology into Critical Medical Anthropology: A Challenge to Biocultural Approaches." *Medical Anthropology* 17 (2): 129–41. https://doi.org/10.1080/01459740.1996.9966132.

Baer, Hans A., Merrill Singer, and Ida Susser. 2003. *Medical Anthropology and the World System*. 2nd ed. Westport: Praeger.

Bagde, A.B., et al. 2013. "Charaka Samhita—Complete Encyclopedia of Ayurvedic Science." *International Journal of Ayurveda & Alternative Medicine* 1 (1): 12–20.

Band, Isabelle C., and Martin Reichel. 2017. "Al Rhazes and the Beginning of the End of Smallpox." *Journal of American Medical Association Dermatology* 153 (5): 420. https://doi.org/10.1001/jamadermatol.2017.0771.

Banerji, Debabar. 1974. "Social and Cultural Foundations of Health Services Systems." *Economic and Political Weekly* 9: 1333–46. https://www.jstor.org/ stable/4363912.

———. 1981. "The Place of Indigenous and Western Systems of Medicine in the Health Services of India." *Social Science & Medicine* 15 (2): 109–14. https://doi .org/10.1016/0271-7123(81)90030-4.

———. 2004. "The People and Health Service Development in India: A Brief Overview." *International Journal of Health Services* 34 (1): 123–42. https://doi .org/10.2190/9N5U-4NFK-FQDH-J46W.

Bangash, Zahir. 2014. "A Normal Reaction?: Six More Children Faint During Measles Drive." *The Express Tribune*, 22 May 2014. https://tribune.com.pk/story /711380/a-normal-reaction-six-more-children-faint-during-measles-drive/.

Barello, Serena, Tiziana Nania, Federica Dellafiore, Guendalina Graffigna, and Rosario Caruso. 2020. "'Vaccine Hesitancy' among University Students in Italy During the COVID-19 Pandemic." *European Journal of Epidemiology* 35 (8): 781–3.

Barrett, Ronald, et al. 1998. "Emerging and Re-Emerging Infectious Diseases: The Third Epidemiologic Transition." *Annual Review of Anthropology* 27 (1): 247–71. https://doi.org/10.1146/annurev.anthro.27.1.247.

Baxter, David. 2007. "Active and Passive Immunity, Vaccine Types, Excipients and Licensing." *Occupational Medicine* 57: 552–6. https://doi.org/10.1093/occmed/ kqm110.

Becker, Gay, and Robert D. Nachtigall. 1991. "Ambiguous Responsibility in the Doctor-Patient Relationship: The Case of Infertility." *Social Science & Medicine* 32 (8): 875–85.

Beckham, J. David, et al. 2016. "Zika Virus as an Emerging Global Pathogen: Neurological Complications of Zika Virus." *Journal of American Medical Association Neurology* 73 (7): 875–9. https://doi.org/10.1001/jamaneurol.2016.0800.

Behar, Ruth. 2014. *The Vulnerable Observer: Anthropology That Breaks Your Heart.* Boston: Beacon Press.

Benecke, Olivia, and Sarah Elizabeth DeYoung. 2019. "Anti-Vaccine Decision-Making and Measles Resurgence in the United States." *Global Pediatric Health* 6: 2333794X19862949.

Bernard, H. Russell. 2018. *Research Methods in Anthropology: Qualitative and Quantitative Approaches.* 6th ed. New York, London: Rowman & Littlefield.

Bhutta, A. Zafar. 2013. "Pakistan May Face International Travel Ban." *The Express Tribune*, 16 May 2013, 9. https://epaper.tribune.com.pk/DisplayDetails.aspx?ENI_ID=11201305160409&EN_ID=11201305160350&EMID=11201305160037.

Bhutta, Zulfiqar Ahmed. 2001. "Structural Adjustments and Their Impact on Health and Society: A Perspective from Pakistan." *International Journal of Epidemiology* 30 (4): 712–6. https://doi.org/10.1093/ije/30.4.712.

Bibeau, Gilles. 1981. "The Circular Semantic Network in Ngbandi Disease Nosology." *Social Science and Medicine* 15B: 295–307.

Biehl, João. 2016. "Theorizing Global Health." *Medicine Anthropology Theory* 3 (2): 127–42. https://doi.org/10.17157/mat.3.2.434.

Biehl, João, and Adriana Petryna. 2013. "Legal Remedies: Therapeutic Markets and the Judicialization of the Right to Health." In *When People Come First: Critical Studies in Global Health*, edited by João Biehl and Adriana Petryna, 325–46. Princeton, NJ: Princeton University Press.

Biner, Özlem. 2017. "Production of 'Dangerous Knowledge', Violation of Academic Freedom and Precarious Solidarities in the Age of Authoritarianism." On Politics and Precarities in Academia: Anthropological Perspectives, University of Bern, 16 November 2017.

Biruk, Crystal. 2018. *Cooking Data: Culture and Politics in an African Research World.* Durham: Duke University Press.

Bloom, David E., and Daniel Cadarette. 2019. "Infectious Disease Threats in the Twenty-First Century: Strengthening the Global Response." *Frontiers in Immunology* 10 (549). https://doi.org/10.3389/fimmu.2019.00549.

Blume, Stuart. 2006. "Anti-Vaccination Movements and Their Interpretations." *Social Science & Medicine* 62 (3): 628–42. https://doi.org/10.1016/j.socscimed.2005.06.020.

———. 2017. *Immunization: How Vaccines Became Controversial.* London: Reaktion Books.

Boddy, Janice. 1994. "Spirit Possession Revisited: Beyond Instrumentality." *Annual Review of Anthropology* 23 (1): 407–34. https://doi.org/10.1146/annurev.an.23.100194.002203.

Bongaarts, John. 2009. "Human Population Growth and the Demographic Transition." *Philosophical Transactions of the Royal Society B: Biological Sciences* 364 (1532): 2985–90.

Boseley, Sarah. 2018. "Resurgence of Deadly Measles Blamed on Low MMR Vaccination Rates." *The Guardian*, 21 August 2018. Accessed 23 April. https://

www.theguardian.com/society/2018/aug/20/low-mmr-uptake-blamed-for-surge
-in-measles-cases-across-europe.

Boyce-Tillman, June. 2014. "Music and Well-Being." *Journal for Transdisciplinary Research in Southern Africa* 10 (2): 12–33.

Briggs, Charles L. 2005. "Communicability, Racial Discourse, and Disease." *Annual Review of Anthropology* 34 (1): 269–91. https://doi.org/10.1146/annurev.anthro .34.081804.120618.

Briggs, Charles L., and Mark Nichter. 2009. "Biocommunicability and the Biopolitics of Pandemic Threats." *Medical Anthropology* 28 (3): 189–98.

Briggs, Charles, and Richard Bauman. 1999. "'The Foundation of All Future Researches': Franz Boas, George Hunt, Native American Texts, and the Construction of Modernity." *American Quarterly* 51 (3): 479–528. www.jstor .org/stable/30042181.

Brown, Hannah, Ann H. Kelly, Almudena Marí Sáez, et al. 2015. "Extending the 'Social': Anthropological Contributions to the Study of Viral Haemorrhagic Fevers." *PLoS Neglected Tropical Diseases* 9 (4): e0003775.

Brown, Peter J., and Marcia C. Inhorn, eds. 1997. *The Anthropology of Infectious Disease: International Health Perspectives*. 1st ed. London: Routledge.

Brown, Theodore M., Marcos Cueto, and Elizabeth Fee. 2006. "The World Health Organization and the Transition from 'International' to 'Global' Public Health." *American Journal of Public Health* 96 (1): 62–72.

Brumble, H. David. 2008. *American Indian Autobiography*. Lincoln and London: University of Nebraska Press.

Bulled, Nicola, ed. 2017. *Thinking through Resistance: A Study of Public Oppositions to Contemporary Global Health Practice*. New York: Taylor & Francis.

Burawoy, Michael. 1998. "The Extended Case Method." *Sociological Theory* 16 (1): 4–33. https://doi.org/10.1111/0735-2751.00040.

Bürgel, J. Christoph. 1976. "Secular and Religious Features of Medieval Arabic Medicine." In *Asian Medical Systems: A Comparative Study*, edited by Charles Leslie, 44–62. Berkeley: University of California Press.

Burki, Talha. 2020. "The Online Anti-Vaccine Movement in the Age of COVID-19." *The Lancet Digital Health* 2 (10): e504–e505.

Campbell, Elaine. 2016. "Exploring Autoethnography as a Method and Methodology in Legal Education Research." *Asian Journal of Legal Education* 3 (1): 95–105.

Caplan, Pat, ed. 2004. *The Ethics of Anthropology: Debates and Dilemmas*. London and New York: Routledge.

Carr, John, and Peter Vitaliano. 1985. "The Theoritical Implications of Caregiving Research on Depression and the Culture-Bound Syndromes." In *Culture and Depression: Studies in the Anthropology and Cross-Cultural Psychiatry of Affect and Disorder*, edited by Arthur Kleinman and Byron J. Good. Berkeley: University of California Press.

Carspecken, Francis Phil. 2013. *Critical Ethnography in Educational Research: A Theoretical and Practical Guide*. New York: Routledge.

Centers for Disease Control and Prevention. 2021. *Global Measles Outbreaks*. Atlanta, Georgia, USA: Centers for Disease Control and Prevention.

Chang, Heewon. 2016. "Autoethnography in Health Research: Growing Pains?" *Qualitative Health Research* 26 (4): 443–51.

Charles, Shamard. 2019. "Measles Outbreak: CDC Finds 704 Cases Nationwide, Most in 25 Years." *NBCN News*, 29 April 2019. Accessed 13 July 2019. https://

www.nbcnews.com/health/health-news/measles-outbreak-latest-cdc-finds-704
-total-nationwide-most-25-n999586.

Chaudhry, Asif. 2015. "Sindh Transmitting Measles to Other Provinces: Survey."
Dawn, 29 January 2015. Accessed 27 August 2019. https://www.dawn.com/news
/1160140.

———. 2019. "Polio Drive Suspended across Country after Spike in Attacks." *Dawn*,
April 27, 2019. Accessed 28 April 2019. https://www.dawn.com/news/1478637.

Che, Chun-Tao, et al. 2017. "Traditional Medicine." In *Pharmacognosy:
Fundamentals, Applications and Strategies*, edited by Simone Badal McCreath and
Rupika Delgoda, 15–30. London: Academic Press.

Chêne, Marie. 2008. "Overview of Corruption in Pakistan." *Transparency
International*. https://www.u4.no/publications/overview-of-corruption-in-pakistan

Clark, Cindy Dell. 1999. "The Autodriven Interview: A Photographic Viewfinder
into Children's Experience." *Visual Studies* 14 (1): 39–50. https://doi.org/10.1080
/14725869908583801.

———. 2003. In *Sickness and in Play: Children Coping with Chronic Illness*. New
Brunswick and London: Rutgers University Press.

———. 2004. "Visual Metaphor as Method in Interviews with Children." *Journal of
Linguistic Anthropology* 14 (2): 171–85. https://doi.org/10.1525/jlin.2004.14.2.171.

———. 2011. In a *Younger Voice: Doing Child-Centered Qualitative Research*.
Oxford and New York: Oxford University Press.

Closser, Svea. 2010. *Chasing Polio in Pakistan: Why the World's Largest Public
Health Initiative May Fail*. Nashville: Vanderbilt University Press.

———. 2012. "'We Can't Give up Now': Global Health Optimism and Polio
Eradication in Pakistan." *Medical Anthropology* 31 (5): 385–403. https://doi.org
/10.1080/01459740.2011.645927.

Closser, Svea, and Rashid Jooma. 2013. "Why We Must Provide Better Support for
Pakistan's Female Frontline Health Workers." *PLoS Medicine* 10 (10): e1001528.
https://doi.org/10.1371/journal.pmed.1001528.

Closser, Svea, Anat Rosenthal, Kenneth Maes, et al. 2016. "The Global Context
of Vaccine Refusal: Insights from a Systematic Comparative Ethnography of the
Global Polio Eradication Initiative." *Medical Anthropology Quarterly* 30 (3):
321–41. https://doi.org/10.1111/maq.12254.

Cohen, Stephen P. 2004. *The Idea of Pakistan*. Washington, DC: Brookings Institution
Press.

Colgrove, James. 2006. *State of Immunity: The Politics of Vaccination in Twentieth-
Century America*. Vol. 16. Berkeley: University of California Press.

Collier, Stephen J., and Andrew Lakoff. 2008. "The Problem of Securing Health."
In *Biosecurity Interventions: Global Health and Security in Question*, edited by
Andrew Lakoff and Stephen J. Collier, 7–32. New York: Columbia University
Press.

Collier, Stephen J., and Aihwa Ong. 2005. "Global Assemblages, Anthropological
Problems." In *Global Assemblages: Technology, Politics, and Ethics as Anthropological
Problems*, edited by Aihwa Ong and Stephen J. Collier, 3–21. Oxford: Blackwell
Publishing.

Comaroff, Jean. 1982. "Medicine: Symbol and Ideology." In *The Problem of
Medical Knowledge: Examining the Social Construction of Medicine*, edited by
Peter Wright and Arthur Treacher, 49–68. Edinburgh: University of Edinburgh
Press.

Cooper, Kenneth J. 1996. "A Kalashnikov Culture." *The Washington Post*, 14 March 1996. https://www.washingtonpost.com/archive/politics/1996/03/14/a-kalashnikov -culture/3e32ca0c-7f5d-418b-8280-c581d9bbb384/.

Cordovez, Diego, and Selig S. Harrison. 1995. *Out of Afghanistan: The Inside Story of the Soviet Withdrawal*. New York: Oxford University Press.

Corin, Ellen E. 1990. "Facts and Meaning in Psychiatry. An Anthropological Approach to the Lifeworld of Schizophrenics." *Culture, Medicine and Psychiatry* 14: 153–88.

Crilly, Rob. 2014. "100 Children Die of Measles in Pakistan." *The Telegraph*, 24 January 2014. Accessed 27 August 2019. https://www.telegraph.co.uk/news/ worldnews/asia/pakistan/9823377/100-children-die-of-Measles-in-Pakistan.html.

Csordas, Thomas J. 1990. "Embodiment as a Paradigm for Anthropology." *Ethos* 18: 5–47.

———. 2014. "Afterword: Moral Experience in Anthropology." *Ethos* 42 (1): 139–52. https://doi.org/10.1111/etho.12043.

Cunha, Burke A. 2004. "Smallpox and Measles: Historical Aspects and Clinical Differentiation." *Infectious Disease Clinics of North America* 18 (1): 79–100. https://doi.org/10.1016/s0891-5520(03)00091-6.

Cunningham, Andrew, and Bridie Andrews. 1997. *Western Medicine as Contested Knowledge*. Manchester: Manchester University Press.

da Col, Giovanni. 2017. "Two or Three Things I Know About Ethnographic Theory." *HAU: Journal of Ethnographic Theory* 7 (1): 1–8. https://doi.org/10.14318/hau7 .1.002.

Dabbagh, Alya, et al. 2018. "Progress toward Regional Measles Elimination— Worldwide, 2000–2017." *Morbidity and Mortality Weekly Report* 67 (47): 1323.

Das, Veena. 1995. *Critical Events: An Anthropological Perspective on Contemporary India*. New Delhi: Oxford University Press.

Davidson, Michael. 2017. "Vaccination as a Cause of Autism Myths and Controversies." *Dialogues in Clinical Neuroscience* 19 (4): 403.

Davis-Floyd, Robbie E. 1994. "The Technocratic Body: American Childbirth as Cultural Expression." *Social Science & Medicine* 38 (8): 1125–40. https://doi.org /10.1016/0277-9536(94)90228-3.

Davis-Floyd, Robbie, Kim Gutschow, and David A. Schwartz. 2020. "Pregnancy, Birth and the COVID-19 Pandemic in the United States." *Medical Anthropology*: 1–15. https://doi.org/10.1080/01459740.2020.1761804.

Dawn. 2014a. "Polio Cases: WHO Recommends Travel Restrictions on Pakistan." *Dawn*, 5 May 2014. Accessed 18 June 2014. https://www.dawn.com/news /1104346.

———. 2014b. "Two More Children Killed Due to Anti-Measles Vaccine." *Dawn*, 1 June 2014. Accessed 2 June 2014. https://www.dawn.com/news/1109916.

———. 2017a. "KP Declares Public Health Emergency." *Dawn*, 1 September 2017. https://www.dawn.com/news/1355309.

———. 2017b. "Post-Antibiotic Era." *Dawn*, 21 November 2017, 8. Accessed 21 November 2017. https://epaper.dawn.com/?page=21_11_2017_008.

———. 2019. "Peshawar Police Arrest Man Alleging Anti-Polio Vaccines Cause Children to Faint, Die." Accessed 24 April 2019. https://www.dawn.com/news /1477890.

Deleuze, Gilles, and Félix Guattari. 1987. *A Thousand Plateaus: Capitalism and Schizophrenia.* Translated by Brian Massumi. Minnesota: University of Minnesota Press, 1980.

Devisch, René. 1990. "The Therapist and the Source of Healing among the Yaka of Zaire." *Culture, Medicine and Psychiatry* 14: 213–36.

Dicks, Bella. 2005. *Qualitative Research and Hypermedia Ethnography for the Digital Age. New Technologies for Social Research.* London: SAGE.

Diesing, Paul. 1972. "Subjectivity and Objectivity in the Social Sciences." *Philosophy of the Social Sciences* 2 (1): 147–65. https://doi.org/10.1177/004839317200200111.

Dinc, G., and Y. I. Ulman. 2007. "The Introduction of Variolation 'A La Turca' to the West by Lady Mary Montagu and Turkey's Contribution to This." *Vaccine* 25 (21): 4261–5. https://doi.org/10.1016/j.vaccine.2007.02.076.

Domercant, J. Wysler, et al. 2015. "Update on Progress in Selected Public Health Programs after the 2010 Earthquake and Cholera Epidemic—Haiti." *Morbidity and Mortality Weekly Report* 64 (6): 137–40. https://www.ncbi.nlm.nih.gov/pmc/articles/PMC4584701/.

Douglas, Karen M., Robbie M. Sutton, and Aleksandra Cichocka. 2017. "The Psychology of Conspiracy Theories." *Current Directions in Psychological Science* 26 (6): 538–42.

Dowson, John. 2000. *A Classical Dictionary of Hindu Mythology and Religion, Geography, History, and Literature.* New Delhi: D.K. Print World (P) Ltd.

Doyal, Lesley. 1979. *The Political Economy of Health.* Boston: South End Press.

Dubé, Eve, Caroline Laberge, Maryse Guay, et al. 2013. "Vaccine Hesitancy: An Overview." *Human Vaccines & Immunotherapeutics* 9 (8): 1763–73.

Durbach, Nadja. 2000. "'They Might as Well Brand Us': Working-Class Resistance to Compulsory Vaccination in Victorian England." *Social History of Medicine* 13 (1): 45–63.

Düx, Ariane, Sebastian Lequime, Livia Victoria Patrono, et al. 2020. "Measles Virus and Rinderpest Virus Divergence Dated to the Sixth Century BCE." *Science* 368 (6497): 1367. https://doi.org/10.1126/science.aba9411.

Easterly, William. 2006. *The White Man's Burden: Why the West's Efforts to Aid the Rest Have Done So Much Ill and So Little Good.* New York: The Penguin Press.

Ebrahim, Zofeen. 2014. "Polio Exporter: Pakistan Slapped with Travel Restrictions." *MintPress News,* 14 May 2014. Accessed 24 August 2019. https://www.mintpressnews.com/polio-exporter-pakistan-slapped-with-travel-restrictions/190541/.

Edward, Terence Rajivan. 2014. "Anthropology in the Context That Produced It." *Research in Hermeneutics, Phenomenology, and Practical Philosophy* VI (1): 347–60. https://philpapers.org/rec/EDWAIT. https://philpapers.org/rec/EDWAIT.

Edwards, Gareth. 2019. "Anti-vaccine Posts Could Be Banned on Social Media after Measles Outbreak." *Scotsman,* 27 March 2019.

Ehrenreich, John, ed. 1978. *The Cultural Crisis of Modern Medicine.* New York: Monthly Review Press.

Elling, Ray H. 1981. "The Capitalist World-System and International Health." *International Journal of Health Services* 11 (1): 21–51. https://doi.org/10.2190/JWM6-D2JC-RLFW-MWDC.

Ellison, Marcia A. 2003. "Authoritative Knowledge and Single Women's Unintentional Pregnancies, Abortions, Adoption, and Single Motherhood: Social Stigma and

Structural Violence." *Medical Anthropology Quarterly* 17 (3): 322–47. https://doi
.org/10.1525/maq.2003.17.3.322.

El-Mehairy, Theresa. 1984. *Medical Doctors: A Study of Role Concept and Job Satisfaction: The Egyptian Case*. Vol. 33. Leiden, Netherlands: Brill Archive.

Enders, John F., et al. 1957. "Measles Virus: A Summary of Experiments Concerned with Isolation, Properties, and Behavior." *American Journal of Public Health and the Nations Health* 47 (3): 275–82. https://doi.org/10.2105/AJPH.47.3.275.

Engels, Friedrich. 1973. *The Condition of the Working Class in England: From Personal Observations and Authentic Sources*. Moscow: Progress Publishers, 1845.

Eriksen, Thomas Hylland. 2010. *Small Places, Large Issues: An Introduction to Social and Cultural Anthropology (Anthropology, Culture and Society)*. 3rd ed. London: Pluto.

Erwin, Deborah Oates. 1987. "The Military Medicalization of Cancer Treatment." In *Encounters with Biomedicine: Case Studies in Medical Anthropology*, edited by Hans A. Baer, 201–27. New York: Gordon and Breach.

Escobar, Arturo. 1984. "Discourse and Power in Development: Michel Foucault and the Relevance of His Work to the Third World." *Alternatives* 10 (3): 377–400. https://doi.org/10.1177/030437548401000304.

———. 2011. *Encountering Development: The Making and Unmaking of the Third World*. Princeton, NJ: Princeton University Press.

Espeland, Wendy Nelson, and Mitchell L. Stevens. 2008. "A Sociology of Quantification." *European Journal of Sociology* 49 (3): 401–36. https://doi.org/10 .1017/S0003975609000150.

European Centre for Disease Prevention and Control (ECDC). 2018. *Monthly Measles and Rubella Monitoring Report—February 2018*. Stockholm: ECDC. https://ecdc.europa.eu/sites/portal/files/documents/Monthly%20Measles%20and %20Rubella%20monitoring%20report%20%20February%202018.pdf.

Fainzang, Sylvie. 2002. "Lying, Secrecy and Power within the Doctor–Patient Relationship." *Anthropology & Medicine* 9 (2): 117–33.

Fair, C. Christine. 2007. *Vaccine Anxieties: Global Science, Child Health and Society*. London: Earthscan.

———. 2014. "Drones, Spies, Terrorists, and Second-Class Citizenship in Pakistan." *Small Wars & Insurgencies* 25 (1): 205–35. https://doi.org/10.1080/09592318 .2014.894061.

Fairhead, James, and Melissa Leach. 2012. *Vaccine Anxieties: Global Science, Child Health and Society*. New York: Routledge.

Farmer, Paul. 1996a. "On Suffering and Structural Violence: A View from Below." *Race/Ethnicity: Multidisciplinary Global Contexts* 3 (1): 11–28. https://www.jstor .org/stable/25595022.

———. 1996b. "Social Inequalities and Emerging Infectious Diseases." *Emerging Infectious Diseases* 2 (4): 259. https://doi.org/10.3201/eid0204.960402.

———. 1999. *Infections and Inequalities: The Modern Plagues*. Berkeley: University of California Press.

———. 2003. *Pathologies of Power: Health, Human Rights, and the New War on the Poor*. Berkeley: University of California Press.

———. 2006. *AIDS and Accusation: Haiti and the Geography of Blame*. Berkeley: University of California Press.

Farmer, Paul, and Nicole Gastineau Campos. 2004. "Rethinking Medical Ethics: A View from Below." *Developing World Bioethics* 4 (1): 17–41. https://doi.org/10 .1111/j.1471-8731.2004.00065.x.

Farmer, Paul, et al., eds. 2013. *Reimagining Global Health: An Introduction, California Series in Public Anthropology*. Berkeley: University of California Press.

Farmer, Paul, et al. 2006. "Structural Violence and Clinical Medicine." *PLoS Medicine* 3 (10): e449. https://doi.org/10.1371/journal.pmed.0030449.

Farooq, Abdul, et al. 2013. "Does Corruption Impede Economic Growth in Pakistan?" *Economic Modelling* 35: 622–33. https://doi.org/10.1016/j.econmod .2013.08.019.

Fassin, Didier. 2011. *Humanitarian Reason: A Moral History of the Present*. Berkeley: University of California Press.

———. 2012. "That Obscure Object of Global Health." In *Medical Anthropology at the Intersections: Histories, Activisms, and Futures*, edited by Marcia C. Inhorn and Emily A. Wentzell, 95–115. London: Duke University Press.

———. 2014. "The Ethical Turn in Anthropology: Promises and Uncertainties." *HAU: Journal of Ethnographic Theory* 4 (1): 429–35. https://doi.org/10.14318/ hau4.1.025.

———, ed. 2015. *A Companion to Moral Anthropology*. Oxford, UK: John Wiley & Sons.

Faubion, James. 2014. "Anthropologies of Ethics: Where We've Been, Where We Are, Where We Might Go." *HAU: Journal of Ethnographic Theory* 4 (1): 437–42. https://doi.org/10.14318/hau4.1.026.

Feld, Steven, and Aaron A. Fox. 1994. "Music and Language." *Annual Review of Anthropology* 23 (1): 25–53. https://doi.org/10.1146/annurev.an.23.100194 .000325.

Feldman-Savelsberg, Pamela, Flavien T. Ndonko, and Song Yang. 2017. "How Rumor Begets Rumor: Collective Memory, Ethnic Conflict, and Reproductive Rumors in Cameroon." In *Rumor Mills*, edited by Gary Alan Fine, Veronique Campion-Vincent, and Chip Heath, 141–58. London and New York: Routledge.

Feldman-Savelsberg, Pamela, Flavien T. Ndonko, and Bergis Schmidt-Ehry. 2000. "Sterilizing Vaccines or the Politics of the Womb: Retrospective Study of a Rumor in Cameroon." *Medical Anthropology Quarterly* 14 (2): 159–79. https://doi.org /10.1525/maq.2000.14.2.159.

Fenner, Frank. 1982. "Global Eradication of Smallpox." *Clinical Infectious Diseases* 4 (5): 916–30. https://doi.org/10.1093/clinids/4.5.916.

Fenner, Frank, et al. 1988. "The History of Smallpox and Its Spread around the World." In *Smallpox and Its Eradication*, edited by Frank Fenner, D.A. Henderson, I. Arita, Z. Jezek and I.D. Ladnyi, 209–44. Geneva: World Health Organization.

Ferguson, R. Brian. 2004. "Tribal Warfare." In *Violence in War and Peace*, edited by Nancy Scheper-Hughes and San Philippe Bourgois, 69–76. Malden, MA: Blackwell Publishing.

Ferrari, Fabrizio M. 2015. *Religion, Devotion and Medicine in North India: The Healing Power of Sitālā*. London: Bloomsbury.

Fishwick, Carmen. 2014. "Peshawar School Massacre: 'This Is Pakistan's 9/11—Now Is the Time to Act'." *The Guardian*, 19 December 2014. Accessed 20 October 2019. https://www.theguardian.com/world/2014/dec/19/peshawar-school-massacre-pakistans-911.

Flood, Gavin D. 1996. *An Introduction to Hinduism*. New York: Cambridge University Press.

Foley, Douglas E. 2002. "Critical Ethnography: The Reflexive Turn." *International Journal of Qualitative Studies in Education* 15 (4): 469–90.

Foster, G.M., and Bettina G. Anderson. 1978. *Medical Anthropology*. New York: John Wiley & Sons.

Foster, George M. 1987. "Bureaucratic Aspects of International Health Agencies." *Social Science & Medicine* 25 (9): 1039–48. https://doi.org/10.1016/0277 -9536(87)90009-8.

Foucault, Michel. 1980. *Power/Knowledge: Selected Interviews and Other Writings*. Translated by Colin Gordon, Leo Marshal, John Mepham, and Kate Soper, edited by Colin Gordon. New York, NY: Pantheon Books.

———. 1982. "The Subject and Power." *Critical Inquiry* 8 (4): 777–95. https://doi .org/10.1086/448181.

———. 2008. *The Birth of Biopolitics: Lectures at the Collège De France, 1978– 1979*. Translated by Graham Burchell, edited by Arnold Davidson and Alessandro Fontana. New York, NY: Palgrave Macmillan.

Fox News. 2012. "Hero Doctor Who Helped Nail Bin Laden Tortured in Pakistani Prison, Says Family." *Fox News*, 11 December 2012. Accessed 15 January 2016. http://www.foxnews.com/world/2012/12/11/hero-doctor-who-helped-nail-bin -laden-tortured-in-pakistani-prison-says-family.html.

Frank, Gelya. 1986. "On Embodiment: A Case Study of Congenital Limb Deficiency in American Culture." *Culture, Medicine and Psychiatry* 10: 189–219.

Frankenberg, Ronald. 1980. "Medical Anthropology and Development: A Theoretical Perspective." *Social Science & Medicine. Part B: Medical Anthropology* 14 (4): 197–207. https://doi.org/10.1016/0160-7987(80)90045-9.

Frawley, David. 2001. "Editor's Forward." In *Natural Healing through Ayurveda*, edited by David Frawley, 9–11. Delhi: Motilal Banarsidass Publisher.

Freilich, Morris. 1967. "Ecology and Culture: Environmental Determinism and the Ecological Approach in Anthropology." *Anthropological Quarterly* 40 (1): 26–43. https://doi.org/10.2307/3316830.

Frembgen, Jürgen Wasim. 2006. *The Friends of God: Sufi Saints in Islam, Popular Poster Art from Pakistan*. Karachi: Oxford University Press.

———. 2008. *Journey to God: Sufis and Dervishes in Islam*. Oxford: Oxford University Press.

———. 2011. *At the Shrine of the Red Sufi: Five Days and Nights on Pilgrimage in Pakistan*. Karachi: Oxford University Press.

Friedrich, Mary Jane. 2016. "Where Will Zika Spread?" *JAMA* 316 (19): 1956. https://doi.org/10.1001/jama.2016.16151.

———. 2017. "Who Calls Off Global Zika Emergency." *JAMA* 317 (3): 246. https:// doi.org/10.1001/jama.2016.20447.

Friedson, Steven M. 1996. *Dancing Prophets: Musical Experience in Tumbuka Healing*. Berkeley: University of California Press.

Fulginiti, Vincent A., et al. 1967. "Altered Reactivity to Measles Virus: Atypical Measles in Children Previously Immunized with Inactivated Measles Virus Vaccines." *JAMA* 202 (12): 1075–80.

Furuse, Yuki, Akira Suzuki, and Hitoshi Oshitani. 2010. "Origin of Measles Virus: Divergence from Rinderpest Virus between the 11th and 12th Centuries." *Virology Journal* 7 (1): 52.

Galeano, Eduardo H. 1991. *The Book of Embraces*. Translated by Cedric Belfrage. New York: W.W. Norton Inc.

Galpin, Richard. 2013. "Fighting Pakistan's Measles Epidemic." *BBC News.* Accessed 27 August. https://www.bbc.com/news/world-latin-america-22724080.

Galtung, Johan. 1969. "Violence, Peace, and Peace Research." *Journal of Peace Research* 6 (3): 167–91.

Garon, Julie, and Walter Orenstein. 2016. "Improving the Science of Measles Prevention-Will It Make for a Better Immunization Program?" *PLoS Medicine* 13 (10): 1–3. https://doi.org/10.1371/journal.pmed.1002145.

Gayer, Laurent. 2003. "A Divided City: 'Ethnic' and 'Religious' Conflicts in Karachi, Pakistan." 1st Pakistan Seminar.

———. 2014. *Karachi: Ordered Disorder and the Struggle for the City.* Karachi: Oxford University Press.

Geertz, Clifford. 1975. *The Interpretation of Cultures: Selected Essays.* London: Hutchinson.

Geest, Sjaak van der, Susan Reynolds Whyte, and Anita Hardon. 1996. "The Anthropology of Pharmaceuticals: A Biographical Approach." *Annual Review of Anthropology* 25 (1): 153–78.

Gera, Nina. 2007. "Impact of Structural Adjustment Programmes on Overall Social Welfare in Pakistan." *South Asia Economic Journal* 8 (1): 39–64. https://doi.org /10.1177/139156140600800103.

Ghatak, Proggya. 2013. "The *Sitālā* Saga: A Case of Cultural Integration in the Folk Tradition of West Bengal." *Ropkatha Journal on Interdisciplinary Studies in Humanities* 5 (2): 119–31.

Global Polio Eradication Initiative (GPEI). 2011. "Polio Spreads from Pakistan." World Health Organisation. Accessed 27 August. http://polioeradication.org/news -post/polio-spreads-from-pakistan/.

Gluckman, Max. 1961. "Ethnographic Data in British Social Anthropology." *The Sociological Review* 9 (1): 5–17.

Godlee, Fiona, Jane Smith, and Harvey Marcovitch. 2011. "Wakefield's Article Linking MMR Vaccine and Autism was Fraudulent." *British Medical Journal Publishing Group.*

Golovnina, Maria. 2014. "Feared Uzbek *Jihād*ists Behind Deadly Pakistan Airport Attack." *Reuters,* 11 June 2014. Accessed 20 October 2019. https://www.reuters .com/article/us-pakistan-militants/feared-uzbek-jihadists-behind-deadly-pakistan -airport-attack-idUSKBN0EM14L20140611.

Good, Byron. 1977. "The Heart of What's the Matter. The Semantics of Illness in Iran." *Culture, Medicine and Psychiatry* 1: 25–58.

———. 1994. *Medicine, Rationality, and Experience: An Anthropological Perspective.* Cambridge: Cambridge University Press.

Good, Mary-Jo DelVecchio, Byron J. Good, Cynthia Schaffer, and Stuart E. Lind. 1990. "American Oncology and the Discourse on Hope." *Culture, Medicine and Psychiatry* 14: 59–79.

Good, Mary-Jo DelVecchio, Paul E. Brodwin, Byron J. Good, and Arthur Kleinman, eds. 1992. *Pain as Human Experience: An Anthropological Perspective.* Berkeley: University of California Press.

Gordon, Deborah R. 1990. "Embodying Illness, Embodying Cancer." *Culture, Medicine and Psychiatry* 14: 275–97.

Gostin, Lawrence O. 2015. "Law, Ethics, and Public Health in the Vaccination Debates: Politics of the Measles Outbreak." *JAMA* 313 (11): 1099–100. https:// doi.org/10.1001/jama.2015.1518.

Gouk, Penelope, ed. 2017. *Musical Healing in Cultural Contexts.* London: Routledge.

Government of Pakistan. 1952. *The First Five Year Plan: A Draft Outline.* Planning Commission, Ministry of Planning Development & Reform. Islāmābād: Government of Pakistan.

———. 1960. *The Second Five Year Plan 1960–65.* Planning Commission, Ministry of Planning Development & Reform. Islāmābād: Government of Pakistan.

———. 1967. *The Third Five Year Plan, 1965–70.* Planning Commission, Ministry of Planning Development & Reform. Islāmābād: Government of Pakistan.

———. 1970. *The Fourth Five Year Plan 1970–75.* Planning Commission, Ministry of Planning Development & Reform. Islāmābād: Government of Pakistan.

———. 1978. *The Fifth Five Year Plan 1978–83.* Planning Commission, Ministry of Planning Development & Reform. Islāmābād: Government of Pakistan.

———. 1983. *The Sixth Five Year Plan 1983–88.* Planning Commission, Ministry of Planning Development & Reform. Islāmābād: Government of Pakistan. http://121.52.153.178:8080/xmlui/bitstream/handle/123456789/7081/The%20Sixth%20Five%20Year%20Plan%201983-1988.PDF?sequence=1&isAllowed=y.

———. 1988. *Seventh Five-Year Plan 1988–93 & Perspective Plan 1988–2003.* Planning Commission, Ministry of Planning Development & Reform. Islāmābād: Government of Pakistan.

———. 1993. *Eighth Five Year Plan 1993–98.* Planning Commission, Ministry of Planning Development & Reform. Islāmābād: Government of Pakistan.

———. 2011. *Living Standards Measurement Survey (PSLM) 2010–11.* Statistics Division, Pakistan Bureau of Statistics. Islāmābād: Government of Pakistan.

———. 2013. *Report on Measles Outbreak in Pakistan.* Wafaqi Mohtasib (Ombudsman) Secretariat. Islāmābād: Government of Pakistan.

———. 2016a. *Living Standards Measurement Survey (PSLM) 2014–15.* Statistics Division, Pakistan Bureau of Statistics. Islāmābād: Government of Pakistan. file:///D:/PSLM_2014-15_National-Provincial-District_report.pdf.

———. 2016b. *Pakistan Economic Survey 2015–16.* Finance Division, Ministry of Finance. Islāmābād: Government of Pakistan. Accessed 15 July 2020. http://finance.gov.pk/survey/chapters_17/11-Health.pdf

———. 2017a. *6th Population and Housing Census—2017.* Bureau of Statistics. Islāmābād: Government of Pakistan. Accessed 15 July 2020. http://www.pbs.gov.pk/content/block-wise-provisional-summary-results-6th-population-housing-census-2017-january-03-2018.

———. 2017b. *Pakistan Economic Survey 2016–17.* Finance Division, Ministry of Finance. Islāmābād: Government of Pakistan. Accessed 15 July 2020. http://www.finance.gov.pk/survey/chapters_17/Pakistan_ES_2016_17_pdf.pdf.

———. 2018. *Pakistan Economic Survey 2017–18.* Finance Division, Ministry of Finance. Islāmābād: Government of Pakistan. Accessed 15 July 2020. http://finance.gov.pk/survey/chapter_20/11_Health_and_Nutrition.pdf.

———. 2019a. "Overview." Accessed 22 December. https://bisp.gov.pk/who-we-are/.

———. 2019b. *Pakistan Economic Survey 2018–19.* Finance Division, Ministry of Finance. Islāmābād: Government of Pakistan. Accessed 15 July 2020. http://finance.gov.pk/survey/chapters_19/Economic_Survey_2018_19.pdf.

———. 2020. *Pakistan Economic Survey 2019–2020.* Finance Division, Ministry of Finance. Islāmābād: Government of Pakistan. Accessed 15 July 2020. http://finance.gov.pk/survey/chapter_20/11_Health_and_Nutrition.pdf.

———. 2022. *Pakistan Economic Survey 2021–2022.* Finance Division, Ministry of Finance. Islāmābād: Government of Pakistan.

Government of Sindh. 2020. "Sindh Map 2013." Government of Sindh. Accessed 28 February. http://www.pdma.gos.pk/new/resources/maps/SindhMap.jpg.

Gramsci, Antonio. 1971. *Selections from the Prison Notebooks of Antonio Gramsci.* Translated by Quintin Hoare and Geoffrey Nowell-Smith, edited by Quintin Hoare and Geoffrey Nowell-Smith. New York, NY: International Publishers.

Gray, Deven, and Joanna Mishtal. 2019. "Managing an Epidemic: Zika Interventions and Community Responses in Belize." *Global Public Health* 14 (1): 9–22. https://doi.org/10.1080/17441692.2018.1471146.

Green, Linda. 1998. "Lived Lives and Social Suffering: Problems and Concerns in Medical Anthropology." *Medical Anthropology Quarterly* 12 (1): 3–7. https://doi.org/10.1525/maq.1998.12.1.3.

Greenhouse, Carol J. 1985. "Anthropology at Home: Whose Home?" *Human Organization* 44 (3): 261.

Greenough, Paul, Stuart Blume, and Christine Holmberg. 2017. "Introduction." In *The Politics of Vaccination: A Global History*, edited by Paul Greenough, Stuart Blume, and Christine Holmberg, 1–16. Manchester: Manchester University Press.

Greenough, Paul, Christine Holmberg, and Stuart Blume, eds. 2017. *The Politics of Vaccination.* Manchester: Manchester University Press.

Gwaltney, John L. 1976. "On Going Home Again—Some Reflections of a Native Anthropologist." *Phylon* (1960-) 37 (3): 236–42.

Hadolt, Bernhard. 1998. "Locating Difference: A Medical Anthropology 'at Home'?" *Anthropology & Medicine* 5 (3): 311–23.

Hadolt, Bernhard, and Anita Hardon. 2017. "Emerging Socialities in 21st Century Health Care." In *Emerging Socialities in 21st Century Health Care*, edited by Bernhard Hadolt and Anita Hardon, 7–10. Amsterdam: Amsterdam University Press.

Hafner, Tamara, and Jeremy Shiffman. 2012. "The Emergence of Global Attention to Health Systems Strengthening." *Health Policy and Planning* 28 (1): 41–50. https://doi.org/10.1093/heapol/czs023.

Hahn, Robert A., and Arthur Kleinman. 1983. "Biomedical Practice and Anthropological Theory: Frameworks and Directions." *Annual Review of Anthropology* 12 (1): 305–33. https://doi.org/10.1146/annurev.an.12.100183.001513.

Hahn, Robert A., and Atwood Gaines, eds. 1985. *Physicians of Western Medicine.* Dordrecht: D. Reidel Publishing Co.

Hakim, Abdul. 2001. "Population Policy Shifts and Their Implications for Population Stabilisation in Pakistan." *The Pakistan Development Review* (40): 551–73. https://pdfs.semanticscholar.org/d18b/082993b987af64d45484a74699f d295daac2.pdf.

Hamborsky, Jennifer, Andrew Kroger, and Charles Wolfe. 2015. *Epidemiology and Prevention of Vaccine-Preventable Diseases.* 13th ed. Atlanta, Georgia, USA: Public Health Foundation and Centers for Disease Control and Prevention.

Haniff, Nesha Z. 1985. "Toward a Native Anthropology: Methodological Notes on a Study of Successful Caribbean Women by an Insider." *Anthropology and Humanism Quarterly* 10 (4): 107–13.

Hansen, Victoria, et al. 2016. "Infectious Disease Mortality Trends in the United States, 1980–2014." *JAMA* 316 (20): 2149–51. https://doi.org/10.1001/jama.2016.12423.

Harrison, Selig S. 1981. In *Afghanistan's Shadow: Baluch Nationalism and Soviet Temptations.* New York: Carnegie Endowment for International Peace.

Hasan, Q., A.H. Bosan, and K.M. Bile. 2010. "A Review of EPI Progress in Pakistan Towards Achieving Coverage Targets: Present Situation and the Way Forward." *EMHJ-Eastern Mediterranean Health Journal* 16(Supp.): 31–8.

Hein, Alexandria. 2019. "New York County Declares State of Emergency Over Measles Outbreak." *Fox News*, 26 March 2019. Accessed 4 April 2019. https://www.foxnews.com/health/new-york-county-to-declare-state-of-emergency-over-measles-outbreak.

Helman, Cecil. 1984. *Culture, Health and Illness: An Introduction for Health Professionals*. Bristol: The Stonebridge Press.

Herani, Gobind M., et al. 2008. *Livestock: A Reliable Source of Income Generation and Rehabilitation of Environment at Tharparkar*. Munich: University of Munich.

Hewlett, Barry S., and Bonnie L. Hewlett. 2007. *Ebola, Culture and Politics: The Anthropology of an Emerging Disease*. Belmont, CA: Wadsworth Cengage Learning.

Hinton, Alexander Laban. 2002. "Toward an Anthropology of Genocide." In *Annihilating Difference: The Anthropology of Genocide*, edited by Alexander Laban Hinton, 1–40. Berkeley: University of California Press.

Hisam, Zeenat. 2016. "LHWs' Struggle." *Dawn*, 22 December 2016. Accessed 23 December 2016. https://www.dawn.com/news/1303672/lhws-struggle.

Hjorth, Larissa, et al., eds. 2017. *The Routledge Companion to Digital Ethnography*, Routledge Companions. London: Routledge.

Høg, Erling, Guillaume Fournié, Md Ahasanul Hoque, et al. 2019. "Competing Biosecurity and Risk Rationalities in the Chittagong Poultry Commodity Chain, Bangladesh." *BioSocieties* 14 (3): 368–92. https://doi.org/10.1057/s41292-018-0131-2.

Holbraad, Martin, Morten Axel Pedersen, and Eduardo Viveiros de Castro. 2014. "The Politics of Ontology: Anthropological Positions." *Cultural Anthropology* 13. https://culanth.org/fieldsights/series/the-politics-of-ontology.

Holmberg, Christine, Stuart Blume, and Paul Greenough, eds. 2017. *The Politics of Vaccination: A Global History*. Manchester: Manchester University Press.

Hoodbhoy, Pervez, and Abdul Hameed Nayyar. 1985. "Rewriting the History of Pakistan." In *Islam, Politics and the State: The Pakistan Experience*, 164–77. http://eacpe.org/content/uploads/2014/01/Rewriting-The-History-of-Pakistan1.pdf.

Hopkins, Donald R. 1983. *Princes and Peasants: Smallpox in History*. Chicago: University of Chicago Press.

Horowitz, Leonard G. 1996. *Emerging Viruses: AIDS and Ebola: Nature, Accident, or Intentional?* Healthy World Dist. https://lust-for-life.org/Lust-For-Life/EmergingViruses/EmergingViruses.pdf

Hotez, Peter J. 2016. "Texas and Its Measles Epidemics." *PLoS Medicine* 13 (10): e1002153. https://doi.org/10.1371/journal.pmed.1002153.

Howell, Signe. 2017. "Two or Three Things I Love About Ethnography." *HAU: Journal of Ethnographic Theory* 7 (1): 15–20. https://doi.org/10.14318/hau7.1.004.

Hughes, James J. 2006. "Human Enhancement and the Emergent Technopolitics of the 21st Century." In *Managing Nano-bio-info-cogno Innovations*, 285–307. Springer.

Husain, Ahmad, et al. 2010. "Unani System of Medicine—Introduction and Challenges." *Medical Journal of Islamic World Academy of Sciences* 18 (1): 27–30. https://www.journalagent.com/ias/pdfs/IAS_18_1_27_30.pdf.

Hussain, Shoaib Fahad, Peter Boyle, Preeti Patel, and Richard Sullivan. 2016. "Eradicating Polio in Pakistan: An Analysis of the Challenges and Solutions to this Security and Health Issue." *Globalization and Health* 12 (1): 63.

Hussain, Syed A., Sharath B. Nagaraja, and Ritesh G. Menezes. 2015. "Military Intervention: The Last Option for Polio Eradication in Pakistan?" *Journal of Infection and Public Health* 5 (8): 508–9. https://doi.org/10.1016/j.jiph.2015.01.003.

Inayat, Ali. 2022. "Decolonizing Methodology: Proposing Kachaharī as Socio-Culturally Acceptable Qualitative Method." *Antropologija* 22 (1): 105–12.

Information Management and Mine Action Programs (iMMAP). 2014a. *Pakistan Emergency Situational Analysis: District Sukkur*. Islāmābād: iMMAP. https://reliefweb.int/sites/reliefweb.int/files/resources/PESA-DP-Sukkur-Sindh.pdf.

———. 2014b. *Pakistan Emergency Situational Analysis: District Tharparkar*. Islāmābād: iMMAP. https://reliefweb.int/sites/reliefweb.int/files/resources/PESA -DP-Tharparkar-Sindh.pdf.

Ingold, Tim. 2008. "Anthropology Is Not Ethnography." *Proceedings of the British Academy* 154 (11): 69–92.

———. 2014. "That's Enough About Ethnography!" *HAU: Journal of Ethnographic Theory* 4 (1): 383–95. https://doi.org/10.14318/hau4.1.021.

———. 2017. "Anthropology Contra Ethnography." *HAU: Journal of Ethnographic Theory* 7 (1): 21–6. https://doi.org/10.14318/hau7.1.005.

Inhorn, Marcia C., and Peter J. Brown. 1990. "The Anthropology of Infectious Disease." *Annual Review of Anthropology* 19 (1): 89–117.

Iqbal, Nasir. 2014. "Sc Orders Regularisation of 366 LHWs in Capital." *Dawn*, 14 October 2014. Accessed 20 April 2018. https://www.dawn.com/news/1140031.

Iqbal, Sehar, et al. 2019. "Iron and Iodine Status in Pregnant Women from a Developing Country and Its Relation to Pregnancy Outcomes." *International Journal of Environmental Research and Public Health* 16 (22): 4414. https://doi .org/10.3390/ijerph16224414.

Iqbal, Sehar, Inayat Ali, Cem Ekmekcioglu, et al. 2020. "Increasing Frequency of Antenatal Care Visits May Improve Tetanus Toxoid Vaccination Coverage in Pregnant Women in Pakistan." *Human Vaccines & Immunotherapeutics*: 1–4. https://doi.org/10.1080/21645515.2019.1705693.

Iram, Mubashara. 2003. "Water Pollution, Poor Sanitation and Its Impact on Health: A Case Study of Punjabi Village, Chapparan, Tehsil Sarai-Alamgir." M.Sc, Department of Anthropology, Quaid-i-Azam University (410/M.sc).

Israili, A.H. 1981. "Humoral Theory of Unani Tibb." *Indian Journal of History of Science* 16 (1): 95–9. https://www.insa.nic.in/writereaddata/UpLoadedFiles/IJHS/ Vol16_1_14_AHIsraili.pdf.

Jamison, Peter. 2020. "Anti-Vaccination Leaders Seize on Coronavirus to Push Resistance to Inoculation." *The Washington Post*, 5 May.

Janes, Craig R., and Kitty K. Corbett. 2009. "Anthropology and Global Health." *Annual Review of Anthropology* 38 (1): 167–83. https://doi.org/10.1146/annurev -anthro-091908-164314.

Janes, Craig R., Kitty K. Corbett, James H. Jones, et al. 2012. "Emerging Infectious Diseases: The Role of Social Sciences." *The Lancet* 380 (9857): 1884–86. https:// doi.org/10.1016/S0140-6736(12)61725-5.

Javaid, Umbreen. 2010. "Corruption and Its Deep Impact on Good Governance in Pakistan." *Pakistan Economic and Social Review* 48 (1): 123–34. www.jstor.org /stable/41762417.

Jick, Hershel, and James A. Kaye. 2003. "Epidemiology and Possible Causes of Autism." *Pharmacotherapy: The Journal of Human Pharmacology and Drug Therapy* 23 (12): 1524–30.

John, Wilson. 2003. *Karachi, a Terror Capital in the Making*. New Delhi: Rupa & Co.

Johnston, Patrick B., and Anoop K. Sarbahi. 2016. "The Impact of US Drone Strikes on Terrorism in Pakistan." *International Studies Quarterly* 60 (2): 203–19. https://doi.org/10.1093/isq/sqv004.

Jones, Delmos J. 1970. "Towards a Native Anthropology." *Human Organization* 29 (4): 251–9.

———. 1995. "Anthropology and the Oppressed: A Reflection on 'Native' Anthropology." In *Insider Anthropology*, edited by E. L. Liza Cerroni-Long, 58–70. USA: National Association for the Practice of Anthropology.

Jones, Seth G., and C. Christine Fair. 2010. *Counterinsurgency in Pakistan*. Santa Monica: RAND.

Jones, Stacy Holman, Tony E. Adams, and Carolyn Ellis, eds. 2016. *Handbook of Autoethnography*. London: Routledge.

Joralemon, Donald. 2017. *Exploring Medical Anthropology*. 4th ed. London: Routledge.

Jorgensen, Joseph G. 1971. "On Ethics and Anthropology." *Current Anthropology* 12 (3): 321–34. https://www.journals.uchicago.edu/doi/abs/10.1086/201209.

Junaidi, Ikram. 2018. "PM's Health Programme to Cover 15 More Districts." *Dawn*, 3 January 2018. Accessed 20 April 2018. https://www.dawn.com/news/1380466.

Jutel, Annemarie, and Kevin Dew, eds. 2014. *Social Issues in Diagnosis: An Introduction for Students and Clinicians*. Baltimore: Johns Hopkins University Press.

Kaadan, Abdul Nasser. 2000. "Al Raz's Book on Smallpox and Measles." *Qatar Medical Journal* 2000 (2): 7.

Kalhoro, Zulfiqar Ali. 2015. "One Deity, Three Temples: A Typology of Sacred of Spaces in Hariyar Village, Tharparkar Sindh." *Research Deliberation* 1(ii): 19–35.

Kane, Robert. 2005. *A Contemporary Introduction to Free Will*. New York: Oxford University Press.

Karafillakis, E., I. Dinca, F. Apfel, S. Cecconi, A. Wurz, J. Takacs, J. Suk, L. P. Celentano, P. Kramarz, and H. J. Larson. 2016. "Vaccine Hesitancy among Healthcare Workers in Europe: A Qualitative Study." *Vaccine* 34 (41): 5013–20. https://doi.org/10.1016/j.vaccine.2016.08.029.

Katz, Samuel L. 2005. *A Vaccine-Preventable Infectious Disease Kills Half a Million Children Annually*. Berkeley: University of California Press.

———. 2009. "John F. Enders and Measles Virus Vaccine—A Reminiscence." In *Measles: History and Basic Biology*, Edited by Diane E. Griffin, Michael B.A. Oldstone 3–11. Heidelberg: Springer-Verlag.

Katz, Samuel L., John F. Enders, and Ann Holloway. 1960. "Studies on an Attenuated Measles-Virus Vaccine: Clinical, Virologic and Immunologic Effects of Vaccine in Institutionalized Children." *New England Journal of Medicine* 263 (4): 159–61.

Katz, Samuel L., Milan V. Milovanovic, and John F. Enders. 1958. "Propagation of Measles Virus in Cultures of Chick Embryo Cells." *Proceedings of the Society for Experimental Biology and Medicine* 97 (1): 23–9.

Katz, Samuel L., David C. Morley, and Saul Krugman. 1962. "Attenuated Measles Vaccine in Nigerian Children." *American Journal of Diseases of Children* 103 (3): 402–5.

Kaufmann, Judith R., and Harley Feldbaum. 2009. "Diplomacy and the Polio Immunization Boycott in Northern Nigeria." *Health Affairs* 28 (4): 1091–1101.

Kawrani, Sudama. 2013. "Thar Mata Thar Sindhi Bhajan." 05:28. https://www.youtube.com/watch?v=lEKImx12Kr4.

Kazi, Elsa. 2017. "The Neem Tree." In *Secondary Stage English*, edited by Abdul Fahim Noonari, 17. Karachi: Imperial Enterprises.

Keesing, Roger Martin. 1987. "Anthropology as Interpretive Quest." *Current Anthropology* 28 (2): 161–76. https://doi.org/10.1086/203508.

Kennedy, Charles H. 1991. "The Politics of Ethnicity in Sindh." *Asian Survey* 31 (10): 938–55. https://doi.org/10.2307/2645065.

Khaleefathullah, Syed. 2001. "Unani Medicine." In *Traditional Medicine in Asia*, edited by Ranjit Roy Chaudhury and Uton Muchtar Rafei, 31–46. New Delhi: World Health Organization.

Khan, Adeel. 2002. "Pakistan's Sindhi Ethnic Nationalism: Migration, Marginalization, and the Threat of 'Indianization'." *Asian Survey* 42 (2): 213–29. https://doi.org/10.1525/as.2002.42.2.213.

Khan, Aftab, et al. 2015. "Measles in Vaccinated Children 1.5 to 3 Years of Age in Rural Community of District Peshawar, Pakistan." *Journal of Ayub Medical College Abbottabad* 27 (4): 825–8.

Khan, Feisal. 2007. "Corruption and the Decline of the State in Pakistan." *Asian Journal of Political Science* 15 (2): 219–47. https://doi.org/10.1080/02185370701511644.

Khan, Muhammad Hussain. 2014. "Sindh's Measles Nightmare." *Dawn*, 25 May 2014. Accessed 25 May 2014. https://www.dawn.com/news/1107969.

Khan, Nadia Taj. 2003. "The Effects of Water and Sanitation on Health: A Case Study of Village Baffa." Department of Anthropology, Quaid-i-Azam University (392/M.sc).

Khan, Shahrukh Rafi. 2002. "IMF Conditions Stunt Growth." *Economic and Political Weekly* 37 (44/45): 4541–4.

Khan, Tariq, and Javaria Qazi. 2014. "Measles Outbreaks in Pakistan: Causes of the Tragedy and Future Implications." *Epidemiology Reports* 2 (1): 1.

Khatwani, Mukesh, and Ishrat Abbasi. 2014. "Assessment of Socio-Political and Socioeconomic Factors Causing Sindhi-Muhajirs Conflicts in Sindh-Pakistan." *British Journal of Interdisciplinary Studies* 1: 40–51.

Khuhawar, M. Yar, Habib-ul-Rehman Ursani, Taj Muhammad Jahangir Khuhawar, Muhammad Farooque Lanjwani, et al. 2019. "Assessment of Water Quality of Groundwater of Thar Desert, Sindh, Pakistan." *Journal of Hydrogeology & Hydrologic Engineering* 7 (2): 2.

Khwaja, Ghulam Hussain. 2018. "Measles Cases on the Rise in Several Districts." *Dawn*, 4 February 2018. Accessed 27 August 2019. https://epaper.dawn.com/DetailImage.php?StoryImage=02_04_2018_117_003.

Kirmayer, Laurence J. 1988. "Mind and Body as Metaphors: Hidden Values in Biomedicine." In *Biomedicine Examined*, edited by Margaret Lock and Deborah Gordon, 57–93. Dordrecht: Kluwer Academic Publishers.

Kleinman, Arthur. 1977. "Depression, Somatization and the New Cross-Cultural Psychiatry." *Social Science & Medicine* 11: 3–10.

———. 1978. "Concepts and a Model for the Comparison of Medical Systems as Cultural Systems." *Social Science & Medicine* 12: 85–93. https://doi.org/10.1016/0160-7987(78)90014-5.

———. 1980. *Patients and Healers in the Context of Culture: An Exploration of the Border Land between Anthropology, Medicine, and Psychiatry.* Berkeley: University of California Press.

———. 1986. *Social Origins of Distress and Disease: Depression, Neurasthenia, and Pain in Modern China.* New Haven: Yale University Press.

———. 1988. *Rethinking Psychiatry: From Cultural Category to Personal Experience.* New York: The Free Press.

———. 2000. "The Violence of Everyday Life: The Multiple Forms and Dynamics of Social Violence." In *Violence and Subjectivity*, edited by Veena Das, Arthur Kleinman, Mamphela Ramphele, and Pamela Reynolds, 226–41. Berkeley, Los Angeles, London: University of California Press.

———. 2010. "Four Social Theories for Global Health." *Lancet* 375 (9725): 1518–9. https://doi.org/10.1016/S0140-6736(10)60646-0.

Kleinman, Arthur, and Byron J. Good, eds. 1985. *Culture and Depression: Studies in the Anthropology and Cross-Cultural Psychiatry of Affect and Disorder.* Berkeley: University of California Press.

Kleinman, Arthur, Veena Das, and Margaret Lock. 1997. *Social Suffering.* Berkeley: University of California Press.

Koen, Benjamin D. 2006. "Musical Healing in Eastern Tajikistan: Transforming Stress and Depression through Falak Performance." *Asian Music* 37 (2): 58–83.

Koplan, Jeffrey P., et al. 2009. "Towards a Common Definition of Global Health." *Lancet* 373 (9679): 1993–5. https://doi.org/10.1016/S0140-6736(09)60332-9.

Koplik, Henry. 1962. "The Diagnosis of the Invasion of Measles from a Study of the Exanthema as It Appears on the Buccal Mucous Membrane." *Archives of Pediatrics* 79: 162.

Kopytoff, Igor. 1986. "The Cultural Biography of Things: Commoditization as Process." In *The Social Life of Things: Commodities in Cultural Perspective*, edited by Arjun Appadurai, 64–94. Cambridge: Cambridge University Press.

Kuehn, Bridget M. 2014. "World Leaders Push to Prepare for Global Threats." *JAMA* 311 (12): 1189–90. https://doi.org/10.1001/jama.2014.2272.

Kuipers, Joel C. 1989. "'Medical Discourse' in Anthropological Context: Views of Language and Power." *Medical Anthropology Quarterly* 3: 99–123.

Kumar, Deepak. 1997. "Unequal Contenders, Uneven Ground: Medical Encounters in British India, 1820–1920." In *Western Medicine as Contested Knowledge*, edited by Andrew Cunningham and Bridie Andrews, 127–90. Manchester: Manchester University Press.

Kurup, Paneenazhikath Narayana Vasudeva. 1983. "Ayurveda." In *Traditional Medicine and Health Care Coverage: A Reader for Health Administrators and Practitioners*, edited by R.H. Bannerman, J. Burton, and Ch'en Wen-Chieh, 50–60. Geneva: WHO.

Laderman, Carol, and Marina Roseman. 2016. *The Performance of Healing.* New York: Routledge.

Laidlaw, James. 2002. "For an Anthropology of Ethics and Freedom." *Journal of the Royal Anthropological Institute* 8 (2): 311–32.

Lakoff, Andrew. 2010. "Two Regimes of Global Health." *Humanity: An International Journal of Human Rights, Humanitarianism, and Development* 1 (1): 59–79. https://muse.jhu.edu/article/394856.

Lancy, David F. 2014. *The Anthropology of Childhood: Cherubs, Chattel, Changelings.* Cambridge: Cambridge University Press.

Lane, Sandra D., and Robert A. Rubinstein. 1990. "International Health: Problems and Programs in Anthropological Perspective." In *Medical Anthropology: Contemporary Theory and Method*, edited by Thomas Malcolm Johnson and Carolyn Fishel Sargent, 396–423. London: Praeger Publishers.

Langford, Jean. 2002. *Fluent Bodies: Ayurvedic Remedies for Postcolonial Imbalance*. Durham, NC: Duke University Press.

Larkin, Brian. 2013. "The Politics and Poetics of Infrastructure." *Annual Review of Anthropology* 42: 327–43.

Latour, Bruno. 2005. *Reassembling the Social: An Introduction to Actor-Network-Theory*. Oxford: Oxford University Press.

———. 2013. *An Inquiry into Modes of Existence: An Anthropology of the Moderns*. Translated by Catherine Porter. Cambridge: Harvard University Press.

Leach, Melissa, and Mariz Tadros. 2014. "Epidemics and the Politics of Knowledge: Contested Narratives in Egypt's H1N1 Response." *Medical Anthropology* 33 (3): 240–54. https://doi.org/10.1080/01459740.2013.842565.

Leng, Chee Heng. 1982. "Health Status and the Development of Health Services in a Colonial State: The Case of British Malaya." *International Journal of Health Services* 12 (3): 397–417.

Leslie, Charles M. 1963. "The Rehetoric of the Ayurvedic Revival in Modern India." *Man* 63: 72–3.

———. 1989. "Indigenous Pharmaceuticals, the Capitalist World System, and Civilization." *Kroeber Anthropological Society Papers* 69: 23–31.

Lévi-Strauss, Claude. 1963. "The Sorcerer and His Magic." In *Understanding and Applying Medical Anthropology*, edited by Peter J. Brown and Svea Closser, 129–37. London and New York: Routledge.

Lewis, Oscar. 1969. "The Culture of Poverty." In *Anthropological Realities: Readings in the Science of Culture*, edited by Jeanne Guillemin. London: Transaction Books.

Lindmeier, Christian. 29 November 2018. *Measles Cases Spike Globally Due to Gaps in Vaccination Coverage*. Geneva: World Health Organization. https://www.who .int/news-room/detail/29-11-2018-measles-cases-spike-globally-due-to-gaps-in -vaccination-coverage.

Lloyd, Jacqueline, Gregory Barz, and Karen Brummel-Smith. 2008. *The Oxford Handbook of Medical Ethnomusicology*. Oxford: Oxford University Press.

Lock, Margaret. 1980. *East Asian Medicine in Urban Japan: Varieties of Medical Experience*. Berkeley: University of California Press.

Lock, Margaret, and Patricia Kaufert. 2001. "Menopause, Local Biologies, and Cultures of Aging." *American Journal of Human Biology* 13 (4): 494–504. https:// doi.org/10.1002/ajhb.1081.

Lock, Margaret, and Vinh-Kim Nguyen. 2010. *An Anthropology of Biomedicine*. Oxford: Blackwell Publishing.

Lock, Margaret, and Deborah Gordon, eds. 1988. *Biomedicine Examined*. Dordrecht: Kluwer Academic Publishers.

Lock, Margaret, and Nancy Scheper-Hughes. 1990. "A Critical-Interpretive Approach in Medical Anthropology: Rituals and Routines of Discipline and Dissent." In *Medical Anthropology: Contemporary Theory and Method*, edited by Thomas M. Johnson and Carolyn Fishel Sargent, 47–72. New York: Praeger.

Low, Gordon. 1999. "Thomas Sydenham: The English Hippocrates." *Australian and New Zealand Journal of Surgery* 69 (4): 258–62.

Luo, Hui-Ming, et al. 2013. "Identification and Control of a Poliomyelitis Outbreak in Xinjiang, China." *New England Journal of Medicine* 369 (21): 1981–90. https:// doi.org/10.1056/NEJMoa1303368.

MacDonald, Noni E. 2015. "Vaccine Hesitancy: Definition, Scope and Determinants." *Vaccine* 33 (34): 4161–4. https://doi.org/10.1016/j.vaccine.2015.04.036.

Madison, D. Soyini. 2011. *Critical Ethnography: Method, Ethics, and Performance.* London: Sage Publications.

Madsen, Kreesten Meldgaard, Anders Hviid, Mogens Vestergaard, Diana Schendel, Jan Wohlfahrt, Poul Thorsen, Jørn Olsen, and Mads Melbye. 2002. "A Population-Based Study of Measles, Mumps, and Rubella Vaccination and Autism." *New England Journal of Medicine* 347 (19): 1477–82.

Mafigiri, Richardson, Fred Nsubuga, and Alex Riolexus Ario. 2017. "Risk Factors for Measles Death: Kyegegwa District, Western Uganda, February–September, 2015." *BMC Infectious Diseases* 17 (1): 462. https://doi.org/10.1186/s12879-017-2558-7.

Mail Online. 2012. "Pakistani Doctor Who Led U.S. To Bin Laden's Hideout As He Is Jailed for 33 Years for Treason 'as Punishment for Humiliating His Country'." 24 May 2012. Accessed 12 January 2016. https://www.dailymail.co.uk/news /article-2148735/Shakil-Afridi-Osama-bin-Ladens-doctor-jailed-33-YEARS -Pakistan-treason.html.

Malinowski, Bronislaw. 1922. *Argonauts of the Western Pacific: An Account of Native Enterprise and Adventure in the Archipelagoes of Melanesian New Guinea.* London: Routledge and Kegan Paul.

Malkani, Sara. 2016. "Pakistan's Healthcare Crisis." *Dawn,* 27 June 2016. Accessed 27 June 2016. https://www.dawn.com/news/1267410.

Malthus, Thomas Robert. 1872. *An Essay on the Principle of Population.* Edinburgh and London: Ballantyne and Company.

Mandel, Bethany. 2019. "Parenting in the Time of Measles." *New York Times,* 3 April 2019. Accessed 3 April 2019. https://www.nytimes.com/2019/04/03/opinion /parenting-vaccines-measles.html.

Manderson, Lenore. 1998. "Applying Medical Anthropology in the Control of Infectious Disease." *Tropical Medicine & International Health* 3 (12): 1020–7. https://doi.org/10.1046/j.1365-3156.1998.00334.x.

Manderson, Lenore, and Susan Levine. 2020. "C-19, Risk, Fear, and Fall-Out." *Medical Anthropology:* 1–4. https://doi.org/10.1080/01459740.2020.1746301.

Mansoor, Hassan. 2015a. "Heatwave Death Toll in Sindh Tops 1,000." *Dawn,* 25 June 2015. Accessed 25 June 2015. https://www.dawn.com/news/1190267.

———. 2015b. "Over 75,000 Children in Sindh Never Received Polio Vaccine." *Dawn,* 2015. http://www.dawn.com/news/1204954.

———. 2016. "10 Policemen, Seven Polio Volunteers Killed in Sindh since 2012." *Dawn,* 21 April 2016. http://www.dawn.com/news/1253369.

Maqsood, Huma. 2001. "Impact of Potable Water and Sanitation on Health: An Ethnographic Study of Village Arayina Wal." M.Sc, Department of Anthropology, Quaid-i-Azam University (358/M.sc).

Marcus, George E. 1995. "Ethnography in/of the World System: The Emergence of Multi-Sited Ethnography." *Annual Review of Anthropology* 24 (1): 95–117. https://doi.org/10.1146/annurev.an.24.100195.000523.

Marszal, Andrew. 2016. "Doctor Who Helped Cia Track Bin Laden Still Languishes in Pakistan Jail." *The Telegraph,* 2 May 2016. Accessed 12 January 2016. http:// www.telegraph.co.uk/news/2016/05/02/doctor-who-helped-cia-track-bin-laden -still-languishes-in-pakist/.

Massé, Raymond. 2007. "Between Structural Violence and Idioms of Distress: The Case of Social Suffering in the French Caribbean." *Anthropology in Action* 14 (3): 6–17. https://doi.org/10.3167/aia.2007.140303.

Mattingly, Cheryl. 2012. "Two Virtue Ethics and the Anthropology of Morality." *Anthropological Theory* 12 (2): 161–84. https://doi.org/10.1177/1463499612455284.

McClure, Catherine C., Jessica R. Cataldi, and Sean T. O'Leary. 2017. "Vaccine Hesitancy: Where We Are and Where We Are Going." *Clinical Therapeutics* 39 (8): 1550–62.

McCoy, David, Sudeep Chand, and Devi Sridhar. 2009. "Global Health Funding: How Much, Where It Comes From and Where It Goes." *Health Policy and Planning* 24 (6): 407–17. https://doi.org/10.1093/heapol/czp026.

McGirk, Tim. 2015a. *How the Bin Laden Raid Put Vaccinators under the Gun in Pakistan.* National Geographic. http://news.nationalgeographic.com/2015/02/150225-polio-pakistan-vaccination-virus-health/.

———. 25 June 2015b. *Tālibān Assassins Target Pakistan's Polio Vaccinators.* Investigative Reporting Program. National Geographic. https://news.nationalgeographic.com/2015/03/150303-polio-pakistan-islamic-state-refugees-vaccination-health/.

McGranahan, Carole. 2016. "Theorizing Refusal: An Introduction." *Cultural Anthropology* 31 (3): 319–25. https://journal.culanth.org/index.php/ca/article/view/ca31.3.01/367.

McKay, Deirdre. 2014. "Affect: Making the Global through Care." In *Framing the Global: Entry Points for Research*, edited by Hilary E. Kahn and Saskia Sassen, xvii, 332 pages. Bloomington: Indiana University Press.

McLuhan, Marshall, and Bruce R. Powers. 1992. *The Global Village: Transformations in World Life and Media in the 21st Century.* Oxford: Oxford University Press.

Mead, Richard. 1748. *A Discourse on the Small Pox and Measles.* London: Nabu Press.

Measles and Rubella Initiative. 2019. "The Problem." Measles and Rubella Initiative. Last Modified 2019. Accessed 26 November. http://measlesrubellainitiative.org/learn/the-problem/.

Megill, Allan. 1994. *Rethinking Objectivity. Post-Contemporary Interventions*, edited by Allan Megill. Durham: Duke University Press.

Memon, Sarfraz. 2012. "Deadly December: Measles Outbreak Claims 87 Children's Lives in Sindh." *The Express Tribune*, 30 December 2012. https://tribune.com.pk/story/486584/deadly-december-measles-outbreak-claims-87-childrens-lives-in-sindh/.

Mere, Mohammed Osama, et al. 2019. "Progress toward Measles Elimination—Pakistan, 2000–2018." *Morbidity and Mortality Weekly Report* 68 (22): 505.

Mezzofiore, Gianluca. 2018. "Why Italy's U-turn on Mandatory Vaccination Shocks the Scientific Community." *CNN*, 7 August 2018.

Miller, Peggy J. 1994. "Narrative Practices: Their Role in Socialization and Self-Construction." In *The Remembering Self: Construction and Accuracy in the Self-Narrative*, edited by U. Neisser and R. Fivush, 158–79. New York: Cambridge University Press.

Miller, Peggy J., and Barbara Byhouwer Moore. 1989. "Narrative Conjunctions of Caregiver and Child: A Comparative Perspective on Socialization through Stories." *Ethos* 17 (4): 428–49. https://doi.org/10.1525/eth.1989.17.4.02a00020.

Mintz, Sidney W., and Christine M. Du Bois. 2002. "The Anthropology of Food and Eating." *Annual Review of Anthropology* 31 (1): 99–119. https://doi.org/10.1146/annurev.anthro.32.032702.131011.

Modanlou, Houchang D. 2008. "A Tribute to Zakariya Razi (865–925 AD), an Iranian Pioneer Scholar." *Archives of Iranian Medicine* 11 (6): 673–7.

Mohanty, Nirode. 2013. *America, Pakistan, and the India Factor*. New York: Palgrave Macmillan.

Mohsin, Saima, and Euan McKirdy. 2015. "Karachi Heat Wave: Unforgiving Heat Claims More Lives." *CNN*, 25 June 2015. Accessed 25 June 2015. http://edition.cnn.com/2015/06/25/asia/pakistan-heat-wave/index.html.

Morgan, Lynn M. 1987. "Dependency Theory in the Political Economy of Health: An Anthropological Critique." *Medical Anthropology Quarterly* 1 (2): 131–54. https://doi.org/10.1525/maq.1987.1.2.02a00010.

Morley, David. 1969. "Severe Measles in the Tropics. I." *British Medical Journal* 1 (5639): 297–300. https://doi.org/10.1136/bmj.1.5639.297.

Morse, Stephen S. 2001. "Factors in the Emergence of Infectious Diseases." In *Plagues and Politics*, edited by A.T. Price-Smith, 8–26. London: Palgrave Macmillan.

Morsy, Soheir. 1990. "Political Economy in Medical Anthropology." In *Medical Anthropology: A Handbook of Theory and Method*, edited by Carolyn Fishel Sargent and Thomas Malcolm Johnson, 26–46. New York: Prager Publishers.

Motlagh, Jason. 5 March 2015. *Fighting Polio Amid the Chaos of Syria's Civil War*. National Geographic. https://www.nationalgeographic.com/news/2015/03/150305-polio-syria-iraq-islamic-state-refugees-vaccination-virus-jihad/.

Mull, Dorothy S. 1991. "Traditional Perceptions of Marasmus in Pakistan." *Social Science & Medicine* 32 (2): 175–91. https://doi.org/10.1016/0277-9536(91)90058-K.

———. 1997. "The *Sitālā* Syndrome: The Cultural Context of Measles Mortality in Pakistan." In *The Anthropology of Infectious Disease: International Health Perspectives (Theory and Practice in Medical Anthropology and International Health)*, edited by Peter J. Brown and Marcia Claire Inhorn, 299–330. London: Routledge.

Mull, Dorothy S., J. Dennis Mull, M.Z. Malik Kundi, and Muhammad Anjum. 1994. "Mothers' Perceptions of Severe Pneumonia in Their Own Children: A Controlled Study in Pakistan." *Social Science & Medicine* 38 (7): 973–87. https://doi.org/10.1016/0277-9536(94)90429-4.

Mullaney, Alexander, and Syeda Amna Hassan. 25 June 2015. *He Led the CIA to Bin Laden—And Unwittingly Fueled a Vaccine Backlash*. Investigative Reporting Program, National Geographic. https://news.nationalgeographic.com/2015/02/150227-polio-pakistan-vaccination-Tālibān-osama-bin-laden/.

Murakami, Hitoshi, Makoto Kobayashi, Masahiko Hachiya, Zahir S. Khan, Syed Q. Hassan, and Shinsaku Sakurada. 2014. "Refusal of Oral Polio Vaccine in Northwestern Pakistan: A Qualitative and Quantitative Study." *Vaccine* 32 (12): 1382–7. https://doi.org/10.1016/j.vaccine.2014.01.018.

Muscat, Mark. 2019. "Improving Immunization Coverage: A Who Perspective." European Immunization Week 2019 Vaccination: Social Responsibility or Mandatory Obligation? Vienna.

Mushtaq, Asim, Sajid Mehmood, Muhammad Ateeq Ur Rehman, Asma Younas, Muhammad Saif Ur Rehman, Muhammad Faheem Malik, et al. 2015. "Polio in Pakistan: Social Constraints and Travel Implications." *Travel Medicine and Infectious Disease* 13 (5): 360–6. https://doi.org/10.1016/j.tmaid.2015.06.004.

Mussadaq, Maha. 2010. "Cost of Hepatitis Treatment Increases 19 Times." *The Express Tribune*, 11 October 2010. Accessed 23 April 2018. https://tribune.com .pk/story/61026/cost-of-hepatitis-treatment-increases-19-times/.

Nagourney, Adam, and Abby Goodnough. 2015. "Measles Cases Linked to Disneyland Rise, and Debate over Vaccinations Intensifies." *The New York Times*, 21 January 2015. Accessed 21 October 2019. https://www.nytimes.com/2015 /01/22/us/measles-cases-linked-to-disneyland-rise-and-debate-over-vaccinations -intensifies.html.

Nasr, Seyyed Vali Reza. 1992. "Democracy and the Crisis of Governability in Pakistan." *Asian Survey* 32 (6): 521–37. https://doi.org/10.2307/2645158.

———. 1994. *The Vanguard of the Islamic Revolution: The Jama'at-I Islamī of Pakistan*. Vol. 19. Berkeley: University of California Press.

Navarro, Vicente, and Carles Muntaner. 2016. *The Financial and Economic Crises and Their Impact on Health and Social Well-Being*. In *Policy, Politics, Health and Medicine Series*. London: Routledge.

Nichter, Mark. 1981. "Idioms of Distress: Alternatives in the Expression of Psychosocial Distress: A Case Study from South India." *Culture, Medicine and Psychiatry* 5 (4): 379–408. https://doi.org/10.1007/BF00054782.

———. 1989. *Anthropology and International Health: South Asian Case Studies*. Dordrecht: Kluwer Academic Publishers.

———. 1995. "Vaccinations in the Third World: A Consideration of Community Demand." *Social Science & Medicine* 41 (5): 617–32. https://doi.org/10.1016 /0277-9536(95)00034-5.

———. 2008. *Global Health: Why Cultural Perceptions, Social Representations, and Biopolitics Matter*. Tucson: University of Arizona Press.

Nishtar, Sania. 2006. *The Gateway Paper: Health System in Pakistan – A Way Forward*. Islāmābād: Pakistan's Health Policy Forum and Heartfile.

Noor, Muhammad Tahir. 2009. "Institutional Dynamics of Governance and Corruption in Developing World: The Case of Pakistan." Ph.D, Department of Political Science Ruprecht-Karls-Universität Heidelberg. http://archiv.ub.uni-heidelberg.de/ volltextserver/9215/1/Complete_Online_publication_doc_19_3_09.pdf.

O'Donovan, James, Hannes F. Wagner, and Stefan Zeume. 2019. "The Value of Offshore Secrets: Evidence from the Panama Papers." *The Review of Financial Studies* 32 (11): 4117–55. https://doi.org/10.1093/rfs/hhz017.

Offit, Paul A., and Susan E. Coffin. 2003. "Communicating Science to the Public: MMR Vaccine and Autism." *Vaccine* 22 (1): 1–6.

Ohnuki-Tierney, Emiko. 1981. *Illness and Healing among the Sakhalin Ainu–A Symbolic Interpretation*. London and New York: Cambridge University Press.

Oldstone, Michael B.A. 2010. *Viruses, Plagues, and History: Past, Present, and Future*. Rev. and updated ed. Oxford: Oxford University Press.

Ong, Aihwa. 1988. "Colonialism and Modernity: Feminist Re-Presentations of Women in Non-Western Societies." *Inscriptions*: 3 (4): 79–93.

Ong, Aihwa, and Stephen J. Collier. 2005. *Global Assemblages: Technology, Politics, and Ethics as Anthropological Problems*. Malden, MA: Blackwell.

Ortner, Sherry B. 1984. "Theory in Anthropology since the Sixties." *Comparative Studies in Society and History* 26 (1): 126–66. https://doi.org/10.1017/ S0010417500010811.

———. 1995. "Resistance and the Problem of Ethnographic Refusal." *Comparative Studies in Society and History* 37 (1): 173–93.

———. 2016. "Dark Anthropology and Its Others: Theory since the Eighties." *Hau Journal of Ethnographic Theory* 6 (1): 47–73. https://doi.org/10.14318/hau6.1 .004.

Ots, Thomas. 1990. "The Angry Liver, the Anxious Heart and the Melancholy Spleen: The Phenomenology of Perceptions in Chinese Culture." *Culture, Medicine and Psychiatry* 14: 21–58.

Ottenberg, Simon. 1990. "Thirty Years of Fieldnotes: Changing Relationships to the Text." In *Fieldnotes: The Makings of Anthropology*, edited by Roger Sanjek, 139–60. London: Cornell University Press.

Otterbein, Keith F. 1999. "A History of Research on Warfare in Anthropology." *American Anthropologist* 101 (4): 794–805.

Pakistan Initiative for Mothers and Newborns (PAIMAN). 2005. *Health Facility Assessment (HFA).* PAIMAN (Islāmābād: PAIMAN). http://paiman.jsi.com/ Resources/Docs/health-facility-assessment-paiman-original-districts.pdf.

Pakistan Press International (PPI). 2014. "Anti-Measles Drive Rescheduled." *Dawn*, 24 April 2014. Accessed 25 April 2014. https://www.dawn.com/news/1101806.

Palamenghi, Lorenzo, Serena Barello, Stefania Boccia, and Guendalina Graffigna. 2020. "Mistrust in Biomedical Research and Vaccine Hesitancy: The Forefront Challenge in the Battle Against COVID-19 in Italy." *European Journal of Epidemiology* 35 (8): 785–8.

Paleček, Martin, and Mark Risjord. 2013. "Relativism and the Ontological Turn within Anthropology." *Philosophy of the Social Sciences* 43 (1): 3–23. https://doi .org/10.1177/0048393112463335.

Pandolfi, Mariella. 1990. "Boundaries Inside the Body: Women's Sufferings in Southern Peasant Italy." *Culture, Medicine and Psychiatry* 14: 255–73.

Panter-Brick, Catherine, and Mark Eggerman. 2018. "The Field of Medical Anthropology." *Social Science & Medicine* 196: 233–9. https://doi.org/10.1016/j .socscimed.2017.10.033.

Pappas, Gregory. 1990. "Some Implications for the Study of the Doctor–Patient Interaction: Power, Structure, and Agency in the Works of Howard Waitzkin and Arthur Kleinman." *Social Science & Medicine* 30 (2): 199–204.

Paradies, Yin. 2016. "Colonisation, Racism and Indigenous Health." *Journal of Population Research* 33 (1): 83–96. https://doi.org/10.1007/s12546-016-9159-y.

Parker, Amy A., et al. 2006. "Implications of a 2005 Measles Outbreak in Indiana for Sustained Elimination of Measles in the United States." *New England Journal of Medicine* 355 (5): 447–55.

Parker Fiebelkorn, Amy, Susan B. Redd, Kathleen Gallagher, Paul A. Rota, Jennifer Rota, William Bellini, and Jane Seward. 2010. "Measles in the United States during the Postelimination Era." *The Journal of Infectious Diseases* 202 (10): 1520–8. https://doi.org/10.1086/656914.

Patel, Manisha, Adria D. Lee, Nakia S. Clemmons, Susan B. Redd, Sarah Poser, Debra Blog, Jane R. Zucker, Jessica Leung, Ruth Link-Gelles, and Huong Pham. 2019. "National Update on Measles Cases and Outbreaks United States, January 1–October 1, 2019." *Morbidity and Mortality Weekly Report* 68 (40): 893.

Paterson, Chris, and David Domingo. 2008. *Making Online News: The Ethnography of New Media Production.* New York: Peter Lang.

Paules, Catharine I., and Anthony Stephen Fauci. 2017. "Emerging and Reemerging Infectious Diseases: The Dichotomy between Acute Outbreaks and Chronic Endemicity." *JAMA* 317 (7): 691–2. https://doi.org/10.1001/jama.2016.21079.

Peirano, Mariza G.S. 1998. "When Anthropology Is at Home: The Different Contexts of a Single Discipline." *Annual Review of Anthropology* 27 (1): 105–28.

Pfeiffer, James, and Rachel Chapman. 2010. "Anthropological Perspectives on Structural Adjustment and Public Health." *Annual Review of Anthropology* 39: 149–65. https://doi.org10.1146/annurev.anthro.012809.105101.

Pfleiderer, Beatrix. 2006. *The Red Thread: Healing Possession at a Muslim Shrine in North India.* Aakar Books.

Phadke, Varun K., Robert A. Bednarczyk, Daniel A. Salmon, and Saad B. Omer. 2016. "Association Between Vaccine Refusal and Vaccine-Preventable Diseases in the United States: A Review of Measles and Pertussis." *JAMA* 315 (11): 1149–58. https://doi.org/10.1001/jama.2016.1353.

Pink, Sarah. 2015. *Digital Ethnography: Principles and Practice.* Los Angeles: SAGE.

Pinto, Sarah. 2008. *Where There Is No Midwife: Birth and Loss in Rural India.* Vol. 10. New York, Oxford: Berghahn Books.

Pirani, Farida. 2009. "Therapeutic Encounters at a Muslim Shrine in Pakistan: An Ethnographic Study of Understandings and Explanations of Ill Health and Help-Seeking among Attenders." PhD, School of Health and Social Sciences Middlesex University.

Plotkin, Stanley A. 2014. "History of Vaccination." *Proceedings of the National Academy of Sciences* 111 (34): 12283–7. https://doi.org/10.1073/pnas.1400472111.

Plotkin, Stanley A. ed. 2011. *History of Vaccine Development.* New York, NY: Springer.

Plotkin, Susan L., and Stanley A. Plotkin. 2004. "A Short History of Vaccination." *Vaccines* 5: 1–16.

Pogge, Thomas. 2010. *Politics as Usual: What Lies Behind the Pro-Poor Rhetoric.* Cambridge: Polity Press.

Porter, Theodore M. 1995. *Trust in Numbers the Pursuit of Objectivity in Science and Public Life.* Princeton, NJ: Princeton University Press.

Press Trust of India. 2018. "3 Children Die Due to 'Expired' Measles Vaccines in Pakistan." *Business Standard,* 4 March 2018. Accessed 6 March 2018. https://www.business-standard.com/article/pti-stories/3-children-die-due-to-expired-measles-vaccines-in-pakistan-118030400628_1.html.

Quirke, Viviane, and Jean-Paul Gaudillière. 2008. "The Era of Biomedicine: Science, Medicine, and Public Health in Britain and France after the Second World War." *Medical History* 52 (4): 441–52.

Qureshi, Ayaz. 2013. "Structural Violence and the State: HIV and Labour Migration from Pakistan to the Persian Gulf." *Anthropology & Medicine* 20 (3): 209–20. https://doi.org/10.1080/13648470.2013.828274.

———. 2015. "AIDS Activism in Pakistan: Diminishing Funds, Evasive State." *Development and Change* 46 (2): 320–38. https://doi.org/10.1111/dech.12151.

Rabinow, Paul. 2002. "Midst Anthropology's Problems." *Cultural Anthropology* 17 (2): 135–49.

Rabo, Annika. 2005. *A Shop of One's Own: Independence and Reputation among Traders in Aleppo.* London: I.B. Tauris & Co Ltd.

Rafatullah, Syed, and Syed Alqasoumi. 2008. "Unani Medicine: An Integral Part of Health Care System in Indian Subcontinent." *European Journal of Integrative Medicine* 1: 39–40. https://doi.org/10.1016/j.eujim.2008.08.076.

Raja, Sobia. 2003. "Study of Diseases and Remedies Emphasis Women Health in Tatral Khurd." M.Sc, Department of Anthropology, Quaid-i-Azam University (457).

Rampton, Mike. 2019. "Italy Bans Non-Vaccinated Kids from School—And Fines Parents up to €500." *Huffington Post*, 13 March 2019. Accessed 14 March 2019. https://www.huffingtonpost.co.uk/entry/italy-bans-non-vaccinated-kids-from-school_uk_5c88e2dae4b0fbd7661f661b#fb-comments

Rana, M.S., M.M. Alam, A. Ikram, M. Salman, M.O. Mere, M. Usman, et al. 2021. "Emergence of Measles during the COVID-19 Pandemic Threatens Pakistan's Children and the Wider Region." *Nature Medicine* 27 (7): 1127–8.

Ranade, Subhash. 2001. *Natural Healing through Ayurveda*. Delhi, India: Motilal Banarsidass Publisher.

Rao, Mohan. 2004. *From Population Control to Reproductive Health: Malthusian Arithmetic*. New Delhi, India: Sage Publications.

Rao, T.S. Sathyanarayana, and Chittaranjan Andrade. 2011. "The MMR Vaccine and Autism: Sensation, Refutation, Retraction, and Fraud." *Indian Journal of Psychiatry* 53 (2): 95. https://www.ncbi.nlm.nih.gov/pmc/articles/PMC3136032/.

Raza, Mohammad. 2016. "Seven Policemen Guarding Polio Workers Shot Dead in Karachi." *Dawn*, 20 April.

Rāzī, Abū Bakr Muḥammad ibn Zakarīyā. 1848. *A Treatise on the Small-Pox and Measles*. Translated by William Alexander Greenhill, Charles Adlard, and James Adlard. London: Sydenham Society Publications. Printed for the Sydenham Society.

Razzaq, Muhammad. 2004. "Community Preference for Different Health Care Systems in a Village Kotla Panju Baig Sheikhupura." M.Sc, Department of Anthropology, Quaid-i-Azam University (431/M.Sc).

Reiss, Dorit Rubinstein. 2019. "The Law and Vaccine Resistance." *Science* 363 (6429): 795. https://doi.org/10.1126/science.aax0019.

Renne, Elisha P. 2010. *The Politics of Polio in Northern Nigeria*. Bloomington: Indiana University Press.

Reuters. 2016. "Despite Vaccination Efforts Measles Kills 350 Children a Day, Report Says." *The New York Times*, 10 November 2016. Accessed 21 October 2019. https://www.nytimes.com/2016/11/11/world/measles-children-unicef.html.

Rhodes, Lorna Amarasingham. 1990. "Studying Biomedicine as a Cultural System." In *Medical Anthropology: A Handbook of Theory and Method*, edited by Carolyn F. Sargent and Thomas M. Johnson, 159–73. New York: Praeger.

Riaz, Haris. 2013. "Public Health Failings Behind Pakistan's Measles Surge." *The Lancet* 381 (9862): 189. https://doi.org/10.1016/S0140-6736(13)60072-0.

Riedel, Bruce. 2011. *Deadly Embrace: Pakistan, America, and the Future of the Global Jihād*. Washington, DC: Brookings Institution Press.

Rivers, William Halse. 1906. *The Todas*. Vol. 1. London, UK: Macmillan and Company, Limited.

Rizvi, Hasan-Askari. 1989. "The Legacy of Military Rule in Pakistan." *Survival* 31 (3): 255–68. https://doi.org/10.1080/00396338908442470.

Roalkvam, Sidsel, and Desmond McNeill. 2016. "What Counts as Progress? The Contradictions of Global Health Initiatives." *Forum for Development Studies* 43 (1): 69–88. https://doi.org/10.1080/08039410.2015.1134645.

Roberts, Jennafer, and Lisa Mitchell. 2017. "It's Your Body, It's Your Decision": An Anthropological Exploration of Hpv Vaccine Hesitancy." In *Public Health in the Age of Anxiety: Religious and Cultural Roots of Vaccine Hesitancy in Canada*, edited by Paul Bramadat, Maryse Guay, Julie A. Bettinger, and Réal Roy, 293–320. Toronto: University of Toronto Press.

Roberts, Leslie. 2019. "Polio Eradication Campaign Loses Ground." *Science* 365 (6449): 106–7. https://doi.org/10.1126/science.365.6449.106.

Robinson, Warren C. 1966. "Family Planning in Pakistan's Third Five Year Plan." *The Pakistan Development Review* 6 (2): 255–81.

Rogers, James Allen. 1972. "Darwinism and Social Darwinism." *Journal of the History of Ideas* 33 (2): 265–80.

Roos, Raymond P. 2016. "Zika Virus—A Public Health Emergency of International Concern." *JAMA Neurology* 73 (12): 1395–6. https://doi.org/10.1001/jamaneurol .2016.3677.

Roseman, Marina. 1991. *Healing Sounds from the Malaysian Rainforest: Temiar Music and Medicine.* Vol. 28. Berkeley: University of California Press.

Ruger, Jennifer Prah. 2007. "Global Health Governance and the World Bank." *Lancet* 370 (9597): 1471–4. https://doi.org/10.1016/S0140-6736(07)61619-5.

Rylko-Bauer, Barbara, and Paul Farmer, eds. 2016. "Structural Violence, Poverty, and Social Suffering." In *The Oxford Handbook of the Social Science of Poverty*, edited by David Brady and Linda M. Burton. London: Oxford University Press.

Sachanandbaghzai. 2011. "Mata Jo Orado." 05:42. https://www.youtube.com/watch ?v=zNvS__Kp2wY.

Saiman, Lisa, Amy S. Arrington, and Michael Bell. 2017. "Preparing for Emerging Infectious Diseases." *JAMA Pediatrics* 171 (5): 411–2. https://doi.org/10.1001/ jamapediatrics.2016.4947.

Samad, Yunas. 1994. "The Military and Democracy in Pakistan." *Contemporary South Asia* 3 (3): 189–201. https://doi.org/10.1080/09584939408719741.

Sarwar, Mahrukh. 2017. "How Pakistan Turned around Its Vaccination Programme Using Technology." *Dawn*, 31 January 2017. Accessed 20 December 2018. https:// www.dawn.com/news/1311870.

Scheper-Hughes, Nancy. 1996. "Theft of Life: The Globalization of Organ Stealing Rumours." *Anthropology Today* 12 (3): 3–11. https://doi.org/10.2307/2783143.

Scheper-Hughes, Nancy, and Philippe Bourgois, eds. 2004. *Violence in War and Peace: An Anthology.* Malden, MA: Blackwell Publishing.

Scheper-Hughes, Nancy, and San Philippe Bourgois. 2004. "Introduction: Making Sense of Violence." In *Violence in War and Peace: An Anthology*, edited by Nancy Scheper-Hughes and San Philippe Bourgois, 1–32. Malden, MA: Blackwell Publishing.

Scheper-Hughes, Nancy, and Margaret Lock. 1987. "The Mindful Body: A Prolegomenon to Future Work in Medical Anthropology." *Medical Anthropology Quarterly* 1 (1): 6–41. https://doi.org/10.1525/maq.1987.1.1.02a00020.

Schuster, Melanie, Juhani Eskola, and Philippe Duclos. 2015. "Review of Vaccine Hesitancy: Rationale, Remit and Methods." *Vaccine* 33 (34): 4157–60.

Sehgal, Ikram. 2017. "Corruption without Borders." *Defence Journal* 21 (5): 84–5. https://search.proquest.com/openview/02c3073d90f7aaba6fe158b8c3cee65a/1 ?pq-origsite=gscholar&cbl=616545.

Shah, Charmaine. 1999. "Effect of Socio-Cultural Belief Practices and Rituals on Maternal Health of Women in Village Jhang Bhagiyal." M.Sc, Department of Anthropology, Quaid-i-Azam University (292/M.sc).

Shah, Mazhar H. 1966. *The General Principles of Avicenna's Canon of Medicine.* Vol. 1. Karachi, Pakistan: Naveed Clinic.

Shah, Nafisa. 2007. "Making of Crime, Custom and Culture: The Case of Karo Kari Killings of Upper Sindh." In *Scratching the Surface: Democracy, Traditions, Gender*, 135. https://www.boell.de/sites/default/files/scratching_the_surface_commentary.pdf #page=145.

Shah, Saeed. 2011. "CIA Organised Fake Vaccination Drive to Get Osama Bin Laden's Family DNA." *The Guardian*, 11 July 2011. Accessed 12 January 2016. https://www.theguardian.com/world/2011/jul/11/cia-fake-vaccinations-osama-bin-ladens-dna.

Shahzadi, Noshina. 1999. "Local Perception of Health and Hygiene in Potohari." M.Sc, Department of Anthropology, Quaid-i-Azam University (259/M.sc).

Shaikh, Babar T., and Juanita Hatcher. 2004. "Health Seeking Behaviour and Health Service Utilization in Pakistan: Challenging the Policy Makers." *Journal of Public Health* 27 (1): 49–54. https://doi.org/10.1093/pubmed/fdh207.

———. 2005. "Complementary and Alternative Medicine in Pakistan: Prospects and Limitations." *Evidence-Based Complementary and Alternative Medicine* 2 (2): 139–42.

Sheehan, Helen E., and S.J. Hussain. 2002. "Unani Tibb: History, Theory, and Contemporary Practice in South Asia." *The Annals of the American Academy of Political and Social Science* 583 (1): 122–35. https://doi.org/10.1177/000271620258300108.

Siani, Alessandro. 2019. "Measles Outbreaks in Italy: A Paradigm of the Re-Emergence of Vaccine-Preventable Diseases in Developed Countries." *Preventive Medicine* 121: 99–104. https://doi.org/10.1016/j.ypmed.2019.02.011.

Siddiq, Maria. 1998. "Socio-Cultural Factors Underlying the Structure and Dynamics of Interface between the Pluralistic Health Care System in Pari Derveizan with Reference to Children Diseases." M.Sc, Department of Anthropology, Quaid-i-Azam University (251/M.sc).

Sinclair, Vicky. 2016. *Lady Montagu and the Introduction of Inoculation*. Wellcome Library.

Singer, Merrill. 1989. "The Coming of Age of Critical Medical Anthropology." *Social Science & Medicine* 28 (11): 1193–203. https://doi.org/10.1016/0277-9536(89)90012-9.

———. 1990a. "Postmodernism and Medical Anthropology: Words of Caution." *Medical Anthropology* 12 (3): 289–304. https://doi.org/10.1080/01459740.1990.9966027.

———. 1990b. "Reinventing Medical Anthropology: Toward a Critical Realignment." *Social Science & Medicine* 30 (2): 179–87. https://doi.org/10.1016/0277-9536(90)90078-7.

———. 1995. *Critical Medical Anthropology*. Amityville, NY: Baywood.

———. 2015. *Anthropology of Infectious Disease*. London: Routledge.

Singer, Merrill, and Pamela Erickson. 2013. *Global Health: An Anthropological Perspective*. Long Grove, IL: Waveland Press.

Singer, M, F. Valentín, H. Baer, and Z. Jia. 1992. "Why Does Juan García have a Drinking Problem? The Perspective of Critical Medical Anthropology." *Medical Anthropology* 14 (1): 77–108. https://doi.org/10.1080/01459740.1992.9966067. PMID: 1294865.

Sirajuddin. 2019. "Peshawar Police Arrest Man Alleging Anti-Polio Vaccines Cause Children to Faint, Die." *Dawn*, April 23, 2019. Accessed 23 April. https://

www.dawn.com/news/1477890/peshawar-police-arrest-man-alleging-anti-polio -vaccines-cause-children-to-faint-die.

Sobo, Elisa Janine. 2016. "Theorizing (Vaccine) Refusal: Through the Looking Glass." *Cultural Anthropology* 31 (3): 342–50. https://journal.culanth.org/index .php/ca/article/view/ca31.3.04/373.

Sodhar, Zain-ul Abdin, and Abdul Ghani Shaikh. 2015. "The Hur Movement: A Foundation for Independent Muslim State." *Journal of Grassroots* 49 (2): 152–62.

Sohail, Munnal. 1999. "Cultural Construction of the Congenital Illness of Children and Relevant Pluralistic Health Care System Existing in the Village Mohra." M.Sc, Department of Anthropology, Quaid-i-Azam University (381/M.sc).

Soomro, Faisal, et al. 2017. "Occurrence and Delineation of High Nitrate Contamination in the Groundwater of Mithi Sub-District, Thar Desert, Pakistan." *Environmental Earth Sciences* 76 (10): 355.

Stewardson, Andrew J., et al. 2009. "Imported Case of Poliomyelitis, Melbourne, Australia, 2007." *Emerging Infectious Diseases* 15 (1): 63–5. https://doi.org/10 .3201/eid1501.080791.

Stewart, Tony K. 1995. "Encountering the Smallpox Goddess: The Auspicious Song of *Sitalā.*" In *Religions of India in Practice*, edited by Donald S. Lopez Jr, 389–98. Princeton: Princeton University Press.

Stiglitz, Joseph. 2000. "What I Learned at the World Economic Crisis." In *Globalization and the Poor: Exploitation or Equalizer?*, edited by Julie Clark and William J. Driscoll, 195–204. New York: International Debate Education Association.

Stöckl, Andrea, and Anna Smajdor. 2017. "The MMR Debate in the United Kingdom Vaccine Scares, Statesmanship and the Media." In *The Politics of Vaccination*, edited by Christine Holmberg, Stuart Blume, and Paul Greenough, 239–59. Manchester: Manchester University Press.

Stoller, Paul. 1989. *The Taste of Ethnographic Things: The Senses in Anthropology.* Philadelphia: University of Pennsylvania Press.

Strassburg, Marc A. 1982. "The Global Eradication of Smallpox." *American Journal of Infection Control* 10 (2): 53–9. https://doi.org/10.1016/0196-6553(82)90003-7.

Strathern, Marilyn. 1987. "The Limits of Auto-Anthropology." In *Anthropology at Home*, edited by Anthony Jackson, pp. 59–67. London: Tavistock Publications.

Strebel, Peter M., et al. 2011. "A World without Measles." *The Journal of Infectious Diseases* 204 (1): S1–S3. https://doi.org/10.1093/infdis/jir111.

Strebel, Peter M., et al. 2012. "Measles Vaccine." In *Vaccines*, edited by Stanley A. Plotkin, Walter A. Orenstein, and Paul A. Offit, 352–87. Elsevier Saunders.

Strebel, Peter M., Mark J. Papania, Amy Parker Fiebelkorn, and Neal A. Halsey. 2013. "Measles Vaccine." In *Vaccines*, edited by Stanley A. Plotkin, Walter Orenstein, and Paul A. Offit, 352–87. Elsevier Saunders.

Subbarayappa, Bidare Venkatasubbaiah. 2001. "The Roots of Ancient Medicine: An Historical Outline." *Journal of Biosciences* 26 (2). https://doi.org/10.1007/ BF02703637.

Sudarshan, S.R., ed. 2005. *Encyclopaedia of Indian Medicine: Basic Concepts.* Bangalore: Taj Press.

Sultana, Farhat. 2013. "Ethnicity and Healing Rituals in Gwadar, Balochistan, Pakistan." *The Journal of the Middle East and Africa* 4 (2): 169–85. https://doi .org/10.1080/21520844.2013.831020.

Tafuri, Silvio, et al. 2014. "Addressing the Anti-Vaccination Movement and the Role of Hcws." *Vaccine* 32 (38): 4860–5. https://doi.org/10.1016/j.vaccine.2013.11.006.

Tariq, Parveen. 2003. "Assessment of Coverage Levels of Single Dose Measles Vaccine." *Journal of the College of Physicians and Surgeons–Pakistan: JCPSP* 13 (9): 507–10. https://doi.org/09.2003/JCPSP.506509.

Tepu, Imran Ali. 2012. "American NGOs Assail CIA over Fake Polio Drive." *Dawn,* 2 March 2012. http://www.dawn.com/news/699586/american-ngos-assail-cia -over-fake-polio-drive.

Thapan, Meenakshi, ed. 1998. *Anthropological Journeys: Reflections on Fieldwork.* New Delhi, India: Orient Longman.

The Express Tribune. 2012a. "Cleric Declares Jihād against Polio Campaign." *The Express Tribune,* 13 June 2012. Accessed 26 May 2015. https://tribune.com.pk/story /392939/obstacles-for-immunisation-cleric-declares-jihad-against-polio-campaign/.

———. 2012b. "Measles Epidemic Sweeps through Sindh Unchecked." *The Express Tribune,* 27 December 2012. Accessed 25 July 2014. https://tribune.com.pk/story /485042/measles-epidemic-sweeps-through-sindh-unchecked/.

———. 2012c. "Measles Outbreak in Sindh: More Than 30 Children Died in 20 Days." *The Express Tribune,* 23 December 2012. Accessed 14 July 2016. https://tribune.com.pk/story/483201/measles-outbreak-in-sindh-more-than-30 -children-died-in-20-days/.

———. 2014a. "30 Children Fall Sick in Swat Upon Receiving Measles Vaccinations." *The Express Tribune,* 24 May 2014. Accessed 25 May 2014. https://tribune.com .pk/story/712501/30-children-fall-sick-upon-receiving-measles-vaccinations/.

———. 2014b. "Alarming Situation: Four Children Reportedly Die from Measles Vaccine." *The Express Tribune,* 29 May 2014. Accessed 20 December 2014. https://tribune.com.pk/story/714649/alarming-situation-four-children-reportedly -die-from-measles-vaccine/.

———. 2015. "Falling on Deaf Ears: Lady Health Workers Take to the Streets over Unfulfilled Demands." *The Express Tribune,* 31 August 2015. Accessed 20 April 2018. https://tribune.com.pk/story/948363/falling-on-deaf-ears-lady-health -workers-take-to-the-streets-over-unfulfilled-demands/.

———. 2017. "Lady Health Workers to Receive Salaries by Next Week." *The Express Tribune,* 17 November 2017. Accessed 20 April 2018. https://tribune.com .pk/story/1560420/1-lady-health-workers-receive-salaries-next-week/.

Thomas, Jim. 1993. *Doing Critical Ethnography.* Vol. 26. London: Sage Publications.

Turner, Patricia A. 1993. *I Heard It Through the Grapevine: Rumor in African-American Culture.* Berkeley: University of California Press.

Turner, Richard. 2019. "Measles Vaccination: A Matter of Confidence and Commitment." *PLoS Medicine*: 1–3.

Turner, V. 1974. *Dramas, Fields, and Metaphors: Symbolic Action in Human Society.* Ithaca, NY: Cornell University Press.

ul Haque, Minhaj, et al. 2016. *The Pakistan Expanded Program on Immunization and the National Immunization Support Project: An Economic Analysis.* Washington, DC: The World Bank.

Underberg, Natalie M., and Elayne Zorn. 2013. *Digital Ethnography: Anthropology, Narrative, and New Media.* Still Image. Austin: University of Texas Press.

United Nations (UN). 2005. *Report on the World Social Situation 2005: The Inequality Predicament.* New York: United Nations Publications.

———. 2013. *Inequality Matters: Report on the World Social Situation 2013*. New York: UN. https://www.un.org/esa/socdev/documents/reports/InequalityMatters.pdf.

———. 2021. *Inequality in a Rapidly Changing World*. New York: UN. https://www.un.org/development/desa/dspd/wp-content/uploads/sites/22/2020/01/World-Social-Report-2020-FullReport.pdf.

Van Dongen, Els, and Sylvie Fainzang. 1998. "Medical Anthropology at Home: Creating." *Anthropology & Medicine* 5 (3): 245.

Van Gennep, Arnold. 2013. *The Rites of Passage*. Translated by Monika B. Yizedom and Gabrielle L. Caffee. Illinois: University of Chicago Press, 1960.

Van Velsen, Jaap. 1967. "The Extended-Case Method and Situational Analysis." In *The Craft of Social Anthropology*, edited by A.L. Epstein, 129–49. London: Tavistock.

Vanderlinden, Lisa K. 2011. "Left in the Dust: Negotiating Environmental Illness in the Aftermath of 9/11." *Medical Anthropology* 30 (1): 30–55. https://doi.org/10.1080/01459740.2010.531067.

Verkaaik, Oskar. 2016. "Violence and Ethnic Identity Politics in Karachi and Hyderabad." *South Asia: Journal of South Asian Studies* 39 (4): 841–54.

Vitale, Geoffrey. 2014. *Anthropology of Childhood and Youth: International and Historical Perspectives*. Lanham: Lexington Books.

Wakefield, Andrew J., et al. 1999. "MMR Vaccination and Autism." *The Lancet* 354 (9182): 950. https://doi.org/10.1016/S0140-6736(05)75696-8.

Wakefield, Andrew J. 2010. *Callous Disregard: Autism and Vaccines—The Truth Behind a Tragedy*. New York, NY: Skyhorse Publications.

Wall, Sarah. 2008. "Easier Said Than Done: Writing an Autoethnography." *International Journal of Qualitative Methods* 7 (1): 38–53. https://doi.org/10.1177/160940690800700103.

Wallerstein, Immanuel Maurice. 1991. *Geopolitics and Geoculture: Essays on the Changing World-System*. Cambridge: Cambridge University Press.

———. 1998. *Utopistics, or, Historical Choices of the Twenty-First Century*. New York: New Press.

Walsh, Declan. 2007. "Polio Cases Jump in Pakistan as Clerics Declare Vaccination an American Plot." *The Guardian*, 15 February 2007. Accessed 16 September 2019. https://www.theguardian.com/world/2007/feb/15/pakistan.topstories3.

Warraich, Haider J. 2009. "Religious Opposition to Polio Vaccination." *Emerging Infectious Diseases* 15 (6): 978. https://doi.org/dx.doi.org/10.3201/eid1506.090087.

Wasim, Amir. 2013. "232 Deaths in Sindh: Poor Handling Led to Measles Outbreak: Minister." *Dawn*, 24 January 2013. Accessed 17 June 2013. https://www.dawn.com/news/781251.

Weiss, Richard S. 2008. "Divorcing Ayurveda: Siddha Medicine and the Quest for Uniqueness." In *Modern and Global Ayurveda: Pluralism and Paradigms*, edited by Dagmar Wujastyk and Frederick M. Smith, 77–99. Albany, NY: State University of New York Press.

Weiss, Robin A., and José Esparza. 2015. "The Prevention and Eradication of Smallpox: A Commentary on Sloane (1755) 'An Account of Inoculation'." *Philosophical Transactions of the Royal Society of London. Series B, Biological Sciences* 370 (1666): 20140378. https://doi.org/10.1098/rstb.2014.0378.

White, Sarah J., et al. 2012. "Measles, Mumps, and Rubella." *Clinical Obstetrics and Gynecology* 55 (2): 550. https://doi.org/10.1097/GRF.0b013e31824df256.

Whitehead, Harry. 2000. "The Hunt for Quesalid: Tracking Léevi-Strauss' Shaman." *Anthropology & Medicine* 7 (2): 149–68.

Whitehead, Neil L. 2004. "Cultures, Conflicts, and the Poetics of Violent Practice." In *Violence*, edited by Neil L. Whitehead, 3–24. Santa Fe, NM: School of American Research.

Wickramanayaka, Sarath Sisara Kumara. 1992. "The Management of Official Records in Public Institutions in Sri Lanka 1802–1990." University of London.

Wikan, Unni. 1991. "Toward an Experience-Near Anthropology." *Cultural Anthropology* 6: 285–305.

Wolfe, Nathan D., Claire Panosian Dunavan, and Jared Diamond. 2007. "Origins of Major Human Infectious Diseases." *Nature* 447 (7142): 279. https://10.1038/nature05775.

Wolfe, Robert M., and Lisa K. Sharp. 2002. "Anti-Vaccinationists Past and Present." *The British Medical Journal* 325 (7361): 430–2.

Woolf, Steven H., Derek A. Chapman, Roy T. Sabo, Daniel M. Weinberger, Latoya Hill, and DaShaunda D.H. Taylor. 2020. "Excess Deaths From COVID-19 and Other Causes, March–July 2020." *JAMA* 324 (15): 1562–4. https://doi.org/10.1001/jama.2020.19545.

World Health Organization (WHO). 2007a. *Health System Profile Pakistan*. WHO (WHO). http://apps.who.int/medicinedocs/documents/s17305e/s17305e.pdf.

———. 2007b. *Manual for the Laboratory Diagnosis of Measles and Rubella Virus Infection*. Geneva: WHO.

———. 2012. *Global Measles and Rubella Strategic Plan: 2012–2020*. Geneva: WHO. https://apps.who.int/iris/rest/bitstreams/53400/retrieve.

———. 2013a. *Annual Report of Measles and Rubella Initiative*. Geneva: WHO. https://www.who.int/immunization/diseases/measles/mri_annual-report_2013.pdf?ua=1.

———. 2013b. *Measles Elimination Field Guide*. Geneva: WHO.

———. 2016a. *Austria: Measles in the Spotlight*. Geneva: WHO. https://www.who.int/news-room/feature-stories/detail/austria-measles-in-the-spotlight.

———. 2016b. "Expanded Programme on Immunization – Pakistan." WHO. Last Modified 26 April. Accessed 17 July. http://www.emro.who.int/pak/programmes/expanded-programme-on-immunization.html.

———. 2016c. "International Health Regulations and Emergency Committees." WHO. Last Modified June 2016. Accessed 20 November. https://www.who.int/features/qa/emergency-committees/en/.

———. 2017. *Substantial Decline in Global Measles Deaths, but Disease Still Kills 90 000 Per Year*. Geneva: WHO. https://www.who.int/news-room/detail/26-10-2017-substantial-decline-in-global-measles-deaths-but-disease-still-kills-90-000-per-year.

———. 2019. "New Measles Surveillance Data for 2019." *Immunization, Vaccines and Biologicals*. Geneva: WHO. Accessed 3 December. https://www.who.int/immunization/newsroom/measles-data-2019/en/.

———. 2019a. "Expanded Programme on Immunization." Geneva: WHO. Accessed 9 December. http://www.emro.who.int/pak/programmes/expanded-programme-on-immunization.html.

———. 2019b. "Measles." Geneva: WHO. Accessed 3 December. who.int/en/news-room/fact-sheets/detail/measles.

———. 2019c. "Measles Reported Cases." Incidence Series WHO. Last Modified 15 July 2019. Accessed 4 December. http://apps.who.int/immunization_monitoring/ globalsummary/timeseries/tsincidencemeasles.html.

———. 2019d. "New Measles Surveillance Data for 2019." *Immunization, Vaccines and Biologicals.* Geneva: WHO. Accessed 3 December https://www.who.int/ immunization/newsroom/measles-data-2019/en/.

———. 2020a. *Reported Measles Cases and Incidence Rates by WHO Member States, as of 8 June 2020.* Geneva: WHO. Accessed 25 June 2020. who.int/im munization/monitoring_surveillance/burden/vpd/surveillance_type/active/measles _monthlydata/en/.

———. 2020b. "Dependence Syndrome." World Health Organization. Accessed 10 August. https://www.who.int/substance_abuse/terminology/definition1/en/.

Wright, Peter, and Andrew Treacher. 1982. *The Problem of Medical Knowledge: Examining the Social Construction of Medicine.* Edinburgh: Edinburgh University Press.

Wynbrandt, James. 2009. *A Brief History of Pakistan.* New York: Facts On File.

Yaseen, Ghulam, et al. 2015. "Ethnobotany of Medicinal Plants in the Thar Desert (Sindh) of Pakistan." *Journal of Ethnopharmacology* 163: 43–59.

Young, Allan. 1976. "Some Implications of Medical Beliefs and Practices for Social Anthropology." *American Anthropologist* 78: 5–24.

———. 1980. "The Discourse on Stress and the Reproduction of Conventional Knowledge." *Social Science & Medicine. Part B: Medical Anthropology* 14 (3): 133–46.

———. 1981. "The Creation of Medical Knowledge: Some Problems in Interpretation." *Social Science & Medicine* 15 (3): 379–86.

Yousaf, Mohammad, and Mark Adkin. 1992. *Afghanistan—The Bear Trap: The Defeat of a Superpower.* Barnsley, UK: Casemate.

Yusuf, Huma. 2012. *Conflict Dynamics in Karachi.* Vol. 19. The United States Institute of Peace.

Yusufzai, Ashfaq. 2014. "Anti-Measles Vaccine Safe but Negligence Causing Complications." *Dawn,* 29 May.

Zaidi, Syed Akbar. 1988. *The Political Economy of Health Care in Pakistan.* Lahore: Vanguard.

Zehra, Nasreen. 1991. "Traditional Health Practices in a Village of Hazara." M.Sc, Department of Anthropology, Quaid-i-Azam University (323/M.sc).

Zimmerman, Francis. 1987. *The Jungle and the Aroma of Meats: An Ecological Theme in Hindu Medicine.* Berkeley: University of California Press.

Zipprich, Jennifer, et al. 2015. "Measles Outbreak—California, December 2014– February 2015." *MMWR. Morbidity and Mortality Weekly Report* 64 (6): 153.

Zoellner, Danielle. 2020. "The Impact of the Anti-vaxx Movement: What Happens if Only Half the Country Gets the Covid Vaccine?." *The Independent,* 18 December.

Index

Note: Pages in *italics* represent figures and pages in bold represent tables.
Pages followed by n denote endnotes.

For Product Safety Concerns and Information please contact our EU
representative GPSR@taylorandfrancis.com
Taylor & Francis Verlag GmbH, Kaufingerstraße 24, 80331 München, Germany